Achieving Professional Excellence and Career Satisfaction in the Dental Hygiene Profession

Volume I of Three Volumes

AuthorHouse™
1663 Liberty Drive
Bloomington, IN 47403
www.authorhouse.com
Phone: 1-800-839-8640

Published by AuthorHouse 08/30/2012

ISBN: 978-1-4772-0582-2 (sc)
*   978-1-4772-5360-1 (e)*

Library of Congress Control Number: 2012908969

Any people depicted in stock imagery provided by Thinkstock are models,
and such images are being used for illustrative purposes only.
Certain stock imagery © Thinkstock.

This book is printed on acid-free paper.

SAVVY SUCCESS Code - 103   authorHOUSE®

SAVVY SUCCESS

Achieving Professional Excellence and
Career Satisfaction in the Dental Hygiene Profession

First Edition

Volume I of Three Volumes

Christine A. Hovliaras, RDH, BS, MBA, CDE
President, Professional Savvy, LLC
Flanders, New Jersey
Adjunct Faculty
Department of Dental Hygiene
New York University
College of Dentistry
New York, New York

Dedication

The first edition of **SAVVY SUCCESS – Achieving Professional Excellence and Career Satisfaction in the Dental Hygiene Profession Volume I of Three Volumes** is dedicated to my loving parents, Ruth Ann and Crist Dimetrios Hovliaras and the biggest blessing of my life, my son, Jarod Crist Delozier.

The biggest dedication goes to my wonderful mother and best friend who passed away on Memorial Day in 2008 from metastatic breast cancer after she was a cancer survivor for 26 years. I want to thank her for everything she did for my sister, Pamela, and me during our lifetime together with her. She encouraged us to set goals, take opportunities that would come our way and to get a college education. She encouraged us to be truthful and respectful of others and treat people like we would always want to be treated. *Proceeds from the sale of* **SAVVY SUCCESS** *will go to the Susan Komen Breast Cancer Research Foundation in my mother's name to find a cure for cancer and offer hope to the dental hygienists I know who are affected by this terrible disease.*

My second dedication is to my son, Jarod, who is going to be 12 in September. He continues to be the driving force in my life to be the best mother I can be. I continually strive to provide him with everything he needs to be successful as a young man. "Jarod, I am so proud of you every day and for being by my side during the good and challenging times. You are the greatest gift I have received in my life."

My last dedication in **SAVVY SUCCESS** goes out to all the dental hygiene students in colleges/universities and to the practicing dental hygienists across the country and globally who are working hard each and every day with the patients they treat to inform, educate and provide valuable professional skills and techniques to improve their patients overall health and wellness. I trust the information you read in this textbook, Volume I, and in Volume II and III, will help give you a renewal and appreciation for everything dental hygienists can do in their careers. The art and science of the dental hygiene profession will continue to grow and expand with your involvement in the profession and participation in the communities you live in providing the utmost of care for your patients.

"You can be anything you want to be, if only you believe with sufficient conviction and act in accordance with your faith; for whatever the mind can conceive and believe, the mind can achieve."

NAPOLEON HILL
Best-selling author of *Think and Grow Rich*

Dental Hygienists Interviewed
for SAVVY SUCCESS

Achieving Professional Excellence and
Career Satisfaction in the Dental Hygiene Profession
Volume I – Volume III

Cynthia C. Amyot, MSDH, EdD
Interim Associate Vice Provost, Online Education
University of Missouri-Kansas City
Director, Distance Education & Faculty Development
School of Dentistry
University of Missouri-Kansas City
Kansas City, Missouri

Jane A. Balavage, RDH, BS
Registered Dental Hygienist
Educator
Entrepreneur
Motivational Specialist
Dallas, Pennsylvania

Linda K. Bohacek, RDH, MA, CDHC, FAADH
Oral Health Consultant
Independent Contractor
Eau Claire, Wisconsin

Justin Bordessa, RDH
Registered Dental Hygienist
Santa Rosa, California

Colleen M. Brickle RDH, RF, EdD
Dean of Health Sciences
Normandale Community College
Bloomington, Minnesota

Mary Calka, RDH
Registered Dental Hygienist
Assistant Clinical Supervisor
All About Kids Pediatric Dentistry
Stamford, Connecticut
Administrative Assistant
American Academy of Dental Hygiene
New York, New York

Christine Charles, RDH, BS
Registered Dental Hygienist
Director, Scientific and Professional Affairs
Johnson & Johnson Consumer and Personal Products Worldwide
Division of Johnson & Johnson Consumer Companies, Inc.
Morris Plains, New Jersey

Mary Ann Cugini, RDH, MHP
Senior Clinical Investigator
Center for Clinical and Translational Research
The Forsyth Institute
Boston, Massachusetts

Gina Dellanina, RDH, BS, MS
Registered Dental Hygienist
Owner of Bubble Gum Smiles and the Prophy Aid®
Newport Coast, California

Ann-Marie C. DePalma, CDA, RDH, FADIA, FAADH
Continuing Education Speaker
Stoneham, Massachusetts

Diane Dornisch, RDH, MBA
Registered Dental Hygienist
Professional Educator
OraPharma, Inc.
Horsham, Pennsylvania

Claudine Paula Drew, RDH, CDA, MS, EdD
Chair, Department of Dental Hygiene
Eastern International College
Belleville, New Jersey

Tammy L. Filipiak, RDH, MS
Director of Clinical Development
Midwest Dental and Mountain Dental
Mosinee, Wisconsin

Jane L. Forrest, RDH, EdD
Professor of Clinical Dentistry
Section Chair, Behavioral Science & Practice Management
Division of Dental Public Health & Pediatric Dentistry
Director, National Center for Dental Hygiene Research & Practice
Ostrow School of Dentistry
University of Southern California
Los Angeles, California

Winnie Furnari, RDH, MS, FAADH
Registered Dental Hygienist
Yonkers, New York
Associate Professor
Department of Dental Hygiene
New York University
College of Dentistry
New York, New York

Peter M. Gangi, RDH, BSED
Registered Dental Hygienist
Office of P.M. Gangi, DMD
Methuen, Massachusetts
Adjunct Clinical Faculty Professor
Department of Dental Hygiene
Middlesex Community College
Lowell, Massachusetts

Kathy Voigt Geurink, RDH, MA
Clinical Associate Professor
Department of Dental Hygiene
The University of Texas Health Science
Center at San Antonio
Public Health Consultant
Association of State and Territorial Dental Directors
Granite Shoals, Texas

Teresa M. Graham, RDH
Registered Dental Hygienist
Brick, New Jersey

Donna M. Grzegorek, RDH
Registered Dental Hygienist
Speaker and Consultant
Barrington, Illinois

JoAnn R. Gurenlian, RDH, PhD
President, Gurenlian and Associates
President-Elect, International Federation of Dental Hygienists'
Haddonfield, New Jersey
Professor and Interim Graduate Program Director
Department of Dental Hygiene
Idaho State University
Pocatello, Idaho

Harold A. Henson, RDH, MEd
Associate Professor
Director, Clinical Simulation
The University of Texas School of Dentistry at Houston
Department of Periodontics and Dental Hygiene
Houston, Texas

Hope-Claire Holbeck, RDH, MS
Registered Dental Hygienist
Chairperson and Assistant Professor
Department of Dental Auxiliaries Education
Middlesex County College
Edison, New Jersey

Janet Kinney, RDH, MS, MS
Assistant Clinical Professor
Periodontics and Oral Medicine
University of Michigan
School of Dentistry
Ann Arbor, Michigan

Robyn Klose, RDH
Registered Dental Hygienist
Owner/Director – NC Dental U
Owner/Director – The Dental Assistant Academy
Director of Clinical Operations – Carolina Dental Management, Inc.
Wake Forest, North Carolina

Elizabeth Lopez, RDH
Registered Dental Hygienist
San Gabriel, California

Stephanie Maddox, RDH, MALD
Registered Dental Hygienist
Master, Academy of Laser Dentistry
Private Practice of Steven Holbrook, DMD
Albuquerque, New Mexico

Pamela J. Myers, RDH
University of Texas Medical Branch
Correctional Managed Care
Manager, Dental Hygiene Program
Huntsville Unit Infirmary
Huntsville, Texas

Vickie Orsini Nardello, RDH MS
State Representative
89th District Connecticut General Assembly
Prospect, Connecticut

Karen Neiner, RDH, MBA
Vice President
Corporate Development and Professional Relations
Hu-Friedy Manufacturing Company, Inc.
Chicago, Illinois

Debra Olsen, RDH, RDHAP
Registered Dental Hygienist in Alternative Practice
Smile Partners
Dental Hygiene Care for California's Seniors & Special Needs
Los Angeles, California

Judith Dember-Paige RDH
Registered Dental Hygienist
Intern, Orofacial Myologist
Author
Westchester, New York

Michelle Panico, RDH, MA
Registered Dental Hygienist
Associate Director, Dentistry in the Community
A.T. Still University of Health Sciences
Arizona School of Dentistry & Oral Health
Community Partnerships & Public Health
Mesa, Arizona

Karen A. Raposa, RDH, MBA
Clinical Education Manager
Hu-Friedy Manufacturing Company, Inc.
Speaker and Author
Raynham, Massachusetts

Jill Rethman, RDH, BA
Editorial Director
Dimensions® of Dental Hygiene
Santa Ana, California
Adjunct Assistant Professor
Department of Dental Hygiene
Ohio State University College of Dentistry
Columbus, Ohio
Adjunct Instructor
Department of Dental Hygiene
University of Pittsburgh School of Dental Medicine
Pittsburgh, Pennsylvania

Candy B. Ross, RDH, BS
Director of Industry and Professional Relations
DEXIS, Gendex, i-CAT, Instrumentarium, KaVo,
Marus, Pelton & Crane and SOREDEX
Marietta, Georgia

Carlos Sanchez, RDH, BSDH, MPH
Registered Dental Hygienist
Los Angeles and Ventura, California
President, Hispanic Dental Association – Los Angeles
Co-Director, University of Southern California
Neighborhood Mobile Dental Van Prevention Program
Clinical Instructor, Division of Dental Public Health and Pediatric Dentistry
Herman Ostrow School of Dentistry
University of Southern California
Center for Community Oral Health Programs
Los Angeles, California

Mary Semancik, RDH
Registered Dental Hygienist
Herndon, Virginia

Jammie Shaughnessy, RDH
Owner, North Valley Comprehensive & Aesthetic Dentistry
Anthem, Arizona

Peggy J. Simonson, RDH, BS
Clinical Teaching Specialist
Candidate, Master in Dental Hygiene
University of Minnesota School of Dentistry
Oral Health Services for Older Adults Program and Division of Dental Hygiene
Department of Primary Care
Minneapolis, Minnesota

Rene Stephenson RDH, BSDH
Sales Representative
Daiichi Sankyo
Lufkin, Texas

Angie Stone, RDH, BS
President, HyLife LLC
Co-Founder, Adopt a Nursing Home
Training Manager, Florida Probe
Xylitol Educator, Wasatch Sales
Edgerton, Wisconsin

Gail Roitman-Trauger, RDH, BA
Territory Manager
Premier Dental Products
Evanston, Illinois

Joyce Turcotte, RDH, MEd, FAADH
President, Professional Learning Services, LLS
Clinical Instructor, Tunxis Community College
Farmington, Connecticut
Practicing Dental Hygienist
BLS Instructor Faculty, American Heart Association
Fairfield, Connecticut

Rebecca Van Horn RDH, BA
Dental Science Liaison Midwest
Procter & Gamble Company
Crest/Oral-B Oral Care Products
Chicago, Illinois

Margaret Walsh, RDH, MA, MS, EdD
Professor
Department of Preventive and Restorative Dental Sciences
University of California
School of Dentistry
San Francisco, California

Cheryl Westphal Theile, RDH, EdD
Assistant Dean for Allied Health Programs
Director, Dental Hygiene Programs
New York University
College of Dentistry
New York, New York

Esther M. Wilkins, BS, RDH, DMD
Department of Periodontology
Tufts University, School of Dental Medicine
Boston, Massachusetts
Forsyth School of Dental Hygiene
Massachusetts College of Pharmacy and Health Sciences
Boston, Massachusetts

Textbooks & Faculty Guide Contributors for
SAVVY SUCCESS

**Achieving Professional Excellence and
Career Satisfaction in the Dental Hygiene Profession
Volume I – Volume III**

Pamela L. Alberto, DMD
Clinical Associate Professor
Department of Oral and Maxillofacial Surgery
New Jersey Dental School
University of Medicine and Dentistry of New Jersey
Sparta, New Jersey

Kenneth Aschheim, DDS, FACD, FAGD
Associate Clinical Professor
New York University
School of Dentistry
New York, New York
Associate Clinical Professor
Mount Sinai School of Medicine
New York, New York

LaVon F. Blaesi, PhD
Faculty Member
Colorado State University
Department of Design & Merchandising
Fort Collins, Colorado

Kathleen Bokrossy, RDH
Registered Dental Hygienist
Business Director, D-Sharp Dental Instruments and *rdhu*
Burlington, Ontario
Canada

Denise M. Bowen, RDH, MS
Professor Emerita
Department of Dental Hygiene
Idaho State University
Pocatella, Idaho

Leanne Carlson, RDT, RDH
Clinical Training Manager
Ondine Biomedical and Periowave Dental Technologies
Vancouver, British Columbia
Canada

Christine Charles, RDH, BS
Registered Dental Hygienist
Director, Scientific and Professional Affairs
Johnson & Johnson Consumer and Personal Products Worldwide
Division of Johnson & Johnson Consumer Companies, Inc.
Morris Plains, New Jersey

Hong Chen, DDS, MS
Clinical Assistant Professor
Department of Endodontics
University of North Carolina – Chapel Hill
School of Dentistry
Chapel Hill, North Carolina

Xi Chen, DDS, PhD
Assistant Professor
University of North Carolina at Chapel Hill
School of Dentistry
Department of Dental Ecology
Chapel Hill, North Carolina

Louis G. DePaola, DDS, MS
Chairman, Clinical Operations Board
Professor, Department of Oncology & Diagnostic Sciences
University of Maryland School of Dentistry
Baltimore, Maryland

James Burke Fine, DMD
Assistant Dean for Postdoctoral Programs
Professor of Clinical Dental Medicine
Director, Postdoctoral Periodontics
Columbia University College of Dental Medicine
New York, New York
Attending Dental Surgeon, Presbyterian Hospital Dental Service
New York, New York

Jacqueline Freudenthal, RDH, MHE
Associate Professor
Department of Dental Hygiene
Idaho State University
Pocatello, Idaho

James Fricton, DDS, MS
Professor
University of Minnesota School of Dentistry and School of Public Health
Senior Researcher, HealthPartners Research Foundation
University of Minnesota
Minneapolis, Minnesota

Jacquelyn L. Fried, RDH, BA, MS
Associate Professor
Director of Inter-Professional Initiative
Department of Periodontology
University of Maryland School of Dentistry
Baltimore, Maryland

Jeffrey Gruneich, PhD
Co-Founder, Vice President
Provia Laboratories, LLC
Lexington, Massachusetts

Harold A. Henson, RDH, MEd
Associate Professor
Director, Clinical Simulation
The University of Texas School of Dentistry at Houston
Department of Periodontics and Dental Hygiene
Houston, Texas

Christine A. Hovliaras, RDH, BS, MBA, CDE
President, Professional Savvy, LLC
Adjunct Faculty, Department of Dental Hygiene
New York University College of Dentistry
New York, New York
Editor Emeritus, *Access Magazine*, 2009-2010
Editor-in-Chief, *Access Magazine*, 2005-2008
Flanders, New Jersey

Richard A. Huot, DDS
Private Practice
CEO, Beachside Dental Consultants, Inc.
Vero Beach, Florida

Claude G. Ibbott DMD, FRCD(c)
Private Practice Periodontist
Pasqua South Oral Health Centre
Regina, Saskatchewan
Canada

Olga A. C. Ibsen RDH, MS, FAADH
Adjunct Professor
Department of Oral and Maxillofacial Pathology, Radiology and Medicine
New York University College of Dentistry
New York, New York
Adjunct Professor
Department of Dental Hygiene
Fones School
University of Bridgeport
Bridgeport, Connecticut

Carol A. Jahn, RDH, MS
Senior Professional Relations Manager
Water Pik, Inc.
Warrenville, Illinois

Shelby L. Kahl, RDH, PC
Registered Dental Hygienist
CEO, Owner, Integrated Oral Health Practice
Shelby Kahl, RDH PC
Fort Collins, Colorado

Lorne Lavine, DMD
President, The Digital Dentist
Burbank, California

Mannie Levi, DDS
Adjunct Faculty
University of Medicine and Dentistry of New Jersey
School of Dentistry
Department of Pediatric Dentistry
West Caldwell, New Jersey

Risa H. Levi, RDH, MS
Assistant Professor
Middlesex County College
Department of Dental Auxiliaries
Division of Dental Hygiene
West Caldwell, New Jersey

Deborah S. Manne, RDH, RN, MSN, OCN®
Registered Dental Hygienist / Head and Neck Oncology Nurse
Adjunct Instructor, Department of Otolaryngology-Head and Surgery
Saint Louis University School of Medicine and Saint Louis University Cancer Center
St. Louis, Missouri
Doctoral Student, PhD in Nursing Program
Sinclair School of Nursing
University of Missouri
Columbia, Missouri

Aaron Mannella, DMD
Private Practice
Pediatric Dental Associates of Randolph
Randolph, New Jersey
Attending Dentist at Morristown Memorial Hospital
Morristown, New Jersey

Renee Marchant, RDH
Registered Dental Hygienist
Owner, Hands-On-Hygiene
Santa Rosa, California

Faith Y. Miller, RDH, MSEd
Associate Professor, Dental Hygiene
School of Allied Health
College of Applied Sciences and Arts
Southern Illinois University, Carbondale
Carbondale, Illinois

Angela Morris, RDH, MS, CCRA, CCRP
Neuroscience Graduate Student
University of Virginia
Charlottesville, Virginia

Angie Mott, RDH
Registered Dental Hygienist
Regulatory Chair, Academy of Laser Dentistry
Owasso, Oklahoma

Brian B. Nový, DDS
Assistant Professor
Department of Restorative Dentistry
Loma Linda University
School of Dentistry
Loma Linda, California

Carole A. Palmer, EdD, RD
Professor and Head, Division of Nutrition and Oral Health Promotion
Department of Public Health and Community Service
Tufts University School of Dental Medicine
Boston, Massachusetts
Professor and Head of the Master's Program
Frances Stern Combined Dietetic Internship/Master's Program
Tufts Medical Center and Friedman School of Nutrition Science and Policy
Tufts University
Boston, Massachusetts
Adjunct Professor, Public Health
Tufts University School of Medicine
Boston, Massachusetts

Edwin T. Parks, DMD, MS
Diplomate, American Academy Board of
Oral and Maxillofacial Radiology
Professor of Diagnostic Sciences
Indiana University School of Dentistry
Indianapolis, Indiana

Frieda A. Pickett, RDH, MS
Adjunct Associate Professor
Idaho State University
Graduate Dental Hygiene Division (Online Program)
Butler, Tennessee

Ellen J. Rogo, RDH, PhD
Registered Dental Hygienist
Associate Professor
Graduate Faculty Member
Department of Dental Hygiene
Idaho State University
Pocatello, Idaho

Colleen Rutledge, RDH
Owner of *Perio-Therapeutics & Beyond*
Dental Hygiene Consultant
National Speaker
Glenside, Pennsylvania

Sylvia L. Santos, RDH, MS
Associate Director
Oral Care Clinical Research
Johnson & Johnson Consumer & Personal Products Worldwide
Division of Johnson & Johnson Consumer Companies, Inc.
Morris Plains, New Jersey

Dianne L. Sefo, RDH, BA
Dental Hygiene Instructor
Concorde Career College
San Diego, California

Ann Eshenaur Spolarich, RDH, PhD
Clinical Associate Professor
Ostrow School of Dentistry of University of Southern California
Division of Dental Public Health and Pediatric Dentistry
Los Angeles, California
Adjunct Associate Professor and Course Director
Clinical Medicine and Pharmacology
Arizona School of Dentistry and Oral Health
Phoenix, Arizona

Lisa B. Stefanou, RDH, BS, MPH
Assistant Director Dental Hygiene Programs
Director of Admissions
Clinical Associate Professor
New York University College of Dentistry
New York, New York

Sharon C. Stull, CDA, BSDH, MS
Lecturer, BSDH Degree Completion Program Director
Community Outreach Coordinator and
Chief Department Advisor
Gene W. Hirschfeld School of Dental Hygiene
Norfolk, Virginia

Janice Hurley-Trailor, BS
Dentistry's Image Expert
Dental Consultant
International Speaker and Author
Scottsdale, Arizona

Bethany Valachi, PT, MS, CEAS
Founder and CEO, Posturedontics, LLC
Dental Ergonomic Speaker, Consultant and Author
Clinical Instructor of Ergonomics
Oregon Health Sciences University
School of Dentistry
Portland, Oregon

Mark A. Varvares, MD, FACS
Professor and Chairman,
Department of Otolaryngology,
Head and Neck Surgery
The Donald and Marlene Jerome Endowed Chair in Otolaryngology
Director, The Saint Louis University Cancer Center
Saint Louis, Missouri

Lisa D. Vaughn, RDH, BS, MSA
Registered Dental Hygienist
Mount Holly Family Dentistry
Mount Holly, New Jersey
Dental Advisory Board Member
Camden County College
Camden, New Jersey

Gail F. Williamson, RDH, MS
Professor of Dental Diagnostic Sciences
Oral Pathology, Medicine and Radiology
Indiana University School of Dentistry
Indianapolis, Indiana

Textbooks & Faculty Guide Reviewers for
SAVVY SUCCESS

**Achieving Professional Excellence and
Career Satisfaction in the Dental Hygiene Profession
Volume I – Volume III**

Joanna Allaire, RDH, MDH
Assistant Professor
Department of Periodontics and Dental Hygiene
The University of Texas School of Dentistry at Houston
Houston, Texas

Meg D. Atwood, RDH, MPS
Associate Professor
Department of Dental Hygiene
Orange County Community College
Middletown, New York

Phebe Blitz, RDH, MS
Interim Dean of Instruction
Career and Technical Programs
Mesa Community College
Mesa, Arizona

Nancy T. Brohawn, RDH, BSDH
Registered Dental Hygienist
Newark, Delaware

Maria Delis, RDH, BS
Registered Dental Hygienist
Laguna Niguel, California

JoAnn R. Gurenlian, RDH, PhD
President, Gurenlian and Associates
President-Elect, International Federation of Dental Hygienists'
Haddonfield, New Jersey
Professor and Interim Graduate Program Director
Department of Dental Hygiene
Idaho State University
Pocatello, Idaho

Pamela A. Hovliaras, DMD, PA
Private Practice Dentist
Hovliaras & Guarnieri, PA
Sparta, New Jersey

Allyson Luckman, RDH, BS
Registered Dental Hygienist
Baltimore, Maryland

Eva M. Lupovici, RDH, MS
Clinical Professor
Department of Dental Hygiene
New York University
College of Dentistry
New York, New York

Oksana P. Mishler, RDH, BS
Clinical Instructor
Department of Periodontics
Division of Dental Hygiene
University of Maryland School of Dentistry
Baltimore, Maryland

Patricia Crane Ramsay, RDH
Director of Alumni Relations
Office of Development
Massachusetts College of Pharmacy and Health Sciences
Boston, Massachusetts

A. Lynn Tobin, RDH, MA
Adjunct Lecturer and Clinical Instructor
Department of Dental Hygiene
Middlesex County College
Edison, New Jersey

Diana Tosuni-O'Neill, RDH, BS
Registered Dental Hygienist
New City, New York

Preface

The first edition of **SAVVY SUCCESS – Achieving Professional Excellence and Career Satisfaction in the Dental Hygiene Profession (Volume I – Volume III)** is for student dental hygienists, dental hygiene faculty members and practicing dental hygienists in the United States and the international community. These textbooks offer new, refreshing information on professional competencies, evidence-based decision making, technology and the ethical responsibilities that should be considered and conducted in the professional careers of dental hygienists and applied into practice every day.

SAVVY SUCCESS has 3-Volume Textbooks and an accompanying Faculty Guide. The 3-Volume Textbooks are as follows:

- Volume I: You-Roles-Practice Environment

- Volume II: Patient Care

- Volume III: Technology-Ethics-Career Success

For **Volume I of the three new textbooks,** I interviewed over 45 dental hygienists who participated in hours of interviews designed to encourage and enlighten the profession about:

- Why they choose a career in dental hygiene;

- How they have helped their patients achieve improved oral care practices;

- What the dental hygiene profession has done for them as a person;

- What qualities do they feel that a dental hygienist must have to be successful;

- The importance of having a mentor; and

- How achieving career success can happen.

Additionally, **SAVVY SUCCESS** discusses the professional roles defined for dental hygiene as administrative/manager, advocate, clinician, educator, public health, research and the addition role of working in a corporate position. The dental hygienists chosen for Chapter 2: Professional Roles represent the five roles with the inclusion of public health being a part of them. These dental hygiene professionals provide their insights on what skills, education and experience is needed to be in each of these roles. It is an enlightening chapter that will provide both students and practicing dental hygienists a view of the other opportunities worth pursuing outside of clinical practice. In Chapter 3: Mentoring, I selected four dental hygienists who serve as mentors and role models in the dental hygiene profession. Their insights will help to spark that passion to get a mentor if one does not have one already.

In Chapter 5: Career Opportunities in Dental Hygiene, I interviewed 10 clinicians who have pursued other roles outside of those discussed in Chapter 2. The ten women highlighted in this chapter will enlighten the readers with other opportunities that a dental hygienist can pursue when they have the vision to pursue additional professional skills and education to obtain these other opportunities.

The goals of the new textbooks (Volume I – Volume III) and the accompanying faculty guide are to provide:
1. Student dental hygienists with the professional skill set they need to enter dental hygiene practice;

2. The professional competencies utilized in practice;

3. An overview of evidence-based decision making to identify the accurate decisions or diagnosis of issues with which patients may appear in practice; and

4. Career opportunities that can be pursued as dental hygienists gain their clinical and professional expertise in practice, as well as the confidence to be the best dental hygienist they can.

The practicing dental hygienists will be: 1) updated on clinical competencies in the delivery of patient care, 2) utilizing technologies to enhance practice-like functions, 3) informed about trends occurring in practice and the importance of ethical decision making and 4) pursuing career opportunities and career satisfaction in their dental hygiene careers.

The Three Textbooks Layout and Units

The units included in the three textbooks cover seven areas of topics that are important in pursuing a career as a dental hygienist. **SAVVY SUCCESS Volume I: You-Roles-Practice Environment** highlights defining who you are, professional roles and career opportunities in the dental hygiene profession, and the practice environment which includes the vision and future of dental hygiene, populations health considerations, business etiquette, leadership, the business of dental hygiene and assisted dental hygiene.

SAVVY SUCCESS Volume II: Patient Care discusses patient care and clinical competencies in the practice of dental hygiene which covers 18 chapters. **SAVVY SUCCESS Volume III: Technology-Ethics-Career Success** focuses on trends and technology (digital radiography, ergonomics, technology in practice, polishing procedures, oral-systemic disease link, teledentistry), ethical responsibility and patient intervention, lifelong learning, balancing work and life and finding career satisfaction to achieve career success as a dental hygiene professional.

The units of the three Savvy Success™ Textbooks (Volume I – III) are as follows:
Volume I: You-Roles-Practice Environment includes:
- **Unit One**: The Dental Hygiene Profession and Your Role in It (Chapters 1 – 5)

- **Unit Two**: Tools and Techniques for Career and Professional Development (Chapters 6 – 10)

- **Unit Three**: Practice Environment (Chapters 11 – 16)

Volume II: Patient Care includes:

- **Unit Four**: Patient Care (Chapters 17 – 34)

Volume III: Technology-Ethics-Career Success includes:

- **Unit Five**: Trends and Technology (Chapters 35 – 40)

- **Unit Six**: Ethical Decision Making (Chapters 41 – 45)

- **Unit Seven**: Securing Professional Career Satisfaction (Chapters 46 – 48)

Each of the 48 chapters in the **first edition textbook, Volume I – Volume III of SAVVY SUCCESS** contain Learning Objectives that will identify competencies that will be gained; a Chapter Overview; Critical Thinking Exercises to assist the student and dental hygiene professional in executing the learning strategies through independent thought and evidence based-decision making; Key Concepts that summarize the main learning objectives from the chapter; Chapter Text which may include tables, diagrams, boxes, sidebars, scripts, figures and suggested readings; and a Summary or Conclusion that provides closing remarks for chapters in **SAVVY SUCCESS**.

There is also an accompanying **SAVVY SUCCESS** Faculty Guide that has also been developed for the 3-Volume textbooks to assist dental hygiene educators in bringing this relevant information into their dental hygiene programs to educate dental hygiene students.

Overview of Seven Units of SAVVY SUCCESS
(Volume I – III)

Volume I: You-Roles-Practice Environment

Unit One: The Dental Hygiene Profession and Your Role in It

*This unit begins the **new Volume I SAVVY SUCCESS™ textbook** with interviews that I conducted with dental hygienists from across the United States who have had experience in the dental hygiene profession. These professionals provide their insights on what made them go into this career, who influenced them to choose dental hygiene and the skills and experiences that are important to be a successful dental hygiene professional.*

Over 45 dental hygienists were interviewed by telephone or by email to share their expertise in the six professional roles in dental hygiene, as well as other roles dental hygienists can pursue to expand their learning, education, professional skills and competencies. A turn-key point in most dental hygienists' careers occurs if they have a mentor who can work with them. Someone to whom they can turn to for guidance, assistance and discussion to identify career opportunities and avenues one may want to pursue in their dental hygiene career.

Career success and expanded opportunities are discussed with insights from ten dental hygienists who have pursued other career opportunities in the profession such as: inventor, forensic dentistry, veterinary dentistry, owning a dental practice, public health, public speaking, editorial director of a peer-reviewed journal, continuing education business owner, book author and a dental hygienist working in a prison facility.

Unit Two: Tools and Techniques for Career Development

This unit will be of great assistance to new graduates writing cover letters and resumes and developing interview skills to get their first dental hygiene position. Practicing dental hygienists can also use this information to update their resumes and cover letters and help to communicate their expertise during these challenging times when the job market has been affected by the economic climate. This unit also discusses the importance of having disability and liability/ malpractice insurance and ensuring that dental hygienists protect themselves during their careers from a job-related injury or ethical situation that may occur in their work environment.

Unit Three: Practice Environment

Topics in this unit discuss the vision and future of the dental hygiene profession; population health considerations; business etiquette in practice; the dental hygienist as a leader; dental hygiene is a business of dentistry; and the important role that dental hygienists play in practice utilizing not only a recare, but a periodontal therapy approach with their patients as well as the use of a dental hygiene assistant to affect overall productivity and profitability in the practice.

Volume II: Patient Care

Unit Four: Patient Care

This unit of **Volume II** *has 18 chapters that focus on elements and competencies of providing patient care, assessment and diagnosis; review of pharmacologic medications; identifying the key oral pathology conditions that occur intraorally/extraorally; oral cancer detection, prevention and treatment; dental caries/minimally invasive dentistry; infection control practices; instrumentation; ultrasonic periodontal therapy; laser therapy in practice; usage of oral hygiene and preventive therapy; mouthrinse usage to maintain oral health; use of anesthesia in dental hygiene practice; nutritional counseling and education with patients; the dental hygienist's role in esthetic dentistry; pediatric concerns for the dental hygienist; and working with patients who have developmental disabilities. It is clinical and scientific information that can be educational for both the student and practicing seasoned dental hygiene professionals.*

Volume III: Technology-Ethics-Career Success

Unit Five: Trends and Technology

In this unit, the **Volume III textbook** *covers new trends occurring in practice to help dental hygienists in time management and efficiency in their positions; use of technology such as digital radiography in practice; trends in polishing practices; the oral-systemic link and its connection to overall wellness; and the use of teledentistry. Teledentistry, in particular, is intriguing as it offers treatment of access to care populations of people who face time and travel issues. This chapter shares how dental and medical professionals can provide treatment and care for these access to care patients through any dental clinic or oral care facility via phone and computer. These professionals provide the care necessary to treat these patients oral healthcare concerns from a remote location in order to provide oral wellness and optimal health considerations.*

Unit Six: Ethical Decision Making

Being a dental hygiene professional requires a college education and a sense of understanding of what is required professionally to make sound ethical decisions in practice to protect the dental hygienist, the patients they treat and the colleagues in the practice. Use of a risk management approach for documentation of records that are hand written or are on the computer must be completed accurately with patient updates and signatures. Medical emergencies are another area that is discussed to provide dental hygienists with a plan that can be shared with their dentist and the team to ensure that the next medical emergency is not a tragedy. Tobacco cessation principles are also discussed with patients who have an addiction to smoking. The chapter covers how the dental hygienist can intervene in education to inform the patient that now may be time to think about stopping this unhealthy habit.

Unit Seven: Dental Hygiene and Securing Career Satisfaction

This last unit of **Volume III of SAVVY SUCCESS** *concludes the thoughts of how important it is to continue lifelong learning in one's dental hygiene career. Taking continuing education courses, becoming certified in local anesthesia, nitrous oxide or laser therapy pending your state practice regulations are just a few of the areas to consider. Setting goals and objectives so a plan of action is in place and staying abreast of the scientific literature in peer reviewed journals and magazines are a sampling of methods the dental professionals may employ to stay in touch* with new news and trends going on in the profession. Balancing work and life can sometimes be complicated and Chapter 47 will provide insights for **SAVVY SUCCESS** readers to consider how to do this in a successful and non-stressful way. The last chapter on dental hygiene and career satisfaction focuses on insights that I and other dental hygienists I have interviewed provide on how to achieve career satisfaction and what skills and attributes can assist dental hygienists in reaching this level of happiness and success in their professional careers.

Appendix and Glossary of Terms

The appendix which is included in **Volume III of SAVVY SUCCESS** highlights information from a chapter author on the ADHA Code of Ethics. The glossary of terms which is included in **Volumes I – III of SAVVY SUCCESS** defines key terms utilized in the 48 chapters that students, faculty members and practicing dental hygienists can review to define the use of them. An index is also included in the three volumes as well.

SAVVY SUCCESS Faculty Guide

The accompanying Faculty Guide contains the Learning Objectives, Chapter Overviews, Critical Thinking Exercises, Key Concepts and a question-and-answer section that dental hygiene faculty members can use in their curriculum with dental hygiene students from the entire 48 chapters included in Volume I - Volume III. I interviewed key educators in the dental professional to get their insights of what a textbook like this should include in order to bring these three textbooks (Volume I – Volume III) into dental hygiene programs nationally and internationally.

Acknowledgements

I would like to thank the 47 dental hygienists who I interviewed by telephone and email for **SAVVY SUCCESS - Achieving Professional Excellence and Career Satisfaction in the Dental Hygiene Profession** to provide a different and exciting niche for the **Volume I and III textbooks** and the associated **Faculty Guide**. Their thoughts and advice that I am sharing with the dental hygiene community will provide information to students, faculty colleagues and practicing dental hygienists to assist them in setting goals and objectives and putting a plan of action into place for their professional careers.

In my 28 years in the dental hygiene profession, I have met many outstanding leaders in dental hygiene, dentistry and medicine. I have worked with these individuals in business, professional organizations and business relationships as well as professional friendships. I want to thank the 46 authors who have written 35 informative and interesting chapters in the new textbooks Volume I – Volume III and Faculty Guide and shared their photographs/figures with our readers. These chapter authors were selected for their expertise in their topic areas included in Volume I – Unit 3: Practice Environment, Volume II – Unit 4: Patient Care, Volume III – Unit 5: Trends and Technology in Practice and Volume III – Unit 6: Ethical Decision Making. Their professional insights have provided a unique, evidence-based approach that is directly applicable to dental hygiene practice. Thank you for taking time out of your work and personal schedules to work with me. I am honored to have you be a part of this endeavor.

Many chapter authors utilized tables, diagrams, boxes, forms etc. from organizations, agencies and universities in dentistry and medicine. I would like to acknowledge the following organizations who granted permission to use this information: American Cancer Institute; American Dental Association (ADA); ADA Center for Evidence-Based Dentistry; American Dental Hygienists' Association; Academy of Laser Dentistry; American Society of Anesthesiologists; Bureau of Labor Statistics; Centers for Disease Control and Prevention; Healthcare Infection Control Practices Advisory Committee; Joint National Committee on Prevention, Detection, Evaluation, and Treatment of High Blood Pressure; National Audiovisual Center; National Cancer Institute; National Institute of Dental Craniofacial Research; National Institute for Occupational Safety and Health; U.S. Preventive Services Task Force, U.S. Public Health Service; and Yale University.

I would also like to acknowledge the following companies who granted permission to me for the use of photographs/figures in **SAVVY SUCCESS - Achieving Professional Excellence and Career Satisfaction in the Dental Hygiene Profession Volume I – Volume III**:

Adrian Pharmaceuticals, Spring Hill, Florida; Air Techniques, Hicksville, New York; Colgate-Palmolive Company, New York, New York; Dentsply International, York, Pennsylvania; D-Sharp Dental, Inc., Burlington, Ontario, Canada; GC America, Alsip, Illinois; Hu-Friedy Manufacturing Company, Inc., Chicago, Illinois; LED Dental, Inc., Burnaby, British Columbia, Canada; Mad Ultrasonics, Yonkers, New York; Milestone Scientific, Inc., Livingston, New Jersey; Oral Biotech, Albany, Oregon; OraPharma, Inc., Warminster, Pennsylvania; Orian Diagnostica, Espoo, Finland; Parkell, Inc., Edgewood, New York; Sirona Dental Systems, Charlotte, North Carolina; Tony Riso Company, Margate, Florida; Ultrasonic Services, Inc., Houston, Texas; and Zila Inc., Fort Collins, Colorado.

The Academy of Laser Dentistry has provided photographs/figures from the following companies: Biolase Technology, Inc., Irvine, California; Hoya ConBio, Fremont, California; Ivoclar Vivadent, Inc., Amherst, New York; KaVo Dental, Charlotte, North Carolina; King Dental Company, Prospect, Kentucky; LED Dental, Inc., Burnaby, British Columbia, Canada; Sirona Dental Systems, Inc., Charlotte, North Carolina; Technology 4 Medicine, San Clemente, California; and Zila, Inc., Fort Collins, Colorado.

I want to thank the 13 book reviewers who did a very thorough review of the units of the three new textbooks and faculty guide and provided valuable feedback to me. Thank you for your time and effort in this process.

I want to thank Nicole Harrison for working with me to make each of the author's tables, boxes, diagram, scripts, forms, etc., to look professional and easy to read. Nikki – you did a great job and I appreciate you being there when I needed you. A big thank you goes out to my business colleague and friend, Tim Breiding, President of Breiding Marketing, for assisting me with all the photographs/figures to look clear and publishable and for working with me to design my front and back covers of the three Textbooks and Faculty Guide. You did a fabulous job!

I want to thank and acknowledge the hard work and long hours that Donna Rounsaville, RDH, BS, who was an intern working with me in 2010-2011 who provided professional relations and marketing efforts for the new three Textbooks and Faculty Guide. I was blessed that you contacted me to work as an intern while you were going for your bachelor of science degree in dental hygiene online.

To my dear friends and neighbors, Debbie and Frank DelPesce, for allowing me to do the front cover photo shoot in their beautiful study. Thank you to my photographer and high school friend, Jim Kapinos, for taking the photographs for the front and back cover of the Textbooks and Faculty Guide.

To my sister, Dr. Pamela Hovliaras, for giving me great insights on questions I ran by her during the years I worked on this project. You are a great friend and I am so thankful to have you as my sister.

My last and final thank you is for my handsome, loving and funny son, Jarod Crist. Thank you for being so patient and giving me your support while Mom was working tirelessly on these three Textbooks and Faculty Guide.

I look forward to any insights and thoughts from our readers on their recommendations on future chapters or modifications I should consider for the second edition of these new Textbooks and Faculty Guide.

Regards,
Christine A. Hovliaras

Table of Contents
SAVVY SUCCESS

Achieving Professional Excellence and
Career Satisfaction in the Dental Hygiene Profession
Volume I

UNIT ONE:

The Dental Hygiene Profession and Your Role in It

Chapter 1: Defining Who You Are

By Christine A. Hovliaras, RDH, BS, MBA, CDE

Learning Objectives

The student dental hygienist and dental hygiene professional will learn the following key objectives from this chapter:

1. Identify who you are, what made you select the dental hygiene position you currently hold, determine the type of dental hygiene professional you want to become and what it takes to continue to empower yourself in the profession.
2. Identify the key elements that allow dental hygienists to continue to work in the dental hygiene profession.
3. Create a list of personal and professional traits that you believe will help you to continue your career as a dental hygienist.

Overview

Discovering a path in the dental hygiene profession does not end in dental hygiene school. It is a life-long journey that requires some introspection, research and personal and professional development. It is a wonderful journey that connects professionals in a diverse and dynamic field that offers new opportunity to expand one's career and provide our patients an environment of health and oral wellness. Those who have lost that spark of passion and inspiration in this field for dental hygiene may find renewal in taking continuing education courses to enhance their knowledge base and by researching new roles that will assist their pursuit of the right avenue in the dental hygiene profession.

Dame Margot Fonteyn was once quoted: "The one important thing I have learned over the years is the difference between taking one's work seriously and taking one's self seriously. The first is imperative and the second disastrous."

We may not all agree that taking one's self seriously is disastrous. In my career, it has proved necessary in order to take myself seriously many times to achieve goals and access opportunities that I felt I had to achieve.

Most dental hygiene professionals and those pursuing a degree in it are serious about work. From the first day of the first course dental hygiene students take in approved dental hygiene programs, they know that this is a healthcare profession that requires its practitioners to have knowledge of gross anatomy, oral-systemic link, pharmacology and dental-medical recommendations, to name but a few fields of study it encompasses. It is a serious profession; one in which practitioners have the power to influence outcomes of either one patient at a time or entire communities. What is required to prepare for this responsibility and the exciting challenges ahead? Dental hygiene professionals need to spend time considering where their careers might go and who those careers might influence.

Defining Who You Are

"Compassionate, caring and kind?"
"Optimistic, energetic and persuasive?"
"Diplomatic, reserved and flexible?"

What short strand of words defines each individual? Everyone at one point or another in their personal development considers who they are. If they don't spend time thinking about it, a wise parent, friend or teacher along the way is certain to introduce the topic!

If professionals could engage someone else to write about them, that story would emerge quite different from the one they would write on their own. In order, to be accurate and true to ambitions that best fit individual personality, it is good to do some self-searching.

No matter in what area of the profession a dental hygienist resides – a student, a new clinician, or an experienced professional – it is certain that the individual probably entered the profession with a lot of curiosity, a measure of ambition and a desire to help others. These were some of the top characteristics mentioned to me as I conducted interviews with more than 45 dental hygiene professionals for this new first edition textbook. These are the characteristics that led many individuals into the profession and helped them keep their careers fresh and exciting.

Why Become a Dental Hygienist?

Mary Calka, RDH, a graduate of the Fones School of Dental Hygiene at the University of Bridgeport, Bridgeport, CT, recalled that her earliest career goal was to help others.

"I wanted to work with people and do something that would help improve their health or quality of life," said Calka, who started her career as a dental assistant following high school. After working as a dental assistant for a few years, she decided she wanted to do more. "I became a dental hygienist," Calka continued.

Carlos Sanchez, RDH, BSDH, MPH, a 2008 graduate of the dental hygiene program at the University of Southern California School of Dentistry, also started as a dental assistant – 12 years before he graduated from dental hygiene school.

"As early as I can recall, my niche has always been helping people out, particularly in a medical sense. I grew up in a family of dental healthcare professionals," Sanchez commented. His father and brother are dentists and a few aunts are dental hygienists. The family didn't force him into the field, Sanchez noted; he was just exposed to it at an early age.

"I wanted to place myself in a unique situation to enrich the lives of others," he said.

Justin Bordessa, RDH, who has practiced since 2004, felt drawn to dental hygiene after struggling with oral health issues in his teens. He noticed during numerous recall visits "that the employees at the dental practice liked their positions and being at work. That initially sparked my interest." He eventually took a position as a sterilization assistant in a private dental practice to further explore oral healthcare options.

What fired his ambition was his interest "to help people not go through the problems I went through." It was the same year that a dental hygiene school opened at Santa Rosa Junior College (CA), in his home town – talk about coincidence.

For 29-year career veteran Donna Grzegorek, RDH, a person entering dental hygiene should be a health advocate.

"We have to practice what we preach. As healthcare providers, we must be committed to life-long learning. We have to have a burning desire to provide the most effective, comprehensive and updated therapies available and that requires a constant search for new information,"
Grzegorek said.

"The most successful dental hygienists I have encountered were enthusiastic, passionate and responsible. I viewed them as very intelligent, detailed individuals who were able to communicate effectively and who provided leadership when called upon to do so," Grzegorek concluded.

These stories are similar to my own. My passion for the dental hygiene profession began when I was 14 years old and in stainless-steel braces on my maxillary arch. I had a wonderful orthodontist who had a dynamic dental team, and they took great pride in reinforcing good oral hygiene habits with their patients. Besides their never-ending encouragement to keep my mouth biofilm-free, the thing that most influenced me to become a dental hygienist was a before-and-after picture on the operatory wall that said it all.

The picture revealed several things. First, it showed before-and-after shots of a patient with good oral hygiene; one side captured her tenure with orthodontics, and the other side showed her smile after the orthodontics were removed. In this picture, there was no gingivitis or development of plaque biofilm on the orthodontic bands and wires, and after the braces were removed, the teeth were beautiful and straight. The other picture was of another patient who did not conduct good oral hygiene practices at home. There was gingivitis and an accumulation of plaque biofilm on every tooth, the orthodontic bands and wires. In the shot showing when the braces were removed, there was decalcification on the enamel and a significant amount of gingivitis. I only had to see that picture once! I became a fanatic about cleaning my teeth. I used a floss threader and performed fabulous brushing technique so I would not look like the patient with poor oral hygiene. My smile and having healthy teeth were very important to me.

After my braces were removed, my teeth looked fabulous and white, and I was proud that I took very good care of them. At that time in high school, my aspiration was to be a lawyer. After my experience with braces, becoming a dental hygiene professional overcame the desire for a law degree.

I actually applied to two dental hygiene programs – one was at the Forsyth School in Boston and the other was at Fairleigh S. Dickinson, Jr., College of Dental Medicine (FDUCDM) in New Jersey. I was accepted to Forsyth, but didn't know if I wanted to go to Boston to go to school. I did not get accepted to Fairleigh Dickinson's Dental Hygiene Program that year, but decided to begin my prerequisite courses for the four-year degree at Fairleigh Dickinson University (FDU). After a year, I reapplied to the dental hygiene program. I did get accepted for the dental hygiene program in September 1982 and jumped in with both feet to become the best dental hygiene student I could become. It was a big "status thing" to become accepted in dental hygiene on our campus. There were a lot of applicants, and only a small number of dental hygiene students were accepted into the program. Plus, we had a wonderful dental school program, and the dental students worked with the dental hygiene students on certain rotations. It was a fabulous place to go to college.

It was in the plan for me to go to FDUCDM and through that decision, the rest of my opportunities followed me. Prior to beginning my first year of dental hygiene school, my mother, Ruth Ann, suggested that I get a job as a dental assistant to make sure that dentistry was the right career option for me. I agreed with her and began working part time during the summer at the lucrative dental practice of Drs. Cohen and Schwartz in Budd Lake, NJ. Little did I know they had a periodontist in the practice with whom I would become friends. His name was Dr. Jeffrey M. Gordon and he also worked as faculty in the Department of Periodontology at FDUCDM.

Dr. Gordon was the best mentor I could ever have. He is a fabulous periodontist, great dental researcher and a wonderful role model. I also worked with Dr. Ira Lamster in the FDUCDM Dental Research Center, with Dr. Gordon. When they started a practice together in 1983, I had the honor of working with them the first year as their receptionist and dental assistant. Dr. Lamster left the practice after a year, Dr. Gordon took it over, and I continued to work with him for 16 years.

Interestingly enough, Dr. Gordon had trained with Dr. Socransky at Forsyth School of Dental Medicine. He left Boston and came to New Jersey. Talk about timing and making decisions. If I had not met Dr. Gordon, I would not have gained the opportunities in dental research and periodontology as a dental hygienist. My experiences starting in his practice as his receptionist, dental assistant and then dental hygienist, paired well with making it a success through hard work and perseverance. I began working as a research dental hygienist at FDUCDM for five years testing an antibiotic, clindamycin, on refractory periodontitis patients and then testing oral care products on reducing plaque and gingivitis. These research efforts led to publishing and presenting our research at the American Association and International Association for Dental Research Meetings from 1984-1989. It was an exciting time, and our research center at FDUCDM was well respected. I accomplished all of this while pursuing a Masters in Business Administration at night at FDU School of Business for four years and working two jobs in clinical practice and research and a part-time clinical instructor position in the dental hygiene department.

After five years at FDUCDM, I left my position in 1989 to pursue a Clinical Research Scientist position with the Warner-Lambert Company. The dental school closed in 1990. I closed one door, and another door of opportunity opened for me. I continued to work with Dr. Gordon for 16 years as his dental hygienist – what a great journey it was!

Keeping Professionals in the Dental Hygiene Field

Opportunity is the primary element that keeps professionals in any line of work, and it is no different for careers in dental hygiene.

Grzegorek described her personal success story as an evolutionary process "that will continue to unfold until the day I retire!" She added: "I have said yes to every professional opportunity that came my way." A life-long learner, Grzegorek's desire to persistently improve herself professionally "has put me in proximity with some of the brightest leaders in the profession."

When asked how she achieved career success, Grzegorek described it like this: "I consider myself to be at the helm of my ship sailing the sea. I am determined to dock at every destination point. I want to experience it all!"

Calka, who has been an RDH for 28 years, always felt there were other aspects of the profession to explore and let her curiosity guide her information gathering. This willingness to ask questions and provide her own input led her to many wonderful opportunities.

"When I was a dental hygienist in private practice, one of the sales representatives had complimented me saying that every time she sent me product samples, I was the only one who called her back to let her know that something had changed," Calka shared. "That was when I was invited to be on the Oral-B advisory board. It was a two-year commitment that allowed me to learn more about corporate integration and how corporate and dental hygiene work together."

The board was comprised of 10 dental hygienists from across the country who met twice a year with the upper management and development staff. Calka enjoyed the interaction on marketing strategies and new developments.

Calka's experience on the Oral-B advisory board further fueled exploration of other areas of dental hygiene. She eventually took a part-time position in product education with OraPharma, Inc. "My role was to go into various dental practices and teach the staff the proper use of the product, ARESTIN®," she commented.
Everyone could benefit by following Calka and Grzegorek's examples. As opportunities arise, take them. One never knows where opportunities will lead and what lessons may be learned along the way. A chance opportunity may lead dental hygiene professionals to meet someone they otherwise may not have encountered. It is good to be confident about capabilities and experience, but I have learned it is also good to be humble at the same time. I always am learning something from others within the dental profession and in business.

The Dental Hygiene Position You Hold

The many options available in dental hygiene today will be covered in Chapters 2 and 5, however, it bears mention at this point that roles in this profession suit a variety of professional work styles.

Calka, for example, wanted to get into a community health setting. "It was the only part of the dental hygiene career path I had not touched on at that time," she recalled. With some help from colleagues and friends in the profession, she found entry into community health centers.

"Now I manage and work with the public school system in a mobile dental hygiene program," she said, explaining that she and her team move the equipment during the school year from school to school. The program delivers a variety of preventive care from examinations and fluoride treatments to applying dental sealants. In the months when school is not in session, Calka works in the community health center in Norwalk, CT, treating a variety of patients from children to the elderly to those who have been diagnosed as HIV positive.

Sanchez, who is currently working as a clinical dental hygienist in a private dental practice and as a clinical instructor at the USC School of Dentistry, is plotting a similar course. He recently completed a Master in Public Health degree.

"I want to reach out to some of these communities and populations that are underprivileged," he commented. "Dental hygiene offers a unique ability to interact with individuals. I am constantly interacting with people from all walks of life. You get different perspectives on life. You get to know your patients. I hope to be a positive impact on them – and vice versa."

Bordessa daily makes in-roads to understanding patient reaction to treatment as a clinician in a general practice that offers sedation dentistry.

"Sedation dentistry attracts patients who can be fearful or phobic. By developing my verbal and non-verbal skills and clinical approach, I have improved their attitudes toward oral health in general, making their visits easier. This helps to ensure a long-term professional relationship in which I can do my best to keep them healthy. Along with this comes the reputation of being gentle," Bordessa explained.

Grzegorek works in a private practice and also offers dental hygiene consulting services when called upon by dentists who know of her work. In addition, she is a myofunctional therapist and uses that expertise in conjunction with her dental hygiene work in an orthodontic practice. She works five days in dental hygiene, splitting her time between the orthodontic and a general practice. She also lectures for VELscope, an oral cancer detection device manufacturer, and offers consulting to other private practices and some corporations.

"Although we have to be able to operate autonomously, dental hygienists also have to be able to function within the dynamic of the team environment," Grzegorek commented. "Often dental hygienists are leaders, so it can be a challenge to shift into being a total team player. I feel the dental hygienist is called upon to be the glue that keeps a dental office functioning. The dental hygienist is frequently the go-to person who is capable of providing common sense, logic and problem resolution."

The Importance of Professional Relationships and Organizations

No professional should think of themselves as alone, even if he or she is the only dental hygienist in the practice. Professional relationships, developed with the help of professional organizations, are important to maintain perspective in the field of dental hygiene.

"For me professional relationships have played an important role in my development as a dental hygienist," said Sanchez. "I've been fortunate to be surrounded by a very influential social and professional network that has empowered me to continue to grow as a dental hygienist. In terms of school, I have been fortunate there, too. USC has well respected dentists and dental hygienists in the field. Some of those mentors continue to be friends now that I have graduated."

Sanchez observed that the profession has gained more and more respect throughout the years, and that as a young dental hygienist, he has a personal obligation to continue building that respect by being involved in professional organizations and in the community.

"I want to be an agent for the oral health care profession," commented Sanchez, who was a member of the Student American Dental Hygienists' Association (SADHA), a group that eventually was absorbed into the American Dental Hygienists' Association (ADHA) membership. In addition, he was a co-founder of Student Professionalism in Ethics Club (SPEC), an organization unique to USC, which he hopes will be adopted on a national level in dental and dental hygiene schools. Sanchez also acts as a board member for Latinos for Dental Careers – a not-for-profit organization that promotes and represents minorities in the dental field.

"I have always felt there is a sense of family in the dental hygiene community. That is something that I have really enjoyed. There is a lot of professional interaction," Sanchez concluded.

Calka echoed this sentiment: "Dental hygiene introduced me to people who have really become friends who supported me through the years. Personally, I have really been enriched by the relationships I have gained through the profession."

Calka firmly believes in the importance that mentors have in professional relationships. "Everybody needs a mentor," she asserted. "Find someone who believes in you – that support from a mentor and the networks we belong to encourage us to grow. I know that opportunities that might not have become available to me opened up because I knew so many people. A simple conversation with a colleague leads to an opportunity."

One of Calka's mentors shared that every time the two climbed into the car to go to a meeting, Mary hatched a new plan. "She said that before our next drive, I would have implemented the plan," she said, chuckling. "All you have to do is pick up the phone or send a couple of emails and before you know it someone is reaching out to you."

Bordessa also values mentorship in the profession. "When we as hygienists get out of school and move into the workplace, we have a lot of information. Sometimes we have an idea about what to do, but the idea of how to go about doing it is kind of a question mark," he commented. He continued, describing how the dentist with whom he practices provides an excellent example on a daily basis of patient communications and interaction.

"I've been able to pick up on a lot of his dialogue with patients and use that when I communicate with them," said Bordessa, who also values the work he does with the other dental hygienist in the practice.

It is this connection and willingness to share knowledge that has meant the most to Grzegorek. "I have been amazed at the honest desire that my mentors and role models have displayed in wanting to assist me in becoming a better dental hygienist."

What Does It Take to be a Dental Hygienist?

I shudder to think that someone may have been practicing for five years in the profession and may still ask themselves the question: What does it take to be a dental hygienist? Or worse, maybe that person moved to another profession and still wonders what it takes. This is what motivated me to write this book. I wanted to share with those new to or ready to move within the profession what roles were available and what a career in dental hygiene would take. For seasoned professionals, especially, I want to share the continuing promise that the dental hygiene profession can be anything that they have the passion and commitment to undertake.

When I put the question of what it takes to be a dental hygienist to the many professionals I interviewed for this text, I received a variety of answers.

Sanchez admitted that he is not sure that everyone is cut out for the dental hygiene field – it takes someone special. "I think one of the most important things is you have to be compassionate and be in tune with others. I think you need to have drive and determination to be the best you can be in the field."

He added that being really successful in the profession takes a different approach. "You have to be passionate about the work that you are doing. You must want to make a difference in the lives of patients, to the office in which you practice, to your peers and colleagues," he said. "There can be a high rate of burn out." To circumvent that burn out, Sanchez asserted that dental hygienists need to get involved, be proactive and not limit the profession to clinical work.

Calka created a list when asked what it takes to be a dental hygienist. "Self-motivated, compassionate and a good communicator. Someone who feels comfortable working with people and working with them in a close proximity," she said, adding that the profession also requires people who don't quit easily and have the ability to think outside the box. "Patience, understanding and good listening," she concluded.

Bordessa placed organizational and communications skills at the top of his list of important dental hygiene characteristics. "You need a certain level of verbal communication skills because you need to translate technical language into layman's terms," he said. "You need to be a goal setter, too. Sometimes there are road blocks that can be frustrating, but keeping long-range goals in mind helps you understand the process."

Dental hygiene is a profession that requires constant self improvement, Bordessa has found. "You can't get to a point where you feel your work is good enough. That is a good recipe for stagnation and burnout. To be an optimal dental hygienist, you need to be involved in the professional organizations, ADHA, for example, and you have to keep up with healthcare science as a whole. There are so many systemic issues affecting patients, we have to know how to approach a variety of medical issues and talk to our patients about how oral and medical diseases may affect their health."

This range of health issues and a continuing desire to understand them made Grzegorek wish she had continued on into dental school.

"I came to the realization a few years ago that I could have a much greater impact on the health and wellness of my patients as a dental hygienist than I could as a dentist," she commented. "I feel the way the profession has evolved I am in the forefront, I am the gatekeeper for oral health and hence full body wellness."

Educating the rest of the population to this point of view also tops the list of what it takes to be a dental hygienist. It is a process that occurs sometimes one patient at a time.

"In terms of my professional life, there is a certain satisfaction I get from working in private practice settings. I like to hear that people call in requesting appointments 'with that happy hygienist – the one who sings!'" Calka laughed.

"I always spend 10 or 15 minutes talking to patients before I begin work with them. As a dental hygienist and provider of care, you need to build a certain amount of trust. That trust comes from listening and understanding."

Calka concluded: "My responsibility to my profession is to be a member who is active. If you want to facilitate change, you have to first be involved."

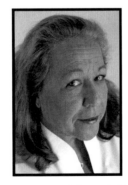

Figure 1.1. Mary Calka

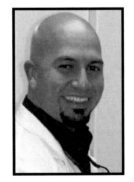

Figure 1.2. Carlos Sanchez

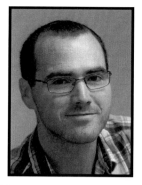 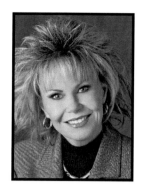

Figure 1.3. Justin Bordessa   **Figure 1.4.** Donna Grzegorek

Professional Savvy, LLC, wants to thank Mary, Carlos, Justin and Donna for being interviewed for the SAVVY SUCCESS™ textbook for dental hygienists. I greatly appreciate the thoughts and insights you have shared with our readers on what dental hygiene means to you and the role you play with your patients. Thank you very much for being a part of this new textbook.

Critical Thinking Exercises

1. Using the characteristics described in this chapter, build a list of desirable characteristics found in most successful dental hygienists. Consider which of these characteristics fit with your own personal and professional traits.

Key Concepts

1. Discovering a path in the dental hygiene profession is a life-long journey that requires some introspection, research and personal and professional development.

2. All professionals should contemplate who they are at various points in their personal/professional development.

3. Some key characteristics of dental hygiene professionals include: a desire to improve the health or quality of life of others; a commitment to life-long learning; further education and a deep sense of enthusiasm, scientific curiosity, passion and personal responsibility.

4. Dental hygiene professionals tend to be highly intelligent, detail oriented and effective communicators.

5. The primary elements that help dental hygiene professionals retain their enthusiasm for the profession are the new and diverse opportunities available.

6. Professional relationships, developed with the help of professional organizations, are important in the field of dental hygiene because they help the dental hygiene professional: maintain perspective; connect to new opportunities; provide information, education and support; and assist in professional and personal development.

Chapter 2: Professional Roles in Dental Hygiene

By Christine A. Hovliaras, RDH, BS, MBA, CDE

Learning Objectives

The student dental hygienist and dental hygiene professional will learn the following key objectives from this chapter:

1. Describe the seven roles that define the dental hygiene profession.
2. Identify key professional characteristics that make one suitable for a dental hygiene position within these roles.
3. Create a profile of a job the reader would like to hold within one of these roles.
4. Develop a plan for achieving a desired position after learning about the structure of the dental hygiene profession.

Overview

The dental hygiene profession is rich with possibilities and potential for those willing to research positions, tackle projects and take charge of their careers. This growing field, defined by the American Dental Hygienists' Association (ADHA)'s six professional roles and Professional Savvy, LLC,'s seventh category, possesses a vibrancy that keeps professionals enthused about their work many years into their careers.

When "Tanya" entered dental hygiene school, she considered that she might work for someone like her uncle who ran a small-town, family dental practice. During her education, she completed a rotation in an elder-care center. It opened her eyes to the oral healthcare needs of the elderly population and to her natural ability to relate to older people. She could put them at ease quickly once in her care. After graduation, a nursing home that was familiar with Tanya's work approached her about joining their full-time staff. It was an easy decision for the new graduate to make.

Dental hygienists who only ever consider private practice as their primary role miss the depth of roles found within the profession. With such a variety of positions, it is a challenge for the dental hygienist to select only one that suits his or her work ethic, employment needs and goals for the future.

Trends in Dental Hygiene the Past 10 Years

According to the Bureau of Labor Statistics, employment of dental hygienists is expected to grow 36% through 2018, which is much faster than the average for all occupations.[1] This is in response to increasing demands for dental care and the greater utilization of dental hygienists to perform services previously performed by dentists.

Attitudes toward entry-level positions in dental hygiene have evolved in the last 10 years. New entrants to the field want to make the same amount of money as a seasoned dental hygienist. They want benefits, bonuses and all the amenities of a full-time job – luxuries that seasoned professionals may have worked toward for 10 years and have yet to realize.

Counselors in the profession advise new dental hygienists to learn their clinical position and prove their worth in the work place first. New entrants to the profession must establish best-business practices such as maintaining the patient schedule, reviewing medical histories, conducting clinical assessments, planning treatment and then providing clinical dental hygiene services, using new technology, recommending products for home use and working as a team with dental practice colleagues. These duties ensure foundational work ethics, help dental hygienists prove their worth in the practice and lead to various job benefit rewards.

With a focus remaining on disease prevention, the past 10 years have seen an expanded scope of practice for dental hygienists in some states and the development of the Advanced Dental Hygiene Practitioner (ADHP).

The expansion allows dental hygienists to work under general supervision versus direct supervision, conducting activities such as administering local anesthesia or nitrous oxide. Clinicians provide care in nursing homes, assisted livings facilities, long-term care facilities and many settings where they have become the front-line care giver.

It is literally a great time to be a part of this profession.

Review the Professional Roles in Dental Hygiene

ADHA defined five professional roles in dental hygiene, as well as a sixth role, public health, which is such an integral part of the other five that it is considered an over-arching role within the profession. For this text, Professional Savvy, LLC, introduces another over-arching role: dental hygiene in the corporate setting. The five basic roles identified by ADHA include: administrator/manager, advocate, clinician, educator and researcher.

Each of these seven roles assumes elements of the other six, which lends that depth and vibrancy that keeps professionals enthused about their work many years into their careers.

Networking is a powerful tool for learning more about the profession and its roles. I have spent many years interviewing dental hygienists who have successfully moved into every variety of dental hygiene position that one can imagine – and a few roles that these busy, talented professionals forged for themselves.

Many have shared their stories here to help others in the profession understand the role and what elements were necessary to move into it. Review the following seven sections and make notes as to the key professional characteristics that match your personal skill set at this point in your professional development.

Administrator/Manager

Definition: Dental hygienists in the **administrator/manager role** guide and direct the work of others as well as execute a variety of administrative duties. Duties may include everything from supervisory roles for other clinicians in the practice to those who maintain supply inventories or act as the office manager. Responsibilities within this role include utilizing data, communicating objectives, applying organizational skills, identifying and managing resources and billing systems and evaluating and modifying programs for oral health, education or health care.

Educational Requirements: Several professionals sited in this section said that a four-year degree is required in the administrative/managerial role. For at least one of those sources, that four-year degree was in psychology – something she said has helped her both with clinical dental hygiene, in assessing and understanding the patient's mindset, and in consulting for understanding the team dynamic.

Professional Characteristics: Skills important to this role, sources said, include good organization and communications skills, a team focus (as the dental hygienist is typically setting procedures for an entire practice or group of practices), familiarity with current research, ability to network and willingness to accept challenges.

Tammy L. Filipiak, RDH, MS, and Teresa M. Graham, RDH, represent two registered dental hygienists who work in the administrator/manager role.

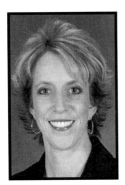 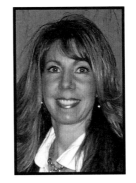

Figure 2.1. Tammy L. Filipiak   **Figure 2.2.** Teresa M. Graham

Since February 2004, Filipiak has worked for Midwest Dental, a dental management company headquartered in Mondovi, WI with more than 90 clinics in Wisconsin, Minnesota, Illinois, Kansas and Iowa, and a Western Division known as Mountain Dental, which currently includes offices in Colorado and New Mexico. She currently holds the position of Director of Clinical Development for the company. What led her to this position? After working for a great prosthodontist for 16 years, Filipiak wanted to have an impact not only in supporting and developing other dental hygienists within the profession, but also with a larger patient audience.

"I saw it as an opportunity for me to give back to other dental hygienists what people had given to me as an individual clinician," commented Filipiak, who received her RDH in 1987 from Northcentral Technical College in Wausau, WI. After completing her Bachelor of Business degree from Upper Iowa University, Filipiak received a Master of Organizational Leadership and Quality degree from Wisconsin's Marian University in 2009.

In her role, Filipiak works in partnership with the dentists and dental hygienists within the practices to identify their specific needs with regard to training/development from the clinical aspect. She also leads the company's clinical team where focus includes developing treatment protocols, clinical orientation, research and planning for continued learning. She also serves as the assistant compliance officer.

She described Midwest Dental's commitment to patient care as a "core philosophy of what we do and who we are. I absolutely have the best job in the world, and the people I get to work with are an added bonus!" Filipiak stated.

A typical day on the job might include traveling within the company's geographical market to visit one of the practices. In a recent visit, she was working with a dentist who had just moved from a private practice location into a Midwest Dental practice. The doctors and dental hygienists were proactive in asking for something of a performance review related to patient care, Filipiak explained.

"The team wanted to develop more consistency in documentation, chart notes and communication with regard to presentation of treatment for patients. We had a round table discussion so everybody had the opportunity to get on the same page. The core focus of my job is to provide support. This can include reviewing research to support clinical care, providing on-site training, investigating changes in clinical technology and working with clinician mentors. I always remind our dental hygienists and dentists that I work for them," Filipiak said.

Filipiak is on call for training and support as the dentists and dental teams need her, and this often includes identifying new areas of opportunity within patient care as well as recognizing the successes once achieved. Filipiak commented that she enjoys working with professionals at different levels in their careers.

For her administrative role, Teresa M. Graham finds employment for dental hygienists, dentists, dental assistants and front office personnel. A practicing clinician since she graduated from Middlesex County College, Middlesex, NJ in 1988, Graham joined leagues with Dental Temps Professional Services, Inc. This move helped her establish Garden State Dental Temps in April 2005. Since then, Graham has worked part time as a dental hygienist and spends the rest of her time placing dental professionals in permanent or temporary positions in practices throughout central New Jersey.

Graham establishes relationships with dental offices through direct mail, website advertising and office visits. She also networks through continuing education classes, oral health conferences and by working in the Dental Temps booth at conference trade shows.

With a position opening in hand, Graham takes detailed information about the practice and personally visits the office to meet their staff. She interviews the office manager and the dentist to find out more about work styles and the type of candidate they seek. With an inventory of required skills, Graham successfully matches the dental candidate's skills and qualifications to the office through a personal interview and thorough a background check.

On the dental hygienist side of the business, Graham carefully reviews resumes and qualifications for the professionals she places, spending an hour to an hour and half with each candidate to build a clinical profile. Before sending a candidate on an interview, she scans cover letters and resumes, reviews with the candidates how to conduct themselves in interviews, and gives them tips on what to ask during their interview time.

Graham saw this service as an extension of her profession. "I didn't have to start a whole new career. I really love being in the dental hygiene field, and I wanted to stay within that field," she shared.

Having performed temping services in the past for other agencies years before, Graham was already familiar with the process.

"I was always interested in the business aspect of the profession. I wanted to share my clinical experience, and skills that I have obtained over the past 23 years with other dental professionals," Graham continued.

While she might have chosen to set up a business on her own, Graham selected a franchised organization because she liked the business support system she received from Dental Temps. She added that continuing education courses in dental hygiene were crucial to conducting successful placement consulting work. "It is critical to your business and to your profession, to always be up-to-date on trends and therapeutic and technological advances in the profession," Graham commented.

Advocate

Definition: Dental hygienists in the role of **advocates** lobby for the healthcare rights of their patients and support the code of ethics, professional standards and goals of their profession. As an advocate, the dental hygiene professional might influence legislators, health agencies and other healthcare organizations to bring existing health problems and available resources together to resolve issues and improve access to care.

Educational Requirements: A four-year degree is required in the advocate role, however, all dental hygienists, regardless of their degree status, have the opportunity to participate in advocacy. To assume leadership roles in advocacy, advanced degrees are helpful. The right candidate must have a large educational background from which to draw because decision making can take so many paths.

Professional Characteristics: The professionals who best fit full-time advocacy roles are able to see the big picture, are independent-minded and have the ability to analyze across a variety of situations.

Both Colleen M. Brickle, RDH, RF, EdD, and Vickie Orsini Nardello, RDH, MS, work in the advocate role. Both strongly state that all clinicians are advocates; it is inherent in the dental hygienists work.

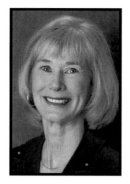 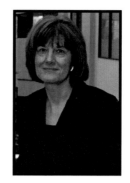

Figure 2.3. Colleen M. Brickle   **Figure 2.4.** Vickie Orsini Nardello

"The desire to help patients who have no voice, to be their voice, and to make a difference in their lives was the primary reason I embraced my role as a patient advocate," said Brickle, who is Dean of Health Sciences at Normandale Community College (NCC) and Program Liaison for dental hygiene at Metropolitan State University (MSU), a position resulting from a partnership between the two institutions. Brickle's administrative duties include the Baccalaureate Degree Completion, Post-Baccalaureate Certificate and Graduate Programs in Dental Hygiene.

"I am still able to spend time mentoring students and dental hygiene professionals toward the future, envisioning a new oral health care delivery system due to this partnership," said Brickle. "Additionally, I now work with nursing students and other healthcare students and professionals to increase their awareness of the challenges of accessing oral health care for underserved populations. Most importantly, I can share my passion for innovation and for creating a future in which dental hygienists and other stakeholders are able to advocate for the rights of the underserved," said Brickle.

Outside of the clinical setting, her advocacy role expanded when she had begun to teach and became more involved in the Minnesota Dental Hygienists' Association (MNDHA). "As an advocate for my patients in the clinical setting, I provided the necessary information so the patients could make an informed choice for their healthcare decisions," said Brickle.

While teaching, Brickle helped get students involved in association activities such as Day at the Capitol.

"We were working on issues such as self regulation and local anesthesia. I wanted students to know that if they took action, their voice would be heard," said Brickle, who graduated with a dental hygiene degree from the University of Minnesota in 1976 and completed her Master in Curriculum and Instructional Design degree in 1988 and her Doctorate in Health Care Education in 2000. She wrote a grant over five years ago that launched a community dental clinic that operates once a week, occasional Saturdays and is housed in the dental hygiene program at Normandale.

"The public clinic is self-sustaining; we don't make money except that which pays the dentist, dental hygienist and office manager and an assistant. We can do the restorative and rotate the students in there to expose them to a different patient population," Brickle explained.

"There are five of us with community clinics housed in our dental hygiene programs. It's huge in our state," she continued. "What they have found is that you can get dental hygienists to volunteer, but you can't get dentists to volunteer."

What drew Brickle into the advocacy role was the desire to help underserved communities find dentists to accept their public program and insurance. "We all have personal stories," she noted. "For me, advocating for the people who come to our community clinic is important. Some of these people drive two and a half to three hours to the cities because we will see them. On another note, we were the first state to mandate continuing education in 1969!"

Orsini Nardello's advocacy took her straight to the state legislature – in a more literal sense.

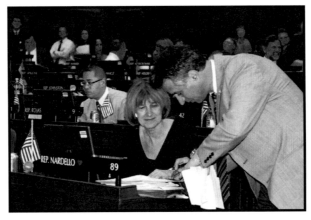

Figure 2.5. Vickie Orsini Nardello working as a State Representative in Connecticut.

A registered dental hygienist for over 41 years and working in a public health role since 1986, Orsini Nardello has served as Majority Whip for the Connecticut House of Representatives. She has been elected State Representative by her constituents for eight consecutive terms.

Currently she chairs the Energy and Technology Committee while serving on the Public Health Committee, Insurance and Real Estate Committee and the Medicaid Managed Care Council. As a member of the Public Health Committee since her election, she has developed policy on scope of practice issues, medical errors, implementing medical quality measures and improving healthcare access. She ran for office to address health issues and despite the demands of being Energy and Technology Chair, she continues to make these issues a priority.

Orsini Nardello graduated with her RDH credential from the Fones School of Dental Hygiene at the University of Bridgeport (CT) in 1971. She went on to earn her Bachelor of Dental Hygiene Education degree from the University of Bridgeport and also received her Master of Health Education degree from Southern Connecticut State University. She credits the Connecticut Dental Hygienists' Association (CDHA) and (ADHA) for her preparation for the legislature.

"As legislative chair of CDHA, I developed first-hand knowledge of how bills are passed. It became clear that ADHA conducts its business in a manner similar to the legislature. The House of Delegates considers resolutions from members, debates resolutions, caucuses and ultimately votes on final policy. Working with other dental hygienists on a national level is excellent preparation for a career in politics. In order for the profession of dental hygiene to advance, dental hygienists must be involved in formulating healthcare policy both on the national and state level.

What has kept Orsini Nardello in office, despite the fact that her party affiliation is different from that of her district, is her hard work and honesty.

"My constituents respect my work ethic, my willingness to work across party lines and the fact that I listen. I am accessible. Those qualities have allowed me to develop a strong base of support among both parties. That support has provided needed funds for campaigns and is the reason why I continue to be elected. People can differ on issues, but honesty, openness and hard work are always valued."

Being an advocate on any level requires dedication. "As a patient advocate, you are also a change agent," Brickle concluded. "It takes commitment and a great deal of dedication and energy to move an initiative forward."

Brickle said what many think about the profession today: It is an exciting time to be a dental hygienist.

"As a profession, dental hygiene has a history of being responsive and sensitive to the needs of the public it serves," she commented. "Dental hygienists, young and old, are dedicated to increasing oral health care access to everyone and now more than ever a shift is occurring for the common good." As mentioned previously, dental hygienists need to be a voice for their patients, especially the underserved and vulnerable populations.

Clinician

Definition: In the profession's most traditional role, **clinicians** communicate with their patients, assess medical and dental histories, take radiographs, conduct a dental hygiene diagnosis, identify the right treatment plan for preventive and restorative services and conduct effective treatment outcome for prevention, intervention or control of oral disease while working independently or in collaboration with other professionals.

Educational Requirements: At this point in time, several sources recommended that all dental hygiene clinicians pursue a bachelor's degree to enhance their knowledge base and credibility in the field. The minimum requirement for international dental hygiene work is the two-year degree with a U.S. dental hygiene license, plus one to two years working experience.

Professional Characteristics: Communication is key to success in dental hygiene whether that is communicating the science of oral health to everyday people or in collaborating with other healthcare professionals. Other characteristics include: listening to patient's needs, communicating effectively, the ability to multi-task, developing a high level of organization skills, possessing a passion for helping others, and cultivating a desire to continue education to learn new technologies and trends in the dental hygiene profession.

What do Claudine Paula Drew, RDH, CDA, MS, EdD, Peter M. Gangi, RDH, BSED, and Rene Stephenson, RDH, BSDH, share in their roles as clinicians? A commitment to what is developing in the traditional role of the dental hygienist.

Claudine Paula Drew, who attended Temple University, School of Oral Hygiene in Philadelphia for her RDH credential, and Columbia University for her bachelor's, master's and doctoral degrees, said she was first taught as a dental hygienist to provide and maintain a healthy oral environment. Later, she was trained to evaluate total patient care and dental hygiene management with its appropriate and anticipated outcomes.

"Temple trained my hands, Columbia trained my mind," she concluded, adding that after more than 40 years as an RDH, she "still has a joy and passion for it." Currently, Drew is the Chair of Dental Hygiene at Eastern International College in Belleville and Jersey City, New Jersey.

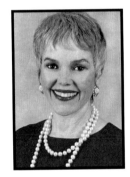

Figure 2.6. Claudine Paula Drew

"I have created my ideal working environment: My enthusiasm for clinic teaching/practice with that of my 'itchy feet' syndrome for travel," commented Drew, who has had several opportunities to see the world and experience diverse cultures. From 1983-84, she practiced dental hygiene in a hospital setting at King Faisal Special Hospital and Research Center in Riyadh, Saudi Arabia. In 1995, she served as a visiting professor in dental hygiene and dental assisting for a year at King Saud University in Riyadh, Kingdom of Saudi Arabia. From 2007-2010, Drew worked at the College of Health Sciences in the Kingdom of Bahrain. Drew commented that her international posts have allowed her to live an enjoyable, interesting life, experience different cultures and "spread my wings."

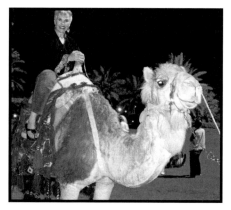

Figure 2.7. Claudine Paula Drew enjoying a ride on a camel in Saudi Arabia.

"Most foreign countries love to have an American licensed healthcare professional," Drew stated. "I believe the United States healthcare licensure system is the best in the world and is recognized as such."

Drew commented that dental hygienists who work abroad are risk takers who leave the safe, secure home situation to experience the unknown. These are individuals who want to expand their world experience, crave change and, she admitted, are easily bored with routine.

To find international employment, Drew suggested that dental hygienists network, attend conferences, seek out foreign dentists and dental hygienists, contact foreign dental and dental hygiene associations, check professional journals for authors who have written about their international experiences, or take out their own classified ad in such journals to find international postings. Another strategy is to contact foreign embassies in Washington, D.C. or the country in which one has an interest.

Rene Stephenson is a 26-year veteran of clinical dental hygiene. She graduated dental hygiene school from Tyler (TX) Junior College in 1986 and then finished her Bachelor of Science in Dental Hygiene degree with East Tennessee State in Johnson City, TN. She also spent five years as a dental assistant before getting her dental hygiene credential.

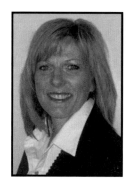

Figure 2.8. Rene Stephenson

"Basically I feel like I have been very instrumental in developing various clinical programs for enhancing the process," Stephenson said. "I have always felt that I am more than just a girl who cleans teeth. I feel like I am an educator. I feel like I am the person who needs to figure out whole body health, going over medical health history, finding out how I can make patients not only healthier with their oral health, but healthier whole body wise."

Stephenson has developed a periodontal therapy program for soft tissue treatment and a dental decay program to determine each patient's propensity for high, medium or low decay evaluation. This aids the dental team in treatment decisions.

"I have different things that I can do to enhance better oral health and get patients to reduce their rate of dental decay," Stephenson commented.

Peter M. Gangi secured his Bachelor of Education degree and simultaneously became a dental hygienist, a role he has filled since 1988. He uses both in his role as a clinician and as a Clinical Instructor at Middlesex Community College in Lowell, MA.

He admitted his dental hygiene position is a bit unique. He has worked in the same practice for more than 20 years – the same one his father started more than 50 years ago. He continues alongside his brother who is a dentist.

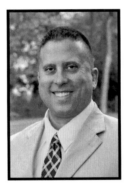

Figure 2.9. Peter M. Gangi

In Gangi's clinical role, he makes certain the tissue is healthy with no signs of gingivitis or periodontitis and then also checks for lesions and completes an oral cancer screening. From this point, Gangi formulates a treatment plan for the patient and sets up any follow-up appointments or referrals.

"I also educate patients on how to prevent oral disease," Gangi explained. "I educate them about what needs to be done to their mouth, whether it is an implant or a root canal, etc. I will discuss exactly what the procedure is while doing my job."

"My responsibilities would be more to prevent oral disease and promote good oral health for each patient and to try to stop the disease process if it's taking place by removing the irritants," Gangi continued, adding that pointing out problem areas that the patient is missing with daily oral care are part of the process, too.

Gangi reported that patient compliance is not as much of an issue as it might be in other practices as he and his family have cared for multiple generations of families in their practice.

"We use digital x-rays, which I love," Gangi said. "I think it is actually a much better tool as far as helping explain to patients what they need, why they need it and actually showing them the disease process, as opposed to holding up an x-ray film up to a light or having it in a light viewer and them trying to look at it. They can't really tell what you are seeing, but with digital x-rays we can actually have a computer screen right next to my operatory. So I just pop it up there, blow it up, magnify it and contrast it to make it look darker or lighter than it is, to show the patient exactly what's going on."

Gangi credits his father's mentoring with leading him into the dental hygiene profession.

"I was going to major in education and teach. Then my father and I had a discussion the summer before my junior year. He knew I was kind of worried about what my future was going to be like," Gangi shared. His father recommended that he teach and use his summers and weekends for dental hygiene – to supplement his teacher's salary – and offered to hire him. When his father shared what he paid a dental hygienist, Gangi realized that he could help people and earn a better salary for his family.

"So when I got out . . . instead of going into teaching I went into full-time hygiene," he continued. Because it's a family practice serving other families, Gangi is now working on some of his father's patient's great-great grandkids.

"Some of those kids that I started working on when they were little are now married and having their own kids, which is pretty unique," Gangi continued. "That is why going to work every day for me is a lot of fun, because every day is different – that is part of being a clinician."

Stephenson agreed. What drew her into the profession and makes her want to stay in the clinician role is her love for people and wanting to communicate good oral hygiene with them.

"I think there is a different personality that walks in the door with each individual patient; it kind of keeps you on your toes. You are able to establish relationships with those people," Stephenson explained. "It gives you the flexibility to kind of be different rather than doing the same mundane thing." She admitted that, for some, clinical work can become stale.

"You feel like you are doing the same thing over and over except when you've got different personalities. You know sometimes I feel like I am 15 different personalities during the day because it changes with each individual patient," Stephenson said.

And the variety does not end with adapting your communications skills to a new patient; variety is inherent to each practice or specialist.

"The beauty of our dental hygiene field as a whole . . . there are so many areas you can go into. You can be a clinical hygienist and working in a private practice, you can be in a periodontal practice, a specialty practice or you can see children all day in a pediatric practice. You could be in a public health setting and do clinical hygiene on the underserved," Stephenson continued. She recommended that others spend a day shadowing a dental hygienist, to get a feel for a typical work day.

At this point in time, Stephenson recommended that all dental hygiene clinicians pursue a bachelor's degree.

Stephenson and Gangi both stressed that communication is key to success in dental hygiene.

"One of the keys is you have to have some social skills to be a dental hygienist, you have to be able to converse with them and find out about their lives as well," said Gangi. "You are making conversation with them for 45 minutes to an hour. It's not all about hygiene."

Gangi, who is also adjunct clinical faculty at Middlesex Community College, continued: "The biggest thing I tell my students in school is that we give you the baseline as far as how to do the job, but your greatest amount of learning is out in private practice. You will learn exponentially every single day. You will see things that you have never seen before."

"You as a dental hygienist owe it to yourself and to your patients to continue to learn and get better at what you do. You just don't survive on what you have been taught in school. You must become a better clinician, you must be a better instructor and you must be a better educator to your patients as you go on," Gangi concluded.

Educator

When dental hygienists take on the role of **educators**, they employ educational theory and methodology to analyze healthcare needs, develop health promotion strategies and deliver and evaluate the results in attaining or maintaining health. Educators reside in every walk of the profession from corporate settings to public health, from faculty positions to clinical roles.

Educational Requirements: Educators need advanced degrees. Particularly for full-time teaching, individuals will need to seek at least a master's degree. However, those with an interest in education may begin with part-time clinical teaching.

Professional Characteristics: A career in dental hygiene education requires the same skill set that dental hygienists bring to the clinical side of the profession: organized, consistent, goal oriented, hard working, flexible, a capable multi-tasker and compassionate.

Dental hygiene educators continually repopulate the intellectual pool of talent in the profession. Cheryl Westphal Theile, RDH, EdD, Cynthia C. Amyot, MSDH, EdD, and Harold A. Henson, RDH, MEd, shared what it takes to educate the next generation of dental hygienists.

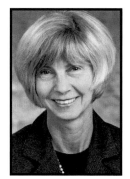

Figure 2.10. Cheryl Westphal Theile

Westphal Theile has worked as a dental hygiene educator since 1976. After she received her bachelor's degree at Fairleigh S. Dickinson, Jr., College of Dental Medicine (FDU), she went on to work in the school's two-year dental hygiene program. Her first teaching position was at FDU, where she eventually became director until the school closed in 1990.

That same year, she started the dental hygiene program at New York University's College of Dentistry, where she is today Assistant Dean for the Allied Health Programs and Director of the Dental Hygiene Departments. Her responsibilities include everything from the admissions process, budgeting, curriculum development, participating in committees that approve curriculum and all certifications for graduation.

Westphal Theile didn't want to describe her move toward education as an evolutionary process, but it worked out that way.

"I think it's because I had the bachelor's degree first. Then when I got the associate's degree, I knew I wanted my master's. I saw myself as an educator, but I also saw myself as an administrator right at the beginning process of getting my master's degree," Westphal Theile explained.

For Cynthia Amyot, the pathway to education was lined with people who saw something in her she had not noticed herself: A passion to teach. She became a dental hygienist in 1976. After spending many years as a clinician, she returned to school at University of Missouri Kansas City (UMKC) in the 1990s to finish her bachelor's and master's degrees. In 2003, she completed her doctorate.

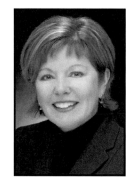

Figure 2.11. Cynthia Amyot

"UMKC faculty were at some of the professional meetings I attended. They approached me and asked if I had considered education. I hadn't, but education runs in our family. The UMKC people recognized that in me. It took a couple of years, but once I got going, I was off and running," said Amyot.

Since 2006, she has served as director of distance education and faculty development in the School of Dentistry at UMKC. She developed two online degree programs over a decade ago – a degree completion and a master's program in dental hygiene. She currently serves as Interim Associate Vice President of Online Education at UMKC.

"I am kind of doing two roles – get people to use more technology, and teaching them how to teach. Right now I feel I have the best of all worlds. I have a hand in all these areas I love," Amyot commented, recommending educational roles to dental hygienists because it opens up so many doors.

"Being in the educational environment, you're the first ones to hear about opportunities out there. It's dynamic. When I came back to school, I barely knew how to turn on a computer. Now I am teaching others about sophisticated technology," she stated.

Harold Henson began teaching before he completed dental hygiene school. He was a substitute teacher in public schools after he completed his bachelor's degree in biology at the University of Houston (TX) before pursuing a dental hygiene certificate in 1995. He began teaching in dental hygiene in 1996.

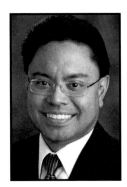

Figure 2.12. Harold A. Henson

"I have always been drawn to education, particularly teaching. It was just something I had an innate ability to do," Henson commented. He started off by volunteer teaching for a year, and later experienced a variety of teaching positions while getting his master's degree at the Baylor College of Medicine at the University of Houston. In 2003, he began full-time teaching. He is currently Associate Professor and Director of Clinical Simulation at The University of Texas School of Dentistry at Houston.

For those interested in teaching, Henson recommended some clinical experience. "You can better understand what a student goes through once you've experienced it yourself," he commented. He also recommends having "a constellation of mentors," to guide your decision making.

"A teacher I think is almost part actor in a way . . . because you are trying to take something that may be a difficult topic and break it down. You have to have a little psychology behind it and of course the methodology," Henson said.

Educators need advanced degrees, said Westphal Theile. For full-time teaching, individuals will need to seek at least a master's degree. However, Westphal Theile encouraged those with an interest in education to start anywhere. "Start by part-time clinical teaching, start by contacting dental hygiene programs; teach in an area in which you have expertise, develop it by giving lectures in continuing education. Start to build your portfolio and experience," she encouraged, stressing that educators eventually will need the credentials to go along with their experience.

"The good news is with so many online educational programs, it becomes easy for anybody anywhere to go on and advance their degrees," Westphal Theile said.

Amyot agreed: "Every degree you get opens new doors. I am amazed at some of the advantages you get – such as grant money – with higher degrees. Advance your degree. Every class I have ever taken applies somewhere else in the profession."

"I have also taught practice management and we taught about alternative careers. The students hadn't thought about anything beyond private practice. There are so many other opportunities out there," Amyot concluded. "We can't box ourselves in; we need to think about what the work world values and realize that dental hygienists already have those qualities."

Researcher

As **researchers**, dental hygienists are not limited to working in laboratory settings but, much as they do in the role of educator, touch a wide spectrum of areas within the profession. In this role dental hygienists apply the scientific method to select appropriate therapies, educational methods or content, interpret and apply findings and solve problems, among other responsibilities.

Educational Requirements: Professionals with an associate's degree will operate in a somewhat limited role in research. To move into it fully, an advanced degree is recommended. If a dental hygienist is pursuing an advanced degree one class at a time, additional science and statistical courses are very helpful.

Professional Characteristics: Work in research requires being a team player, creative, thinking out of the box and sometimes working outside of personal comfort zones. It is critical to have integrity, confidentiality and a strong inclination toward serving others in the professional community.

When dental hygienists begin a career in research, they delve deeply into the science of the profession. Christine Charles, RDH, BS, Mary Ann Cugini, RDH, MHP, Janet Kinney, RDH, MS, MS, and Jane L. Forrest, RDH, EdD, reveal the hours of education necessary to career advancement and success in this important role.

"It was sort of the anomaly, because at that time our choices basically coming out of school were to teach dental hygiene, do public health or work in an office. That was about the extent of our opportunities," Charles commented. Rather than suffering tunnel vision or saying no to anything, Charles took the opportunities that came her way.

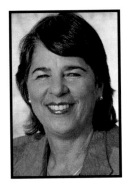

Figure 2.13. Christine Charles

Charles, who became an RDH in 1972, worked as a clinician initially and quickly found her way to research thanks to an advertisement her mother clipped from the New York Times. Charles, who had completed a bachelor's degree at the University of Bridgeport in Bridgeport, CT, replied to the ad for a research and development opening at Lever Brothers, then affiliated with the Unilever Global company, interviewed and got the job.

"Initially I was doing actual clinical evaluations – scoring supragingival plaque and stain and things like that. Over time, I was running clinical studies and caries clinical trials and putting things together for advertising support packages. I also did a few other toiletry evaluations, but primarily, I worked in oral care research," Charles said. "I really didn't know what it would be like. I really didn't have a clue. It was just a matter of they wanted someone who had that . . . science and dental hygiene background and a 'can do' attitude."

Having a dental hygienist on staff was sort of an unheard of thing at that time, according to Charles. "I guess from a business perspective, it was cheaper to hire a dental hygienist than to bring a dentist in every day," she continued.

After 10 years, she moved to Warner-Lambert Company and became the first dental hygienist the company ever hired to work in research.

"I basically worked on LISTERINE® mouthrinse at Warner Lambert," said Charles, who was instrumental in securing the American Dental Association's (ADA) Seal for LISTERINE® in 1989. She now holds the title of Director of Scientific and Professional Affairs for the Global Consumer Healthcare Research, Development and Engineering Division of Johnson & Johnson Consumer and Personal Products Worldwide. Charles is responsible for Latin America and the Asia Pacific Regions in providing professional support for the company's technologies and products, manage scientific affairs and develop long-term relationships with key opinion leaders in dentistry, dental education, dental research, medicine and dental health associations to achieve Johnson & Johnson's key business objectives.

"I am in a corporate setting, but there are many other settings . . . you can work within in research," said Charles. She added that oral health researchers work for clinical research organizations, health insurance companies, academic institutions, government entities, such as the National Institutes for Health (NIH), and, like herself, in corporate settings for well-known oral health product manufacturers.

This variety also extends to the people with whom you work, Charles said. In the course of a research professional's day, he or she may connect with public health officials, academic colleagues, health experts and opinion leaders.

Jane L. Forrest, Professor of Clinical Dentistry, Section Chair of Behavioral Science and Practice Management and Director of the National Center for Dental Hygiene Research & Practice at the Ostrow School of Dentistry at the University of Southern California, recommended that to be competitive in research, dental hygienists should pursue a doctoral degree.

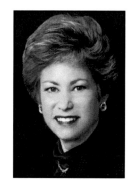

Figure 2.14. Jane L. Forrest

"You don't know what you don't know until you start an advanced degree program," said Forrest, who graduated from Fairleigh S. Dickinson, Jr., College of Dental Medicine in 1972 with a Bachelor of Science in Dental Hygiene. Then she earned a Master of Science in Public Health Dentistry from Boston University in 1976, and in 1994, Forrest received a Doctorate in Higher Education Administration from Nova Southeastern University in Fort Lauderdale, FL.

At the doctoral level, Forrest stated, you develop greater familiarity with the skills in research and the scientific approach. "To help the profession, we need to build the core of researchers. We need to build it so that they will advance dental hygiene. Unfortunately, many dental hygienists with doctoral degrees are no longer in dental hygiene," Forrest commented.

As part of a grant from the Health Resources and Services Administration (HRSA) that Forrest wrote in 1993, the National Center for Dental Hygiene Research was formed. The initial focus of the National Center grant was to validate the ADHA National Dental Hygiene Research Agenda and to train collaborative teams of dental hygienists in the research process. Forrest explained that teams were composed of practitioners, educators and a research mentor, who was typically an educator.

"The teams had to come up with a research topic related to the national dental hygiene research agenda," said Forrest, explaining that another focus of the grant was to use the agenda to advance practice. During a five-day workshop, the program participants attended sessions to prepare and refine their research projects. As part of their project, they also developed an implementation plan so they could begin the project when they returned to their own university.

"Throughout the year we made site visits to each of the universities to review how the teams were doing with their plan," explained Forrest. "It was such a fantastic experience that by the end of the grant we wondered how we could keep all the participants connected. We knew we could not keep flying them in for training without further grant support. It was about that time that people were beginning to use the Internet and email."

"The second grant I wrote dealt with research collaborations through the use of this new Internet technology. We were able to bring the teams back as they were finishing their research projects, and we taught them how to use the Internet. Half of them did not even have email at that time," Forrest explained. The participants received hands-on Internet training and then shared their research information. As another part of this grant, Forrest launched the DHNet (http://www.usc.edu/dhnet). It currently serves as the electronic infrastructure for the National Center. The National Center also serves as a think tank, which sponsors conferences, and through the center, Forrest and her colleagues conduct research on practice behaviors of dental hygienists.

A third grant she wrote involved how to integrate evidence-based decision making into curricula, which also included launching another website, Evidence-Based Decision Making (http://www.usc.edu/ebnet). Integrated into this website is a section on Culturally Competent Care, which was part of a fourth HRSA grant. In 2006, HRSA eliminated grant support for allied health projects, which was the source of funding that Forrest received. She hopes that HRSA will restore the funding, especially since the majority of healthcare workers are in the allied health fields.

Forrest was motivated to become involved in research because not only was it part of her university job to write grants, but also she felt grant funding could provide needed resources to support the advancement of dental hygiene. She is not alone. "There is a whole community of people in dental hygiene education, research and practice who believe this is a need as well, said Forrest, and "our team at the National Center is continually working on ways to contribute to fulfilling this need."

Mary Ann Cugini attended dental hygiene school at Forsyth School for Dental Hygienists in Boston, graduating in 1972. "I started off in private practice actually working for my own dentist for about five years and then went into public health," she explained. She attended Northeastern University and received a bachelor's degree in 1981 and a Master of Health Professions Policy in 1991 with a focus in health.

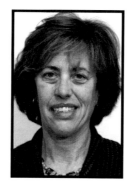

Figure 2.15. Mary Ann Cugini

"Boston in the 1970s had neighborhood health centers that were all linked to the five major hospitals in Boston. So I was a dental hygienist in a comprehensive medical/dental center. We provided clinical care as well as taught oral health education in the schools," Cugini continued.

"I went from that public health experience into my very first research experience. I was working for a contract research organization," she stated, explaining that these private, for-profit companies do clinical trial work for industries for claim support for their products.

"That's where I got my first taste of research – doing clinical trials for claim support for companies such as Warner Lambert," said Cugini, who did clinical studies for over-the-counter products. By 1985, she was involved in clinical trials supported by the National Institutes of Health (NIH). Cugini counted her good fortunes in working with Dr. Max Goodson at the Forsyth Institute in the development of Actisite.

"That's when we did the first multi-center trial for an FDA-approved product for dentistry," she added. A move to Braun in 1997, then a division of Gillette, led Cugini from Clinical Research Manager to overall Manager to Director of Research during the next 10 years of her career.

In 2007, she returned to Forsyth Institute in Boston as Senior Clinical Investigator and Director of External Research Collaboration.

"You always keep your options open, because I am back here at Forsyth where I actually started my research career," said Cugini. "Forsyth, in addition to doing basic science research, has a clinical research facility where we conduct clinical trials for NIH studies and industry here. Forsyth is non-profit so all of us write grants to support ourselves."

In this role, Cugini manages the clinical trials coming into the facility – the study and patient flow, etc. – as well as grant writing to bring in studies and consulting with industry partners that come into Forsyth and want to utilize the institution's expertise in clinical trials.

"I couldn't have gotten where I was in research without having a good foundation in clinical," Cugini said. "Having the experience as a self-starter in private practice gives you an amazing foundation . . . because you can make your own course."

Janet Kinney is an Assistant Clinical Professor and Principal Investigator at the Michigan Center for Oral Health Research (MCOHR), a fairly new entity for the University of Michigan. Kinney received her Bachelor of Science degree in dental hygiene from the University of Michigan in 1983. She spent much of the next 22 years working as a clinician in periodontics.

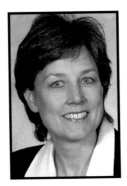

Figure 2.16. Janet Kinney

"My specialty was always periodontics," Kinney explained. "I loved the challenge, the work, the patient rapport, seeing results and behavior change, and knowing I made a difference. I know this happens in other specialties, but for me periodontics was exciting."

She moved around the country, and even overseas for her spouse's job, and eventually, in 2004, came back to the master's degree program she had always desired. She pursued two master's degree programs at the University of Michigan in Dental Hygiene and Clinical Research and Statistical Design. She studied with the intent to eventually train young researchers.

"The brochures to entice people to apply to the clinical research and statistical design program in no way said 'dental hygienist,'" Kinney said, explaining that at first she was scared to death to sell herself as a principal investigator of clinical studies in the program.

"There were medical doctors (MD) and doctors of osteopathy (DO) all around," she recalled. "I was nervous going toe-to-toe with these professionals. However, going through the program reassured my commitment and interest and aptitude in research."

What does Kinney love about research?

"It's never the same. Depending on the project, my responsibilities may include being an examiner, a patient recruiter, or I may collect data from the patient's study visits, notes on care, and studying and delivering protocols.

"If there are multiple examiners, I may go through a calibration exercise with other examiners on the study. As a co-principal investigator, I have been more involved in the regulatory end of it. I submit the research protocol to the Institutional Review Board (IRB). When the IRB has inquiries or amendments, I straighten those out and coordinate with another group on campus." For those less familiar with the research field, Kinney explained that the main purpose of IRB is to protect patients involved in research studies at the university, and the calibration process ensures that all examiners on a given study use the same language, take the same measurements and observe in the same way so there is consistency among examiners.

"The examiners want to agree 95% of the time," Kinney stated. "There are all sorts of activities we must perform on a patient when they are in for the study, and we want to make certain we are all performing it the same way."

Some of the studies in which Kinney has been involved include researching the oral health implications of a drug that had been on the market for five years for the drug's manufacturer, and an NIH study on a collaborative project with Sandia National Laboratory in Livermore, CA.

"I always knew when I worked in clinical practice that results from clinical research guided our practice. We didn't make a change without having some evidence that the change was needed. There was that inner acknowledgement that I had," Kinney noted. When she returned to school in 2004, she was pleased to find that the research program was re-designed for dental hygiene students.

"Before it was very limited. I was lucky enough that not only was that the direction I wanted to go, but that I had a program and phenomenal mentors that supported me," said Kinney.

Those interested in research can explore it in a somewhat limited role with an associate's degree, according to Charles, "but to really move into it fully, I would recommend that you continue your education." She said that science and statistics courses are very helpful.

"When we are filling positions for clinical research associates, we look for people who are not just task-oriented, but those who can look and see the whole picture," stated Cugini.

Work in research also requires a "can do" attitude, said Charles.

"It's a being a team player, sometimes being creative, sometimes working outside of your comfort zone . . . I guess depending on a role that you have within research, it can be as limited or broad as the positions are available," she continued.

Cugini credited the dentist she worked with in private practice. "I was very fortunate in working with a dentist who was very accepting of the role of the dental hygienist as very key and an important position among the team. So I was exposed to forwarding-thinking professionals throughout my career who really embraced the concept of teamwork and that you were expected to perform. Obviously, if you didn't bring anything to the table . . . it didn't look favorably upon your profession let alone yourself," said Cugini. "I always . . . grasped for every opportunity that I had to get involved in the management side as well as the clinician side."

Public Health

Because the dental hygienist's role in **public health** is an integral part of all five others, it spans the spectrum of professional roles. Dental hygienists with roles in public health assist epidemiologists in researching the populations whom they serve, provide clinic and preventive services to schools and other public organizations, act as educators of oral health within their communities, perform administrative and managerial duties within their public health departments and serve as advocates of oral health and ending oral disease-causing behaviors.

Educational Requirements: As with research and educational roles, someone new to the profession with an associate's degree may find entrance positions, but will find that an advanced degree is needed to open more doors and move into leadership positions.

It is wise to pursue some continuing education courses in public health and read important documents such as Healthy People 2010 and the new information coming out on Healthy People 2020 for more education. Those with an inclination in this area might also consider attending the National Oral Health Conference.

Professional Characteristics: Dental hygienists pursuing positions in public health must have the ability to step up and stand up for what they think is right, and be able to present that and be able to interact with some critical thinking skills. Public health is a people-oriented role – even more so than other areas of dental hygiene. It requires compassion for those less fortunate and the ability to collaborate with other healthcare professionals. Public health dental hygienists need to be persistent, patient and motivated; they are the leading oral health providers for their patients.

As explained before, public health is an over-arching role that extends into the other areas of dental hygiene's professional roles. Kathy Voigt Geurink, RDH, MA, Debra Olsen, RDH, RDHAP, Peggy J. Simonson, RDH, BS, Angie Stone, RDH, BS, and Vickie Orsini Nardello, RDH, MS, are excellent examples of the interplay this particular role has with the other five in the profession.

In addition to her role as an advocate, Orsini Nardello has served in a public health position for more than 22 years as a public health dental hygienist in the Hartford (CT) school system. It was the lure of a work schedule that allowed her time with her family that first drew her into public health. However, "once I got here I was very drawn to this because I began to realize the vast discrepancy between the services and the access that was available to the private sector versus the public sector," she asserted. (For reference, see Figure 2.5 on page 48).

She was shocked by disparity between the public health setting and private practice in relation to the number of children with unmet dental needs and realized the potential impact that a school-based program could make.

"Before I came to the public health clinic, I had worked in a pediatric practice. Children in the practice came from families of moderate – to high-income levels and had low decay rates. Then I went to the school-based dental clinic setting and the children had a high incidence of decay, no insurance and many had never had a dental visit. It was as if I had entered a third-world country."

Her responsibilities in the clinic include full administration of the entire clinic from permission slips issued to and record keeping for all the students, to working with teachers and administrators and billing and logging statistics. "Basically I am responsible for all administration because we want our dentists to spend all of their time providing restorative care, and we need to ensure that services are provided in a cost effective manner." The clinic provides all dental services with the exception of orthodontia and offers care to students with or without insurance. Most students are Medicaid eligible.

Angie Stone has been involved in public health for more than eight years. A personal crisis prompted her move from clinical work into nursing homes.

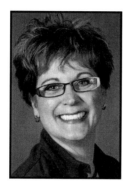

Figure 2.17. Angie Stone

Stone's mother-in-law suffered from both emphysema and chronic periodontal disease. With her mother-in-law confined to a nursing home and too weak to leave the home to seek dental attention, Stone felt helpless to assist her. The laws in Wisconsin prevented Stone from performing any dental hygiene without the supervision of a dentist, and the nursing home staff was too busy with other duties to attend to it.

"I knew her lungs were constantly infected because of her mouth," Stone commented. "But I couldn't do anything because there was no dentist at the nursing home." When her mother-in-law passed away, Stone vowed to do something to make a difference in such situations.

While the laws prevented her from practicing her profession without a dentist's supervision, Stone found that she could provide education to the nursing home staff about the importance of oral care linked with each resident's overall health. She called nursing homes in her area and offered to educate staff about dental hygiene. Many were responsive. Stone offered the education program for free.

"I had a mission. The one particular location I had visited for a couple of years had a dentist on staff who did exams," Stone said, explaining that the dentist came to the in-service training session Stone offered.

"He came up to me at the end and told me that I didn't have a clue as to what these patients were like to get to cooperate," Stone remembered. She decided to do rounds with the dentist and sit in the in-house dental clinic. Although she found the dungeon-like facility archaic, she decided that it was better than nothing and began offering dental hygiene services.

At that same time, the Wisconsin legislature passed a law that dental hygienists could apply for a medical assistance provider number. This allowed Stone to be paid for her dental hygiene services at the nursing home.

Advised by a colleague, Stone called the newspaper and was interviewed about her work at the nursing home. The resulting article led another dental hygienist, who wanted to join Stone's efforts, to contact her about nursing home practice for dental hygienists.

The pair eventually contacted Patterson Dental Supply which linked them to a dentist who was remodeling his offices and getting new furniture. He donated his lightly used dental exam chair to the nursing home.

"The arrangement is nothing that has been scripted," Stone said. "No one told me what to do."

In the effort to educate the Certified Nursing Assistants (CNAs) at the nursing homes, Stone joined forces with Shirley Gutkowski, RDH, BSDH, FACE. Gutkowski and Stone decided that it wasn't right to truck all over Wisconsin for free.

"We decided to do something called 'Adopt-a-Nursing-Home,'" Stone concluded. This program involved dental hygienists presenting themselves to local nursing homes as resources and educational trainers for the nursing staff. Stone assumed the program would sell itself as nursing homes have an annual requirement for in-service oral health training.

Gutkowski had developed content for training sessions for a nursing home in Florida that were available on CD. These became the foundational tools for Adopt-a-Nursing-Home.

The CD-Rom program kit includes three year's worth of training in the form of PowerPoint presentations, slide handouts and speaker notes.

"All the dental hygienist needs to do is read through the presentation a few times, and present it to the nursing home staff. It's very simple compared to what we went through at the beginning," Stone explained. She estimated that over 20 dental hygienists are participating in the program.

"We have a three-hour CE course we require them to take before they can adopt a nursing home. It's a very different approach. We teach them who the CNA is, what their level of education is, and what their day in the nursing home is like. The course is available on Dental Tribune in three, one-hour sessions," Stone said.

Early in the process of establishing the kit for the dental hygienists, Gutkowski contacted Johnson & Johnson and asked for support of the in-service training program. The company offered to purchase 50 of the CD-Rom training kits and supplied toothbrushes. The program continues to gain momentum each year.

"Dental hygienists must approach nursing home workers as an advocate and a resource," said Stone.

Sometimes, she stated, the dental hygienist walking in new to this environment has no concept of what the CNA's day is like. Oral care, Stone noted, frequently gets pushed to the bottom of the list.

"Until you sit in on a shift change, take a complete report and shadow the CNAs, you have no idea," said Stone, who advised the dental hygienists to leave off with the finger wagging and hand slapping until that mile in the CNA's shoes is completed. "They need us to help them."

Stone noted that working with geriatric patients requires patience and a willingness to think outside the box.

"It's not a traditional setting at all," she continued. "The suction I use is one typically used to clear the mouth of people who are unconscious. It's not how we were trained in dental hygiene . . . you need to put perfectionism aside. You want to remove every bit of calculus. You want to do everything how we were taught. However, under these circumstances, you have to focus on biofilm reduction. You do what you can. Thirty minutes is the maximum that one of these patients will be able to sit there. You must be compassionate."

Upon graduation from dental hygiene school, Kathy Voigt Geurink's first dental hygiene position was as a public health hygienist in a school system. "My decision to go into dental hygiene was influenced by a dental hygienist who provided classroom oral health education in my elementary school. At this time, I thought 'what a fun job!'" said Voigt Geurink, who received her dental hygiene degree from the University of Minnesota. She went ahead and completed degrees in a Bachelor in Dental Hygiene Education as well as a Master in Health Programming from the University of Northern Colorado.

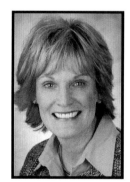

Figure 2.18. Kathy Voigt Geurink

"I continued my education while working as a dental hygienist. I am happy that I did it that way although it can be done in a number of different ways," said Voigt Geurink. She recommends that dental hygienists pursuing public health as a career be able to speak out about what is right for the health of the public. She suggested volunteer work in the community to gain an understanding of the challenges and needs of vulnerable populations such as children and elderly. "Critical thinking is also an important skill and an advanced degree is helpful to professional development," stated Voigt Geurink.

Working in elementary schools, Voigt Geurink provided oral health education, screenings and referrals to the community clinic where she provided preventive services. Her next job took her from the local level to the state level as a public health dental hygienist planning, implementing and evaluating oral health programs for underserved populations in Colorado.

Voigt Geurink did contract work in a nursing home during this time. One day per week, she provided clinical services for elderly patients in an on-site clinic and prevention and educational sessions for the nursing home staff. She also conducted a dental hygiene student rotation at this site to train dental hygiene students in elderly patient care. After 10 years of working in public health, Voigt Geurink accepted a position in the Dental Hygiene Department, School of Allied Health Professionals at the University of Texas Health Science Center in San Antonio (UTHSCSA). She has taught community oral health for over 20 years and wrote a widely used textbook, Community Oral Health Practice for the Dental Hygienist.

"Community projects," Voigt Geurink said, "are very important in a dental hygiene curriculum. They make the connection between what is taught and what can be done to improve the oral health of citizens in our communities."

Voigt Geurink continues teaching public health courses at UTHSCSA, but has also returned to public health practice through consulting work with the Association of State and Territorial Dental Directors (ASTDD). She works with an ASTDD Committee on School and Adolescent Oral Health and a committee on Health Aging, bringing partners together to improve access to care for these populations. She also volunteers at various community health fairs and community organized oral health promotion events.

Peggy J. Simonson, another University of Minnesota graduate, completed her Bachelor of Science degree at night after finishing her dental hygiene degree. She paired her BS with a minor in Gerontology, something that would factor into her future career plans.

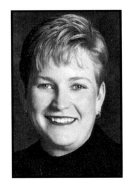

Figure 2.19. Peggy J. Simonson

Simonson did a rotation at the Wilder Senior Dental Clinic, the first full-service dental clinic in Minnesota that exclusively serves older adults that is funded by the Amherst H. Wilder Foundation in St. Paul, MN. From that moment, in 1988, she was hooked.

"I think I was the only one in my class who decided I wanted to work with older patients, but I guess I realized geriatric dental hygiene was really uncharted territory at the time," said Simonson, who now supervises dental hygiene students on clinical rotation and also performs some clinical work with patients.

"I have had some of those patients for more than 22 years now," Simonson commented, adding that she felt she didn't have enough training specific to this population; there just wasn't anything available. This is where her gerontology education became useful: "It gives you a good landscape of aging. I think it was very good background material. It gave me a broad prospective of different issues. We do work in ethnically diverse neighborhoods now, and I am more sensitive to some of those issues, for example, than I would have been."

To help educate others, Simonson works with Dr. Stephen Shuman, associate professor and director, Oral Health Services for Older Adults Program in the Department of Primary Dental Care at the University of Minnesota Graduate School and School of Dentistry, who offers a four-day continuing education course for practicing dental hygienists.

"It is for people out in the community who are already practicing and find themselves not knowing enough about the very old patient. These professionals may be thinking they want to work in a nursing facility," Simonson said.

Debra Olsen is owner of Smile Partners in Los Angeles, CA, a mobile dental hygiene service dedicated to serving patients with a wide variety of physical and intellectual challenges, including those with complex medical conditions. As a mobile service, Olsen travels to patients so that they don't have to move away from any necessary medical equipment or the safety of their familiar environment.

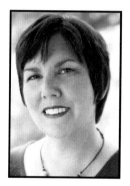

Figure 2.20. Debra Olsen

"I used to babysit for a little girl whose father was a dentist," Olsen shared. She went from family babysitter to front office help in his dental practice and became friends with his dental hygienist. This lady led her to register for dental hygiene classes. "I was going to be a lab tech, but I would have missed out on the people," said Olsen.

Licensed as an RDH in 1991 from Pasadena City College, Pasadena, CA, Olsen had over 16 years experience as a clinician and then applied to a program for the registered dental hygienist in alternative practice (RDHAP) credential from the University of the Pacific (UOP) in San Francisco, CA.

To apply for the RDHAP license, the state requires a dental hygienist to have two years of clinical practice experience. She also took a four-month course from UOP along with a board examination to become an RDHAP. She was inspired to move into this unique role by Marilyn Blackmun and Charlotte Burruso, two of the original 17 women who were part of a Health Manpower pilot project launched in 1981. The project made it possible for dental hygienists to go out into the state of California to provide oral care for those without access to care. By 2004, dental hygienists in California could finally be licensed as RDHAPs.

Olsen currently works four days a week as an RDHAP in her mobile practice and one day in a private practice with a dentist.

"I ended up working under a grant for the local regional center to improve the oral health for some developmentally disabled people in a facility in Glendale (CA)," Olsen said of her mobile practice. "Basically, we were training the direct care staff. I fell into that position and didn't realize that I would be treating a lot of developmentally disabled."

"By going to group homes, some larger facilities – I have a real variety in my practice," she continued, adding that she has a handful of contracts with communities that have skilled nursing, assisted living and memory or Alzheimer's care. "I also go into private homes because I have one particular physician, Dr. Wayne Chen out of Keck Medical Center, who has a geriatric home visit program that still refers me. He gave us many referrals on a regular basis."

In her mobile practice, Olsen performs typical dental hygiene duties such as scaling and root planing, prophylaxis, fluoride varnish and also in-service training for group homes. For those patients who are able-bodied enough, she uses a comfortable folding chair and a mobile dental unit. She tends to not use water for the bed-bound who have inhalation risks. She also spends a good amount of her time working with caregivers.

She must also deal with billing to insurance companies and sending out statements. Along with this, Olsen markets her practice to the community and to other dental hygienists. Her mobile practice business is doing very well.

"I do so much education about what the RDHAP is. I come upon dental hygienists who don't know," Olsen said. "Even though those pilot program women paved the road, we are still clearing the path."

Public health is the perfect setting for professionals who want collaborative practice. "The reality here is that it really is for someone who is self directed, independent and . . . again, wants a position of authority. This is a perfect setting for it because we have a very collaborative team," noted Orsini Nardello.

"The student should understand that public health careers for dental hygienists run the gamut from high-level administrative positions to providing oral hygiene care for the elderly residents in a nursing home as well as doing oral health education in the schools," said Voigt Geurink.
Simonson stated that public health is a field for those with excellent, well developed clinical skills. She felt it could be hard work for newly graduated students.

"Our biggest challenge when we have students on rotation is that they are still learning how to hold a scaler. Then they have to adapt that to someone who is moving around," she commented. "It demands a lot of creative thinking."

Simonson said communicating with the elderly patient frequently involves more layers than the typical clinician-patient dynamic.

"When you get into geriatrics or anyone with special care needs, now you may have family that you have to communicate with, nurses might want to talk to you or maybe you need to call the physician's office because the nurses don't know about the cardiac condition, for example. A social worker might get involved if they feel there's been some issue that might jeopardize the patient's rights. There are a whole lot more players involved when you are in this environment. That's what I love about it. But, for someone who just wants to get the job done, it might not be the calling."

"The rewards that you get back make it valuable. It can be something small – someone says thank you or a child gives a hug. Or it can be that you're on a team of interdisciplinary professionals, and you actually get to see some outcomes, some achievements, in making a difference in the oral health problems that these people experience," Voigt Geurink concluded. "It is not a career that you are going to see results over night, because it has been 30 some years and I am finally now just starting to see that now we are making a difference."

Corporate

Definition: Much like the dental hygienist's role in public health, professionals who move into the corporate realm also perform duties that fall into categories such as research, administrative/managerial, education and clinical work. In addition to this, these dental hygiene professionals perform more corporate-minded activities such as research and development of new products and services, assisting in clinical trials to test those products and services, professional sales, educational management in dental hygiene and dental schools, professional relations and eventually assisting marketing professionals to present those products and services to the public or professional audiences.

Educational Requirements: A master's degree in this day and age is extremely desirable since it would make a difference as the competition in this role has grown. Dental hygienists considering moving into this area, who have a bachelor's degree already, might consider adding continuing education courses in business and business management and marketing. A Masters in Business Administration (MBA) is the entry level qualification in corporate America, and speaking a second language can also move you to the front of the line, as well.

Professional Characteristics: Obvious characteristics that dental hygienists already possess include organization, time management, people skills, effective communication and presentation skills and collaboration with colleagues. Work in the corporate world requires flexibility and a willingness to spend additional hours in the work day, as well as being available via email and phone in off hours and traveling. Business travel is also required. The position also requires professionals to be motivated and excited about products and/or brands they represent. Corporate professionals need to be ambitious and diplomatic. Finding such a role may require moving to a major metropolitan area, such as Chicago, New York, Boston, Los Angeles, Dallas, etc., where major oral healthcare companies are headquartered.

Another career path for dental hygienists that some professionals take is the one leading into the corporate world. Christine Charles, RDH, BS, Diane Dornisch, RDH, MBA, Karen A. Raposa, RDH, MBA, Karen Neiner, RDH, MBA, Candy B. Ross, RDH, BS, and Rebecca Van Horn, RDH, BA, secured their dental hygiene credential and went on to use that knowledge in the oral health corporate environment. Each person's work day is dedicated to improving oral health, developing new and unique products that can help dental professionals recommend quality products to their patients and working with dentists and dental hygienists. And each person interviewed claimed it is not a work environment for which every dental hygienist is cut out.

"There is no nine-to-five in corporate America," commented Diane Dornisch. "I love this position because you are always learning. You don't know it all, you can't know it all." It was the abundance of opportunities that drew Dornisch into the corporate world.

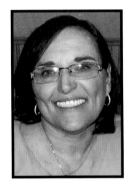

Figure 2.21. Diane Dornisch

"It was growth, it was learning something new . . . I love dentistry and helping dental professionals and patients. That is why I chose to go into a dental corporate setting," explained Dornisch, who graduated from Philadelphia Community College in 1980. It was not her first experience in oral health. She started working as a dental assistant to a dentist who taught at Temple University.

Dornisch worked as a clinician until 1995 and taught at Manor College in Jenkintown, PA for six years. In 1995, Dornisch accepted a Professional Service Representative position with Dentsply, Inc. It was the best of both worlds — she could use her knowledge of science and dental hygiene to work as a specialist who would troubleshoot problems dental offices were having with Dentsply products. She could educate them on the chemistry and proper material placement techniques.

While with Dentsply, Dornisch also worked as a Sales Trainer and in the Clinical Research Department monitoring clinical studies and writing product inserts. She also worked with different teams such as marketing for new product development and assisted in conducting in-house testing.

In 2002, Dornisch moved to a sales position with Pfizer, which was eventually sold to Johnson & Johnson. At the time of the sale, Dornisch was named Senior Account Manager for the Consumer Health Group, eventually she was placed at OraPharma, Inc. (another Johnson & Johnson Company at that time). At OraPharma, she sold ARESTIN® to dental offices; it is a position that she viewed as more of an educational role. She recently accepted the position of a Professional Educator for OraPharma. In this role she will be working with both dental and dental hygiene schools educating students on ARESTIN®. In December 2009, OraPharma was sold to Water Street Health Care Partners.

"My position helps dentists and dental hygienists learn about a product that maybe they don't have time to research," Dornisch continued. "When you have a company representative who knows their product . . . it is a value to any dental professional. You can provide them with a breadth of information that they don't have to go look up. Through this type of education, they can utilize that information to help their patients."

Karen Neiner who has been a dental hygienist since 1980, described the corporate environment in which she works as entrepreneurial. Neiner spent eight years as a clinician before moving into a corporate position with dental instrument manufacturer Hu-Friedy Manufacturing Company, Inc., in 1989.

Neiner described her clinical experience as wonderful. She split her time between a high-profile cosmetic dental practice on Chicago's famed Michigan Avenue and a rural community in Northwestern Indiana mapping naturally occurring water fluoridation in communities with well water to prevent fluorosis and dental decay in the children growing up there.

"There was a desire to make certain we were prescribing the appropriate vitamins and fluoride supplements. It was a very diverse experience," said Neiner, who received her Associate of Science degree from Indiana University. She then went back and worked within a degree completion program to finish her Bachelor of Science in dental hygiene degree at Chicago's Northwestern University in 1988.

"I didn't need the credit hours, however, I knew that I needed some experience in industry, so I negotiated an internship with Hu-Friedy. I paid Northwestern tuition to have an elective and work as an intern at Hu-Friedy [for class credit]. After that, [Hu-Friedy] offered me the first associate product manager position," said Neiner, who completed her MBA at Chicago's DePaul University in 2000.

"I moved into marketing and sales positions throughout the organization," said Neiner, who became an internal architect of new product development process, educating herself to become a lead auditor for EBAR and ISO Certification and Regulatory Requirements for regulatory issues.

She also worked with end users to put together a website, "Friends of Hu-Friedy," that gives benefits and continuing education to end-users to evaluate products.

"Knowing customer requirements and also learning what good manufacturing processes are – because that wasn't necessarily my strength – over time you do develop that. The science aspect of dental hygiene has given me a great background. The scientific process works wherever you apply it.

"I don't know if a different corporate structure would have given me this much pleasure. I am never bored," said Neiner. "Hu-Friedy gives me outlets for creativity." There have been opportunities, too, to mentor the next generation of product managers, something she greatly enjoys. She currently holds the position of Vice President of Corporate

Development and Professional Relations for Hu-Friedy. In this position, she is responsible for seeking business opportunities in new markets for Hu-Friedy. She works with dental professionals and professional associations to facilitate a relationship with them and the company, and continues to develop quality instrumentation to meet the unmet dental needs of the dental profession.

For Karen A. Raposa, Clinical Education Manager with Hu-Friedy Manufacturing Company, Inc., a typical day in the office involves sales calls and public relations activities in all dental programs in the Northeast territory, which includes New England, Manhattan and portions of eastern New York and New Jersey. In addition, Raposa provides lectures and continuing education courses for dental professionals and students and creates marketing strategies to promote use of Hu-Friedy instruments in school curricula, clinics and activities. She started this position with Hu-Friedy in August 2010.

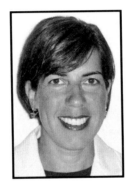

Figure 2.22. Karen A. Raposa

Raposa, who was previously Senior Manager of Professional Relations and Brand Manager on Colgate Total toothpaste with Colgate Oral Pharmaceuticals, spent many office hours reviewing and responding to requests from different associations across the country for support and partnerships. This included sponsoring a meeting speaker and partnering with publications that wanted support for continuing education or mailers, etc. She held this position with Colgate for over four years.

"I was the Brand Manager of everything that had 'Colgate Total' on it whether that was items at conventions, materials that the sales representatives used, samples that went out, advertising or direct mail, it had to come through me before it went out to dental professionals," Raposa continued.

She enjoys the marketing functions that have been a portion of current and past jobs. During her time at Colgate, she tested the advertising messages for the professional audience by holding focus groups to find out what the professional audience wanted and what words and phrases were compelling to them.

"I could get really jazzed when I sat behind the two-way mirror [during product testing and market research focus groups] and watched something I had developed being tested with dental professionals. I loved hearing my colleagues say, 'I never knew this!' or 'I wish I had known this about Colgate before,'" said Raposa.

Raposa feels she is having a significant impact from an educational standpoint. "Even though I was a product manager, I was educating people about products in a meaningful way," she said. She pointed out that it could be frustrating, too, but the rewards far outweigh the burdens.

Raposa came to Colgate after first working as a clinical dental hygienist for 21 years and then holding her first corporate position at Oral-B for five years.

"I had a six-month period as an Assistant Professor at Boston University," said Raposa, who graduated from the University of Rhode Island with her associate's and bachelor's degrees. "My role at Colgate was a combination of all of those things I just mentioned," she continues, noting that she finalized her education for the corporate world by earning an MBA from University of Massachusetts in 2001.

"As a dental hygienist, I always felt I was wearing a lot of hats — I never felt I was just scaling and polishing teeth. I was an educator as a dental hygienist with every patient I saw. I was selling dentistry — certainly not something they didn't need — but you had to learn how to speak to a patient in order to get them to understand what they needed. Very early on as a clinician I realized that I did a lot of different things all day long." The dentist with whom she worked, Dr. Phillip Robitaille of Somerset, MA was a great supporter and sent her to many classes to learn new things. Raposa completed the first phase of her education with a bachelor's degree that opened doors to teach clinical dental hygiene in community colleges. She taught at Bristol Community College as an adjunct professor while in private practice.

Candy B. Ross was wrestling with a career decision: Did she want to pursue dentistry or possibly nursing? A very astute biology professor asked her, "Since you enjoy biology/microbiology so much, why not think about dentistry? Also think about the possibly of expanding to work in dental research."

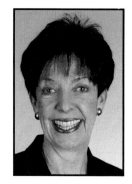

Figure 2.23. Candy B. Ross

"I wish I could have found that professor years later to say thank you," Ross said. "His simple encouragement changed my entire career. With his encouragement, when I graduated from University of Rhode Island, I made an appointment at Forsyth Dental Research Institute in Boston and told them I was interested in working in dental research. I asked what I needed to get started. I left with a new job because one of the researchers had just received a notice for new grant money! That three-year run launched my career in dental research. I had the privilege of working with icons like Drs. Ralph Lobene and Sid Socransky on some of their early work on chlorhexidine. I knew then, I was in the right place at the right time."

She then moved to St. Louis and assumed she would never find another research position as there were no dental institutes in the area. An advertisement in the Sunday newspaper caught her attention as she searched the pages for a private practice job. Monsanto Company, the largest manufacturer of phosphates, had an advertisement for a clinical dental hygienist to conduct research projects on toothpaste. She applied for the job and once again was fortunate enough to be hired. Her job entailed both clinical and laboratory work as well as early testing on sealants.

After seven years at Monsanto, another advertisement in the Sunday newspaper under dental hygiene caught her eye: Hygienist wanted to travel and do educational presentations to dental and dental hygiene schools. This job was with Teledyne WaterPik.

"I had the wonderful opportunity again to get hired. The beauty of this position was the ability to grow into a position where I could use the skill sets I had learned at both Forsyth and Monsanto," Ross stated. The position involved conducting clinical research trials to substantiate therapeutic claims as well as contributing to the overall marketing of the products.

"I had the opportunity to work with many icons in the dental research community along with a variety of professional organizations" she continued. "Keeping my eyes open, working with so many wonderful mentors and being willing to work hard to learn new skills allowed me to have a wonderful and fulfilling career in clinical research."

Ross was originally hired at Teledyne WaterPik as an Educational Consultant to speak to groups of dental and dental hygiene students. This job grew into a Marketing Manager position to drive the professional side of the marketing business. When clinical trials were required to substantiate marketing claims used in advertising, the job title became "Clinical Research Manager."

"The more I worked with top researchers in the country, I became very aware of a need to pull these icons together for strategic discussions. Thus we formed the first domestic Oral Health Advisory Board and then subsequently an International Advisory Board. "My job was to build relationships with our advisors, plan and coordinate our meetings and ensure our advisors were well prepared for any of our meetings. I had the opportunity to frequently travel internationally to do the same for our International Board along with making presentations to our distributor partners.

Ross' job then changed once again to Director of Clinical Research and Professional Relations, Worldwide. "I was so fortunate to be at Teledyne and have the opportunity to work with then President, Mel Cruger. Mel believed in the value of strong professional relations and he supported my work and I was able to grow with this company for 23 years."

And it did not end there; Ross left WaterPik for a small start-up company, DEXIS, in digital radiology in 1999. She was able to use all her skill sets and contacts in the industry and become one of the four directors in the company. Five years later, DEXIS was acquired by a large conglomerate along with many other dental companies. Through a reorganization, Ross' job expanded to Director of Industry and Professional Relations for DEXIS, Gendex, i-CAT, KaVo, Marus, Pelton & Crane, Instrumentarium and Sordex.

"I never expected to be so blessed in my career. My advice is to read, stay alert to new products and new companies. Develop an idea of what you feel you're passionate about. Ask questions. Seek out mentors. Go to dental meetings and introduce yourself to corporate representatives. Volunteer when there are events or charity clinics in your area. Never be afraid to ask . . . . you never know where it will take you! And have faith that if you truly want to grow and change, it will happen" Ross concluded. "The dental industry is small. Be open, seek new contacts and never stop building relationships!"

Following interests and opportunities led Rebecca Van Horn to dental hygiene in a corporate setting. Her family dentist recommended that she go into dental hygiene. A presentation by Candy Ross, however, convinced her to take her talents into corporate.

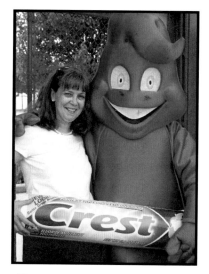
Figure 2.24. Rebecca Van Horn

"A lot of people do not maintain their license in corporate, I do," said Van Horn, who obtained both her Associate of Science and Bachelor of Science degrees in dental hygiene from Ohio State in 1979.

"I saw a presentation in 1984 by Candy Ross – she was the professional educator for Teledyne WaterPik. I had been in clinical hygiene for three or four years. After the presentation, I went up and asked her more about working in corporate," Van Horn said. It immediately attracted her.

"I was single at the time. It was important for me to work for someone who offered a decent benefit package. A lot of positions in clinical at that time didn't offer that," Van Horn said. "The interest I had was in prevention. Oral-B was one of the premier companies in preventive dentistry."

Van Horn was hired by Oral-B in 1987 and has worked in corporate full time ever since. As manager of professional and academic relations, Van Horn gives presentations in dental and dental hygiene schools, makes certain schools have Oral-B products in their clinics, and fulfills a public relations role while at conventions and professional meetings.

Of keeping Crest and Oral-B products in schools, Van Horn said: "We believe that if the product is in front of students while they are learning, there is a greater likelihood that they will go back to that product in private practice."

There is more variety and variability in a corporate setting, Van Horn observed. "I think you take what you learn as a dental hygienist and you build upon it scientifically. I would be a better dental hygienist if I moved back into the clinical role having been in this job. I would be better able to evaluate products and the people selling it."

"I think there is opportunity in corporate to be successful monetarily and have an impact on a business. You are limited only by your energy and ability to get things done," Van Horn continued.

Ross advised those interested in the corporate role to seek a master's degree.

"It has changed dramatically . . . When I first started in a corporate setting there were not many dental hygienists doing that. I think it's very different now that we have had a lot of hygienists to demonstrate their capability in a lot of different areas, so the competition is a little stronger," Ross continued.

"You have to have the education behind you," agreed Dornisch. "Companies will not look at a dental hygienist who only has her associate's degree in dental hygiene. At least that's the way it is now. You have to have a bachelor's degree. Understanding dentistry and what goes on in the office has been invaluable to me. It has made me very successful. You have to have a willingness to step outside your comfort zone. Working in a corporate environment is very different than working in a clinical setting."

Neiner recommended that dental hygienists not only complete their bachelor's degree but also take electives in marketing, economics, accounting and business if they have an interest in corporate settings.

"I took an additional elective in an internship to get that (business) experience," she explained. "It doesn't always have to be formal education." Neiner also recommended that dental hygienists with an interest in business seek out retail sales opportunities that can give them experience, adding that "an organization will look to see how determined you are to develop your professional skills. Did you work to develop sales or marketing skills?"

Neiner also stated that keeping an involvement with professional associations and the oral health community is important. "Be involved with your sales representatives, volunteer for them, be thirsty for knowledge, ask good questions," she listed.

Be aware, too, of the major differences between the clinical and the corporate work days, advised Ross.

"Dental hygiene is such a very clear, delineated day," she observed. "You start and you end and you don't think about it anymore." Corporate positions tend to take more time than the day allows, and you are always thinking about projects being worked on."

Raposa agreed. "You are never done at the end of the day," she said. "You have to be okay with that. You have to be able to end your work day and be self disciplined." And you must be able to manage office politics, she added.

"In corporate, you work with people and you want their buy-in and support, but those people do not report to your position," Raposa continued. "In a corporate position, you roll with the punches and 'put out fires' when you least expect it."

Dornisch described the corporate personality as persistent and capable of taking a 'no' answer. "Just because they say 'no' today doesn't mean they will say no tomorrow. You might be scared to death to pick up your bag and go back in there. That resilience is something some people can't do."

Neiner described it as having "a strong work ethic and a thick skin. The key is that education is life-long. You never have it all. You are always searching."

Being open-minded is another plus said Dornisch. "You have to be a person who likes all different types of people. You deal with a lot of personalities. You need to understand your field. You have to be a good dental hygienist. If something you learned 20 years ago is good enough, and you feel you don't need to update that, you are not going to be successful in the corporate arena," Dornisch commented.

Dornisch also added that a dental hygienist in the corporate arena must learn to admit when he or she does not know an answer.

"I will say 'I will get the answer for you,' to the doctor. Follow up, stick to it and go back in. I earned a lot of respect when I went back with answers to their questions," Dornisch explained. "I have handled dental and dental hygiene schools. The faculty will sometimes ask me to talk to the students about careers in sales or corporate America. I tell them it is a career that I never imagined in a million years."

"It's all about relationships," Ross concluded. "It's pulling out a skill that I already have and that I am able to use in a completely different environment, that's really fun and exciting."

"Dentistry is a great profession," concluded Van Horn. "From a corporate perspective, we saw a presentation that one of the executives within Procter & Gamble presented that focused on oral care and how it is going to grow and grow. I feel fortunate to be where I am right now."

Professional Savvy, LLC, wants to thank these well established dental hygiene professionals who have shared their expertise in their professional roles and the choices they made to establish themselves in their professional careers. Words cannot express my appreciation for the time they committed to be interviewed for this new textbook, SAVVY SUCCESS™, and to share their personal stories with our readers on the many roles dental hygienists can achieve in their career in the dental hygiene profession. Thank you again and my very best wishes to all of you.

References

1. Bureau of Labor Statistics website. Occupational Outlook Handbook, 2010-2011 ed. "Dental Hygienists." Available at http://www.bls.gov/oco/ocos097.htm. Viewed Feb. 1, 2012.

Critical Thinking Exercises

1. Using definitions from the chapter, develop a three-page essay about a future role of interest to you in dental hygiene and how you can shape that role with your own professional interests to serve the profession.

2. Use your essay to create and present a slide show about the dental hygiene role that most interests you at this point in your education/career. Present this information to your class or a group of friends and mentors.

Key Concepts

1. Dental hygienists who only ever consider the private practice as their primary role miss the depth of roles found within the dental hygiene profession.

2. Government statistics reveal that employment of dental hygienists is expected to grow faster than average for all occupations through 2018.

3. The past 10 years have seen an expanded scope of practice for dental hygienists in some states and the development of the Advanced Dental Hygiene Practitioner (ADHP).

4. The American Dental Hygienists' Association (ADHA) defined five professional roles in dental hygiene, as well as a sixth role, public health, which is such an integral part of the other five that it is considered an over-arching role within the profession: administrator/manager, advocate, clinician, educator and researcher.

5. A seventh role, dental hygiene in the corporate setting, has been included by Professional Savvy, LLC.

6. Dental hygienists in the administrator/manager role guide and direct the work of others as well as execute a variety of administrative duties.

7. Dental hygienists in the role of advocate lobby for the healthcare rights of their patients and support the code of ethics, professional standards and goals of their profession.

8. Clinicians participate in communication with their patients, assess medical and dental histories, take radiographs, conduct a dental hygiene diagnosis, identify the right treatment plan for preventive and restorative services and conduct effective treatment outcome for prevention, intervention or control of oral diseases while working independently or in collaboration with other professionals.

9. Dental hygienists as educators employ educational theory and methodology to analyze healthcare needs, develop health promotion strategies and deliver and evaluate the results in attaining or maintaining health.

10. Dental hygienists in research roles apply the scientific method to select appropriate therapies, educational methods or content, interpret and apply findings and solve problems in a wide spectrum of areas within the profession.

11. The dental hygienist's role in public health is an integral part of all five other professional roles.

12. Dental hygienists with roles in public health assist epidemiologists in researching the populations whom they serve, provide clinic and preventive services to schools and other public organizations, act as educators of oral health within their communities, perform administrative and managerial duties within their public health departments and serve as advocates of oral health and ending oral disease-causing behaviors.

13. Dental hygienists involved in corporate settings perform duties that fall into categories such as research, administrative/managerial, education and clinical work, as well as more corporate-minded activities such as research and development of new products and services, assisting in clinical trials to test those products and services, professional sales, educational management with dental hygiene and dental schools, professional relations, and assisting marketing professionals to present those products and services to the public or professional audiences.

Chapter 3: Mentoring

By Christine A. Hovliaras, RDH, BS, MBA, CDE

Learning Objectives

The student dental hygienist and dental hygiene professional will learn the following key objectives from this chapter:

1. Identify the characteristics of a mentor and assess existing relationships for potential and future mentors.
2. Discuss why mentors are important to professional and career development.
3. Create a plan for securing a mentor or mentors to offer career counseling and professional development.
4. Once a mentor or mentors have been identified, describe how to make use of that relationship to develop long-range goals, objectives and a career path.
5. Identify how to give back to the profession by mentoring and contributing to the education of others and professional colleagues.

Overview

While dental hygienists may find opportunities to be mentored by family members, educational seminars or professional publications, the richest, most dynamic experience is found in connecting with other dental hygiene professionals. Mentors exist in all walks of life, from a parent, grandparent or sibling, to college professors, employers or colleagues. In this chapter, some of the most successful dental hygienists in the dental hygiene profession share how mentors changed the course of their careers.

What comes to mind when one reads the word "**mentor**"? A parent or grandparent? Does this person look like an older sibling?

For this chapter, I interviewed a few distinguished names in the dental hygiene field who found mentors in exactly these people early on in their lives. For Jane A. Balavage, RDH, BS, her creative grandmother, who could make something from nothing, was her first mentor. Mary Semancik, RDH, learned to share her knowledge from the example her parents set as she was growing up.

Every professional should have a mentor, or as many as three. This trusted advisor is someone who can offer an objective opinion about another person or his or her work. Ideal mentors are individuals who are close enough to the person being evaluated to know his or her work style, habits and personal life, yet are not so closely related that they cannot offer advice or even criticism. Barnes reports that as the mentorship experience increases so does the level of career satisfaction.[1] Additionally, mentorship can promote one's career, income and job satisfaction.[2] Powerful mentors can provide positive differences in **mentees'** careers and help to grow them professionally.[3]

Margaret Walsh, RDH, MA, MS, EdD, used professional literature to fill the mentor's shoes by walking her through the steps of scientific investigation.

"I turn to **peer-reviewed journals** and I look up articles written in my area of interest," Walsh explained. "I try to find high-quality studies and use them as models for my studies." When she refers to high-quality studies, she means those that are funded by recognized organizations and, of course, that the studies have been printed by respected publications.

Another area in which Walsh found mentoring was in the research field. It's something she recommended to others: "Find somebody with a similar interest to yours. Offer your time to them."

What she discovered is that dental hygienists have a unique perspective in preventive measures. "I was in the field with all kinds of basic and clinical scientists who did not ask the same questions in which I had interest," Walsh stated.

She further observed: "One of the messages I try to impart is, don't be too impatient with yourself. I think the bar is being raised so high. My advice is to align yourself with someone who is already successful, help them, and you will learn; they will teach you. As you work with that individual, you will come to a point where you identify the questions that are most salient to you."

Dental hygiene icon, author and educator Esther M. Wilkins, BS, RDH, DMD, credited both the first dentist with whom she worked, Dr. Frank Willis, and her disciplined older sister as early mentors in her career success.

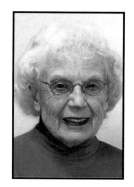

Figure 3.1. Dr. Esther M. Wilkins

"My sister was quite remarkable in terms of mentoring," remarked Wilkins. "She sat me down and said, 'hey, you have to go to college!'" Acting as both mentor and study partner, Wilkins' sister guided her early education and established that foundation of life-long learning that sustained Wilkins' educational pursuits well beyond her dental hygiene degree through master's and doctoral degrees.

Semancik's story is similar. The 2008 Sonicare/*RDH* (magazine) Mentor of the Year Award recipient was born into a professional, mentoring family. Her father, a renowned Kentucky veterinarian who was the first in his state to have his own hospital, mentored several students each year – some of whom lived in the guest house on her family's horse farm. In addition, Semancik's father hosted other veterinarians who came to study at his veterinary practice or use the hospital facilities.

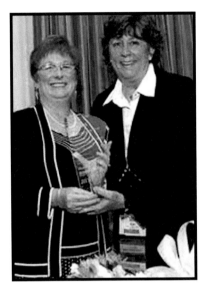

Figure 3.2. Mary Semancik

"My mother was a big influence, too," Semancik added. As wife and mother of seven children, her mother was mentor, coach and teammate.

"I saw how much she took time for each of us. I never heard my mother complain about being a parent. There was always a positive attitude from her about her job," Semancik explained. "It was just part of growing up, that any knowledge you had you passed on to the next person."

Balavage, a 36-year-veteran of dental hygiene and the 2007 RDH Mentor of the Year, described herself as **self-motivated**, and, like Wilkins and Semancik, drew inspiration from a family mentor, her grandmother.

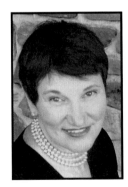

Figure 3.3. Jane A. Balavage

"She could take nothing and make something out of it. She was my best motivator and mentor in my life," said Balavage.

She refers to mentoring as a rewarding experience. "You can teach anybody a skill, but until you bring that skill from the heart, until you have passion about what you do and how you do it and how to get to a patient's heart, until you make that connection – that is where you light the fire."

The inspiration behind Balavage's teaching is to show students how to achieve this level of commitment and connection with their own patients.

"It's exciting. It's a catalystic effect," Balavage said. "Otherwise, you're just doing a job. The real power is getting to the heart and soul of the profession."

If you're just going to a job every day, you're in the wrong job or the wrong profession!

Do You Have a Mentor(s)?

Everyone needs a mentor to grow professionally, and a mentor does not necessarily have to be a teacher, professor or professional contact. Anyone or anything that ignites passion for the profession can be a mentor. This is a firm belief of Walsh, who has mentored professionals in the fields of both research and education.

"If you're not mentored, you cannot progress in your career. If you do not mentor, you can't progress in your career. It's a symbiotic, win-win situation. I learn as much from my protégés as they learn from me, but I won't work with someone if they're not committed, my time is too valuable," she stated.

Good candidates for a mentor include: An alma-mater professor, a past or present boss or supervisor, close colleagues with whom the person works, or others knowledgeable in a specific area in which the person has interest. Dental hygienists might consider seeking mentors from the American Dental Hygienists' Association (ADHA), their constituent (state) organization, or local component (region of state in which they reside), or by contacting dental hygienists who have become well known in an area of expertise in dental hygiene.

Wilkins shared a story of a friend who was both Wilkins' patient and a college student who didn't know what course to pursue with her life. One day while Wilkins had this young woman in her chair, she suggested she try dental hygiene. Many years later, after the lady retired from a long career in dental hygiene, she wrote a thank-you note to Wilkins.

"I was a mentor that early by selling the profession to someone else. A lot of mentoring instances are short-term," Wilkins said.

Balavage also engages in some "**chair-side**" **mentoring** of patients. One such patient, who was also a co-worker with Balavage in a nursing home, had the opportunity to watch Balavage at work and be her patient. She was so impressed with Balavage, she shared stories about Balavage with her daughter, Angie, who was a dental hygiene patient. Angie Yorina, entered the dental hygiene field with a great appreciation of it, and became Balavage's protégé. Yorina nominated her for the 2007 Sonicare/RDH Mentor of the Year Award .

"I finally met Angie at a meeting. She was like a sponge! " shared Balavage, who was deeply honored by Yorina's nomination.

"She was . . . a newbie to the field," Balavage remembered. "Her mother used to share with Angie that there was a dental hygienist who was so excited about her job. She told Angie: 'I hope you become a dental hygienist just like Jane. She does creative things with the patients.' " Balavage said the example that impressed Angie's mother was a time she took off her shoes and used bailer twine to floss between her toes to demonstrate the proper technique to a large group of people.

"In some of my mentoring, I used teaching," Wilkins noted. "All teachers and students have that relationship. Even when I teach continuing education courses, people write me letters or come back to other sessions I teach. The idea is: We need each other. We can certainly benefit from the lives and mistakes of others. Isn't that a basic?"

How Do You Utilize a Mentor in Your Career?

Deciding on a mentor does not necessarily need to be a formal arrangement and a professional's team of mentors should probably grow and change as that person's career grows and changes.

However, in some instances, Walsh advised that "you have to enter into contract with a mentor if you want that mentor to take you seriously." Likewise, she continued, it is important for the mentor to provide concrete guidelines as to what he or she expects to be accomplished and when.

Walsh referred to it as a constant interactive process "where there are deadlines and we are working toward a common goal." When Walsh mentors, she helps her protégés develop a timeline in which certain expectations will be met. Walsh explained that she sets one date in which the **protégé** will have his or her specific aims developed. By another date, that individual will complete a literature review supporting those aims.

"I give them very concrete deadlines that they must meet," said Walsh, who insists that each protégé must agree to publish their data once it's collected and analyzed before she will agree to work with them.

"It is important to me that energy invested in research mentoring ultimately produces outcomes that contribute to the body of knowledge. It's constantly a give and take," Walsh commented. "Those publications, I believe, mentor more people than individual mentors can do on their own. I can mentor three post-doctoral students a year. If each one of those students publish their papers, they can mentor innumerable people to help them with their research efforts in a particular area."

"It's the same thing in education. If you publish a piece in the Journal of Dental Hygiene on special teaching techniques . . . then all of the dental and dental hygiene educators can benefit from that. Every publication is providing mentoring," Walsh concluded.

Identifying a Mentor – The Do's and Don'ts

One of the biggest challenges a professional will face is identifying a mentor. It can be a lot like connecting with someone who becomes a life-long friend or spouse. Much of what makes the relationship work is in the chemistry and dynamic that forms between the two people. A good mentor is an active listener who takes an interest in the mentee's career and goals. This individual will not interrupt while another is talking and asks questions about statements that have been made. Poor candidates do not listen and tend toward self-centeredness.

When dental hygienists are seeking a mentor, they should consider the professionals they know, those in positions of interest or those who have been acknowledged as being a mentor through receiving an award or as a key opinion leader. For dental hygienists, superior mentors are those in the field who have had career success in one or more areas of oral health.

A mentor should be a good communicator and be able to outline steps the mentee needs to take in order to learn a new area of opportunity in the dental hygiene profession. A mentor needs to understand the mentee's goals.

Early in my career, I worked for Dr. Jeffery M. Gordon, as mentioned in Chapter 1. I consider him a mentor in my career. He noticed that I was self-motivated and inquisitive and recommended I pursue becoming a research dental hygienist as another avenue of work. There were very few research dental hygienists in the early 1980s.

Also as mentioned in the first chapter, I began working for Dr. Gordon in his new periodontal practice in 1983 as the office manager and his dental assistant when I was a second-year dental hygiene student in the Fairleigh S. Dickinson Junior College. At that time, Dr. Gordon also was involved in Fairleigh Dickinson's Dental Medicine Research Center. He asked if I would be interested in learning how to become a research dental hygienist and clinical investigator. I jumped at the opportunity and began as a clinical investigator conducting a clinical trial on clindamycin therapy in refractory periodontitis patients for him. Then I became involved in recruiting patients for an upcoming mouthrinse study for which I was trained as the clinical examiner.

My work with Dr. Gordon helped me to attain five years research experience at my alma mater that later assisted me in securing my corporate position with Warner-Lambert Company in 1989. It was exciting and enriching work that I had not considered before Dr. Gordon suggested I pursue it. I am thankful for his mentorship, friendship and professional advice.

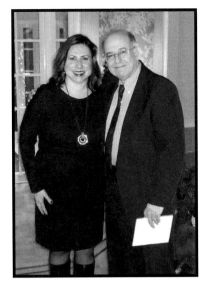

Figure 3.4. Dr. Gordon and I at an office dinner celebration in December 2011.

What is key then is for dental hygienists to develop relationships with those who can offer an objective opinion about their work, strengths and interests. While these may be things professionals can determine on their own, it is helpful to have that support person to reinforce what is already known.

My other mentor in my dental hygiene career was Regina Dreyer Thomas, RDH, BS, MPA. Regina was an unbelievable role model for me. She was a dental hygienist with a master's degree who wrote a book entitled, *CAREER DIRECTIONS for Dental Hygienists –Your Guide to Change and Opportunity.* She wrote three editions of this book, and I had met her after I graduated with a Bachelor of Science degree in Dental Hygiene from Fairleigh Dickinson University College of Dental Medicine. What fascinated me the most about Regina was that she had a level of professionalism all her own; she was very well respected and shared with me the many wonderful roles that dental hygienists could expand their careers in this profession. So being a clinician and educator were not the only roles in the early 1980s. Through reading Regina's three editions of her book over the next 10 years (I wrote a chapter about my role as a research dental hygienist in the early 1990s when I worked for the Warner-Lambert Company), I learned about other dental hygiene professionals working in a variety of roles and learned valuable feedback from each of them. Regina also introduced me into joining the International Federation of Dental Hygiene (IFDH) in 1991 and invited me to be on her career panel presentation that was presented in the Netherlands. I must thank Regina as well as Dr. Gordon for being two unbelievable role models and mentors to me in my dental hygiene career.

Walsh called this determination of interest the first step; the second step is finding someone to serve as a major mentor in that area. She quickly pointed out that every career has its minor mentors; those individuals who offer quick advice over the phone with whom one does not develop an in-depth relationship.

For Balavage, belonging to professional organizations led to mentors. "Get involved in your professional association because that is where the building blocks are – that's how I got started. I got to meet people above me and I wanted to be like them. I absorbed everything I could in those situations. Those are huge building blocks for your career and your profession."

Being a member of a professional organization "was my mentor," Balavage continued. "When I first started out, I wasn't a member. When I got involved, that was the spearhead. I took continuing education courses. Learning above and beyond what you already know is powerful. It's a life-long learning process."

According to Semancik, there are a lot of "everyday mentors" in the profession, who lend a helping hand on a daily basis. Drawing from the foundation of sharing knowledge that her parents established for her, Semancik helped her colleague, Pam Walters, RDH, return to the profession after a 20-year absence. Walters, for a number of reasons, had been out of dental hygiene for a long time. Semancik offered a friendly, open forum in which questions were welcomed. Walters was so thankful, she nominated Semancik for the Sonicare/RDH Mentor of the Year Award.

Semancik said of receiving the award: "I'm just an everyday dental hygienist who just tried to be fair and helpful to her colleagues. There are lots of us who do this!" A greater reward for Semancik was that Walters not only returned to dental hygiene but also got involved in the state organization.

"You think of that professor or teacher who knew all the answers, who you could go to, who was helpful, maybe they lit a little fire under you in school to get you motivated – to me that's what a mentor is, but that's not what I did," Semancik said. "I was just there for my colleague. I let her ask me. You have to back off and let them come to you. You have to be there with very positive responses. When there is a negative, sandwich it between two positives and make certain that the person can learn something from what you have explained."

Giving Back to the Dental Hygiene Profession

Everyone needs to give back to the profession, said Semancik.

"You can't call yourself a professional and not be involved. I don't understand the thought process where you think you could just go to work and then go back home; that you're not active in your community, that you don't volunteer for things, that you're not on your board. You don't have to give 20 hours a week. If you're a busy person, pick one project. Give a day, give half a day."

For experienced professionals, becoming involved may range from volunteering in a public health setting to participating in clinical research trials, or giving time to launch a project for their local component or teaching a continuing education course. For students, it can mean being involved in the student dental hygiene organization, volunteering in a private practice or simply offering some time to their dental hygiene school to help out. Both the student and the professional can contribute their time to local health fairs, community outreach projects and civic organizations.

Semancik suggested that it is the small, daily efforts that make a difference. "When I go into a practice, I always go in and make things a little bit better than I found it. You can't change everything. You shouldn't go in thinking you are going to change everything. You should pick one area and make that better and healthier for patients," she continued.

Walsh concluded: "Whenever I have someone come to me and say they want to work with me, I always say yes. I learn as much from protégés as they will learn from me as a mentor. It's a very interactive kind of relationship. I don't care how far up the ladder you get, if you stop looking for major mentors, you stop growing."

Professional Savvy, LLC, wants to personally thank Esther, Jane, Peg and Mary for being interviewed for this chapter and providing their valuable insights on what mentoring means to them and how our readers could find unique and wonderful mentors to help guide their future to success. My very best regards to all of you for being role models in the dental hygiene profession.

References

1. Barnes, WG. The mentoring experiences and career satisfaction of dental hygiene program directions. J Dent Hyg. 2004;331-9.
2. Chao, GT. Mentoring phases and outcomes. J Voc Behav. 1997;51:15-28.
3. Scanlon, KC. Mentoring women administrators: Breaking through the glass ceiling. Initv. 1997;58:39-59.

Critical Thinking Exercises

1. Create a list of three to five people in your life who could be potential mentors using the criteria described in this chapter. Evaluate the people on that list and pick at least one person to approach and discuss beginning a formal mentoring relationship. Set appointments to consult with your mentor.

2. Make a list of ways to contribute to the dental hygiene profession and discuss that with your mentor. Decide which ways might best contribute to the profession and expand your career opportunities.

Key Concepts

1. Every professional should have a mentor, or as many as three, at various times in his or her dental hygiene career.

2. Mentors offer objective opinions about another person or his or her work, work style, professional strengths or weaknesses, habits and a small part of his or her personal life. A mentor is not so closely related that they cannot offer advice or criticism.

3. Mentorship can take many forms. If a dental hygiene professional can draw information to improve their career from another professional, a professional publication or peer-reviewed journal or a research paper, that is also a form of mentoring.

4. Self-motivation is key in both finding and securing a mentor relationship and committing to its course.

5. Mentors can be found in many areas of the dental hygiene profession from the operatory and classroom, to the professional organization, in a university setting, working in a research laboratory, in public health facilities or in an oral health company.

6. In some instances, the mentee or protégé will want to make the most of the mentor relationship by entering into a formal agreement with the mentor and developing a list of goals, objectives and deadlines.

7. Advancing one's career is a matter of being able to identify likely mentor candidates or subject matter no matter where he or she is on the career path.

8. It is important to not draw from the profession without also contributing – even while still a student. Dental hygienists and dental hygiene students should recognize opportunities to give something back professionally through the community, profession or one-on-one by mentoring.

9. Mentoring relationships strengthen the entire dental hygiene profession.

Chapter 4: Career Success – Elevating Your Dental Hygiene Position

By Christine A. Hovliaras, RDH, BS, MBA, CDE

Learning Objectives

The student dental hygienist and dental hygiene professional will learn the following key objectives from this chapter:

1. Define what career success means to you professionally.
2. Identify the elements that will help you achieve career success.
3. Identify the challenges to your plan and how you can create a strategy to overcome them.
4. Strategize a course of action using three primary elements of career success to help maintain your momentum.
5. Prepare to launch your career success plan.

Overview

Career success takes many different shapes. Its weight can be measured in as many ways as there are dental hygienists to consider it. For some professionals, career success is the culmination of daily successes over the course of months and years. For others, success is measured by the accomplishment of a list of personal goals. To achieve career satisfaction, it is important to measure both those daily and weekly successes against personal and professional goals that have been purposefully chosen and extend over a three-year period. A continual process of reviewing success helps the dental hygienists to see their professional progress.

Gail Roitman-Trauger, RDH, BA, related a story that many in dental hygiene will find familiar.

"I fell into dentistry because of my older sister. Her first job after school and on Saturdays was working for two orthodontists across the street from our high school. My father thought it was great to be able to walk to work from school and have predictable hours; therefore, he encouraged me to find similar work," she explained. More than 30 years later, Roitman-Trauger's after-school-job developed into a territory sales manager position with a major dental product manufacturer.

"The present position I have pulls everything together that I've done in dentistry since I started as a dental assistant in high school," she shared. "Even though I dabbled in various corporate dental jobs during the last 14 years, the constant was working part time as a clinical dental hygienist. I was pleasantly surprised how varied my present position is."

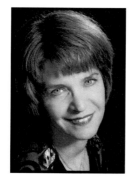

Figure 4.1. Gail Roitman-Trauger

She chose her first position in dental hygiene because it was convenient. It became a profession when Roitman-Trauger decided to invest in it.

Circumstances of life sometimes do require individuals to make convenient decisions. There is nothing really wrong with this approach as long as the individual does not let the pattern guide his or her entire life. To make purposeful, proactive career decisions, consider the **elements of career success.** These include, but are not limited to: a broad system of measuring success, collegial respect, coping skills, team contribution, professional involvement, tenacity, integrity, flexibility, continuing education, networking and retaining a passion for the dental hygiene profession.

Career Success: What Does It Mean To You?

There are many ways to define career success in dental hygiene. For one dental hygienist, it is the opportunity to help an individual. Another might achieve it by influencing a larger population to improved oral health. For yet another, career success is a pyramid in which one accomplishment is layered on another to attain a pinnacle goal. Ann-Marie C. DePalma, CDA, RDH, FADIA, FAADH, a 30-year veteran of the profession, offers an additional idea about career success.

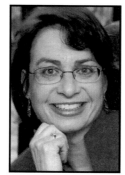

Figure 4.2. Ann-Marie C. DePalma

"I define career success as wanting to get up in the morning to go to work, not dreading the day ahead," she commented. DePalma added that enjoying what the professional does is important because of the amount of time spent at work.

"Success isn't about a monetary amount," DePalma continued. "It is about how you feel about what you are doing."

Elizabeth Lopez, RDH, has been in the dental hygiene field for more than five years and expressed a view of career success similar to DePalma's. "I define career success in the dental hygiene profession several ways," she commented. "It could be when a patient's health is improved because of my ability to teach and communicate what they need to do to achieve better health. Another success is being a member in my professional organizations, the American Dental Hygienists' Association (ADHA) and the California Dental Hygienists' Association (CDHA). I believe being involved is very important. It helps me in many aspects of my career."

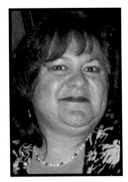

Figure 4.3. Elizabeth Lopez

Robyn Klose, RDH, who has over ten years' experience as a dental hygienist, commented that she believed that the definition of career success in dental hygiene is based on the individual goals of each dental hygienist.

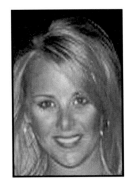

Figure 4.4. Robin Klose

What Do Dental Hygienists Think About Career Success and Do They Have It?

As with so many aspects of one's path in life, the definition of career success, too, lies in the hands of the individual. Those dental hygienists who experience the greatest job satisfaction also try to consciously track success on a regular basis. It's a little like counting one's blessings. The dental hygienist who fails to recognize daily and monthly success could possibly become unsatisfied with their dental hygiene career. The concept of career success must be broad enough to encompass everyday goals, not just lofty five-year plans.

Klose supported this idea, sharing that her career success has bloomed on many levels. First and foremost is successfully guiding patients with diseased tissue to better oral health. "I'm sure I am speaking for all dental hygienists on that one!" she exclaimed.

Gaining **respect** for what one does or says is another aspect of career success, DePalma commented. "When others in the profession look to you to confirm something or to seek your advice, that is a measure of professional success," she said. In a specific instance, DePalma recalled a patient who was unusually quiet during her three-month recare appointment.

"She seemed more subdued than usual that day. When I asked her what was wrong, she broke down in tears. She told me that her adult son, who had a chemical dependency issue, had relapsed and was not doing well. We spent the entire hygiene appointment discussing his situation and where she could get help. I decided that being there for her at that moment was more important than 'cleaning her teeth' that day," DePalma said. Her employer agreed.

When the patient returned for a re-scheduled appointment, she expressed gratitude for the time DePalma took to speak with her that day.

"I felt enormous career success because I was able to help her," DePalma said. "Dental hygienists go the extra mile for their patients in so many ways each day – it proves that they are models of career success." She cautioned that a career in dental hygiene is not all rosy and wonderful. Success also can be measured by the amount and maturity of a dental hygienist's **coping skills** that he or she develops for handling stress, negative outcomes or even job loss.

"There have been setbacks in my career along the way. Losing a job for whatever reason is never easy. Many dental hygienists experience the loss of a job at some point in their career," said DePalma. "Sometimes it is something that was done or not done, but most often it is something completely out of their control. But how one responds and deals with the loss is a measure of career success." She finds truth in the old adage, 'when one door closes, another opens.'

"When one loses a position that one enjoyed, one has to deal with the traumatic event. But often bigger and better things are in store, although at the time of the event that can't be seen," DePalma said. "Career success is accomplished by picking oneself up and finding that new challenge."

Identify The Key Elements of Success

What other elements make up the anatomy of career success? Achieving success in any career or personal endeavor requires a measure of hard work and establishing professional alliances. It also takes commitment, tenacity and a willingness to learn, DePalma offered. For Roitman-Trauger success flows from continuously learning new skills while encouraging and influencing others.

Stephanie Maddox, RDH, MALD, commented that for her career success was a combination of several elements that included making a difference in patient lives and helping them obtain and maintain a healthy oral environment. Her list of elements of success also included educating patients and the community as a whole about the rewards of good oral care and the importance of the dental hygiene profession. Maddox continued, citing the importance of creating an environment of calm friendliness and confidence in the office setting. For her, **team contribution** and being a valuable asset in the practice and for the doctor also held importance. She employs the entire dental hygienists' arsenal of skills and gifts to achieve these goals and is committed to learning new skill sets as warranted.

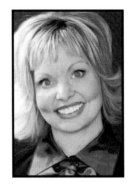

Figure 4.5. Stephanie Maddox

Mentors are another important element, Maddox noted. She counted her father, who inspired her to become a dental hygienist, as her first mentor; her second is the dentist with whom she practices.

"He has a scientific mind and retains every bit of information. He keeps himself current and pushes himself to consistently strive for more. I hope I have even a micron of his drive, intelligence and kindness in me," Maddox said. Her third mentor is fellow dental hygienist, Donna Jarosz, RDH, who Maddox referred to as her "stabilizing force every day."

"Donna treats her patients as family and friends, and that has inspired me to do the same, which our patients truly appreciate," Maddox explained. "We share their highs and lows, and they are treated as individual people, not just mouths. This also helps with burn-out, by the way, because the job isn't just cleaning tooth after tooth. It's seeing new people through the day and learning about each individual."

For Lopez, passion and **professional involvement** are key elements of career success. "Keeping up on current treatment and products to help improve my patient's oral health is what is important," she commented, adding that her involvement with professional organizations helps her to do this.

"I have the opportunity to meet seasoned dental hygienists and share experiences of patient care and job situations," Lopez explained. "I also have the opportunity to meet and learn from the corporate sponsors of the products produced for the dental patient. I believe being a member of ADHA and the opportunities it provides to connect with dental hygienists on so many different levels of expertise have helped me become a better dental hygienist. The leaders in the association have such diverse experiences from which I am able to learn and expand my own experiences and exposures."

Roitman-Trauger also values her involvement in professional organizations and the mentors she has found there.

"Every experience I have had can be attributed to the fantastic network of dental hygienists I've met and worked with over the years," said Roitman-Trauger. "Whenever I have been to a professional meeting, if I'm able to take away one concept or skill, I've been energized and then can influence my patients and colleagues."

Like many of the dental hygienists, Lopez listed **family support** as essential to her career success.

"My father was a mentor to me. He taught me to never give up on my dreams. He instilled a good work ethic and taught me how to be a strong and responsible woman. He knew that dental hygiene was my dream, and so it was his dream for me to complete this, too," Lopez shared. She also named Bernadette Hovland, RDH, as a friend, co-worker and mentor.

"She was the person I would call on those long days of dental hygiene school to share the good and bad days. Bernie set the example of what an exceptional dental hygienist was. She showed me how to treat patients both in and out of the chair with compassion and professionalism," said Lopez, who added that her friend also returned to school after starting her family. This set an example for Lopez that an individual can achieve much by wanting it enough.

Identifying the Challenges of Career Success and How to Overcome Them

For Lopez, the journey from dental assistant to RDH took 10 years and an earnest **tenacity** to see her goal through to the end. "I learned many life lessons throughout those years. Life does not stop just because you are busy trying to achieve a goal. I had several obstacles during school. I lost my father unexpectedly to a cerebral aneurysm. It was the hardest obstacle I had ever experienced," said Lopez, who also overcame an illness serious enough to require surgery during her final year of school. "Because of who I am and my perseverance, I knew dental hygiene was my calling," she observed.

"Graduation day was one of my proudest moments. I knew I had completed this and no one could take that away from me," Lopez concluded.

For Roitman-Trauger, a major challenge was not knowing exactly what she wanted in a full-time job. In the past, she taught in a clinical setting, provided product consulting and sales and even worked in Switzerland as a clinician.

"I enjoy people and welcome interaction," explained Roitman-Trauger, whose network of friends relayed her resume until it reached the desk of her current boss.

"I didn't think I was interested in sales, however, when I interviewed I knew this would be a position that would offer a variety of opportunity and challenge," Roitman-Trauger said. Her two-state territory offered diverse responsibilities, travel and the opportunity to train and support approximately 130 distribution sales representatives about her product line. In addition to these duties, she is responsible for educating the faculty and students of 19 dental hygiene and two dental schools in her territory as to the benefits of the diverse product line she represents.

Klose, who is Regional Director for Carolina Dental Management, cannot recall a particular moment when she decided to try management, but she does not regret accepting the challenge of the position.

"As the company grew, I felt my extensive exposure to most forms of practice management and dental systems, as well as my strong focus on patient satisfaction, would be an asset. I applied for the regional director position, which also involved staying directly involved with their dental hygienists as hygiene director," Klose shared.

"I have worked to advance my knowledge in new science, research and technology training and with that I found that there was so much I could do to add to not only dental hygiene but everything that surrounds it, too. I have combined all this acquired knowledge and personal experience to help create an inspired, effective and motivational curriculum that refines the systems surrounding the patient's total experience with a dental practice," Klose said.

Strategize a Course of Action: How You Can Achieve Career Success

DePalma noted that many clinicians feel "trapped" or experience burnout in the course of their careers.

"However, these same dental hygienists often have not had a willingness to learn something new, to step out of their **comfort zone**. We all get complacent and lazy at various times, but that complacency and laziness can lead to burnout or the trapped feeling," DePalma said. To fight this, she encouraged dental hygienists to select continuing education courses on topics with which they have no familiarity or consider changing their role entirely within dental hygiene.

"Success is measured by being able to step out of that comfort zone and experience new and innovative ideas," DePalma concluded.

Dental hygienists can stretch themselves beyond the four walls of the operatory in a number of ways that include:

The Pursuit of Continuing Education

In the practice in which Maddox works, **continuing education** requirements are triple to those annually outlined by her state. "I always feel the need to push myself more and learn more. This personality trait is perfect for the practice in which I work. New techniques, new technologies and new information drive us and make us better practitioners," said Maddox, who achieved Mastership honors with the Academy of Laser Dentistry when there were no other Master level hygienists in her state and only a very few in the world.

A particular position in DePalma's dental hygiene career path required that she continue her education beyond the bachelor's degree level. "The thought of going back to school was both a thrill and a challenge," said DePalma who pursued a Master in Education degree with a focus on adult learning. The program blended online courses with real class time.

For Klose continuing education and a passion for her profession help her continue to achieve career satisfaction. "While in college I remember someone making a statement that dental hygienists rarely stay in their field due to burnout. I refused to allow that to happen to me, there are too many exciting things about dentistry. This has been a driving factor to achieve success in this profession."

Finding Ways to Network

Most of DePalma's career roles beyond clinical hygiene have come through **networking** with dental hygiene professionals through professional associations.

"I belong to a number of professional associations and each in its own way has provided me with enormous opportunities that I would not have achieved if I had not been an active member and networked. Volunteering in various positions has exposed me to opportunities where I have learned vast knowledge which is useful for not only the association, but me as well," she advised.

"Become active in dental hygiene associations, join online discussion groups, take additional courses, all will help direct you to a mentor. Ask a trusted colleague to recommend someone or ask someone yourself. I always am willing and excited when someone asks me to mentor them," DePalma said. "Helping another professional is a wonderful way to give back to the profession of dental hygiene."

Following Your Passion

Follow your **passion**, said DePalma. "Decide what you enjoy about your current position, what you are passionate about, and what makes you feel good at the end of the day. Then seek a mentor who has experience with your passions."

Maddox agreed, adding: "I would recommend that new dental hygienists find the facets of the profession that they love, and let those fuel their fire. If it's not strictly clinical hygiene, find some other niche in the office that fuels it. Maybe there will be a need to leave clinical hygiene behind and work more in the community care settings, or administratively. Maybe someone looking for a career change would love to educate other hygienists about new technologies. If you look at the avenues, and at yourself, you can find your niche."

Implement Your Career Success Plan

Maddox noted that career success is never complete.

"I have achieved success today. Tomorrow, I must continue to strive," she explained. "I can look at my list (of accomplishments) and feel very satisfied with my successes. I have also been deemed successful by the outside world as well." In 2006, Maddox was one of five dental hygienists selected nationally for the Hygienist of the Year Award through Modern Hygienist Magazine and Discus Dental. She has been featured in two other dental hygiene magazines as a success story, and has been recognized by the Academy of Laser Dentistry.

"Those things are validating, indeed, but only to a certain extent," she admitted. "Those are moments frozen in time." What is a more dynamic and challenging way for her to monitor her feelings of success is to return to her five-point list: making a difference in patients' lives, educating patients, creating an inviting environment in the practice, using her arsenal of skills and gifts and finally avoiding burnout.

"My list is a daily, or even hourly, way to monitor my feelings of success and that is how I will measure my success. The list might change, too, as time goes on and priorities might shift. It is important to self-assess regularly to make sure I am on the track on which I want to be," she said.

Lopez concluded: "I would recommend the profession of dental hygiene to others if they were interested in contributing to improving overall health. They need to realize that they will be an educator, advocate and therapist. The beauty of our profession is also the flexibility we have to schedule our own hours and days in which we wish to work."

Professional Savvy, LLC, offers a thank you to Gail, Ann-Marie, Elizabeth, Robyn and Stephanie for being interviewed and sharing their thoughts on what career success meant to them and the key elements that encompass career success. Thank you for being a part of SAVVY SUCCESS™.

Critical Thinking Exercises

1. Write a paragraph defining career success for yourself, using the broadest possible range of goals from everyday achievements to awards to which you aspire to achieve and a description of your dream job. List the elements that will help you achieve career success (i.e., education, volunteer experiences, mentors, involvement in professional organizations, etc.) and the challenges that need to be overcome (i.e., finances, schedule, family obligations, etc.). Keep this paragraph in a convenient folder or binder for use with the critical thinking exercises found in Chapter 6.

2. Exchange career success paragraphs with a few classmates or colleagues. Note the differences between the definitions. Offer constructive observations (note: not criticism) about each other's definitions.

Key Concepts

1. Success in dental hygiene is not limited solely to monetary or award achievement. Dental hygiene professionals need to develop a broad sense of career success, from everyday success in optimizing patient care to long-range goal achievement.

2. While life circumstances may require professionals to make a decision based on convenience, long-range goal achievement requires them make purposeful decisions and not merely be guided from one position to the next by random incidents.

3. Involvement in dental hygiene's professional organizations is an important key in career success. Membership in an organization opens the door to many elements of success including: networking opportunities, continuing education, access to others who have a great passion for the profession and are willing to share that with others, and a connection point for attaining a mentor.

4. Because of the time a dental hygienist has to spend with patients, career success can be more than just attending to oral health needs. Small victories can be won in counseling a patient with systemic disease and other healthcare issues in order to improve patient compliance with oral care practices at home.

5. Dental hygienists must develop coping skills to manage the disappointment that comes with career setbacks and shortfalls and continue to develop career goals and objectives to inspire them to achieve more.

6. Dental hygienists may experience career success and job satisfaction by contributing to the team in the dental practice. Even small assistance can make a difference in the camaraderie of the team and the overall environment of the practice.

7. Securing a mentor is important to ensuring career success. This individual offers counsel, support and direction to someone who may be too entrenched in his or her daily responsibilities to have an objective view of his or her career. A mentor can be one or several family members early in the professional's or the student's life.

8. When feelings of burnout or boredom set into the professional's daily routine, he or she must re-visit the elements of career success, particularly networking with others in the field, continuing education programs or rediscovering his or her passion for dental hygiene through thoughtfully considering long-range goals.

Chapter 5: Other Career Opportunities in the Dental Hygiene Profession

By Christine A. Hovliaras, RDH, BS, MBA, CDE

Learning Objectives

The student dental hygienist and dental hygiene professional will learn the following key objectives from this chapter:

1. Identify that a variety of other positions for dental hygienists exist beyond strictly clinical work.
2. Identify the professional characteristics and responsibilities necessary to work in these positions.
3. Create a list of your own personal professional characteristics that might be a match for a more interesting and challenging position in the dental hygiene profession.
4. Develop a networking list for the type of position you are interested in pursuing and identify the person or people you could contact to learn more about this career opportunity outside of clinical practice.

Overview

Finding the right dental hygiene position may require dental hygienists to think outside the operatory walls of the dental practice in which they currently work. Those professionals who have found career satisfaction beyond clinical work take education and clinical experience and put it to use in areas that many would not have conceived 20 years ago. It is important to learn as much as possible about all opportunities of the dental hygiene profession and what it takes to succeed in each.

An inventor, a forensic dental team member, an author, an editor, an educator. Many opportunities in dental hygiene lie outside clinical work, yet begin with the same skill set that leads individuals into the profession: Organization, a strong work ethic, the ability to self-motivate, a drive to succeed and the opportunity to provide meaningful service to others. Some enterprising dental hygienists offered their advice and success stories to reveal how these areas may provide new opportunities to other dental hygienists.

"If a dental hygienist is seeking a position that is atypical for the profession, the first step is to identify personal strengths," said Michelle Panico, RDH, MA. She offered a personal inventory that the dental hygienist should assess:

- Am I a creator, implementer, starter or finisher?
- What am I passionate about?
- Do I prefer to provide direct clinical services, manage programs or plan and implement projects?
- What population do I like to work with – children, adolescents, adults, pregnant women, seniors, homebound, intercity or rural communities?

Pursuing positions that are not immediately listed in the professional roles diagram also will require the dental hygienist to expand his or her comfort zone, stated Gina Dellanina, RDH, BS, MS. An entrepreneur-inventor who graduated with a Master of Science in dental hygiene in 2000, Dellanina developed and patented the Prophy Aid, an autoclavable prophy paste holder that attaches to the small suction that simplifies and speeds up the polishing process.

As an inventor, Dellanina is the owner and product designer of the Prophy Aid. As the owner of a company, she markets and learns everything she can about how to successfully operate a business while her idea is developing into a product that is sold globally.

"I have been in this position for more than six years developing the Prophy Aid and only two years selling it," Dellanina explained. "If you become an inventor be prepared to be pushed outside your comfort zone."

JoAnn R. Gurenlian, RDH, PhD, observed that her chosen path – professional speaking – is one that is not easy for most people. In fact, it is a path that doesn't seem to suit her personal characteristics.

"I am by nature a relatively shy person. I am the one who would rather read a book quietly in a room than be the life of a party," Gurenlian commented. "But, my passion for dental hygiene topics such as oral cancer, diabetes, oral medicine, women's health, changing health disparities and improving the health of the public make me forget that I am in front of a group of people. My passion for and interest in these topics takes over, and I am launched into a discussion that makes me forget that I am the one who is speaking."

Winnie Furnari, RDH, MS, FAADH, plunged beyond most professional's comfort zones into one she knew would be a good fit for her: Forensic dental hygiene. Furnari has practiced in this fascinating field since 1989, and she observed that as a member of a forensic identification team, a dental hygienist needs no more than the license to practice.

"Our education provides us with a solid base that allows us to make new opportunities for ourselves," said Furnari. "Many dental hygienists, who practice in forensic dentistry, do expand their knowledge with formal course training and continuing education experiences."

Jammie Shaughnessy, RDH, decided to use her education in a different way and take the reins on a dental business. A business owner since September 2007, Shaughnessy sees patients sporadically throughout the week and spends the balance of the time managing all aspects of human resources for her business (hiring, firing, staffing and delegating tasks and responsibilities).

"I have always had a knack for business, dealing with people and problem solving," Shaughnessy stated. "I like to work autonomously too. So owning a practice fit more into my ideal, rather than consulting, sales or teaching. I don't like to depend on others to make things happen. So I knew I had to be 'in charge,' if you will."

Autonomy is an important factor in moving outside the professional roles grid. At an early age, Jill Rethman, RDH,

BA, and editorial director for *Dimensions® of Dental Hygiene*, realized she was a self-starter and had no fear of working on her own.

"I also realized that I had a need to look around the corner to see what else was waiting for me. I like to take risks. With each position I've held, I was able to pursue it because I didn't fear the unknown. I also have a very supportive husband who always encouraged me to reach for the stars," Rethman said. These are key factors in making a trail-blazing move successful.

One characteristic that helped Joyce Turcotte, RDH, MEd, FAADH, grow her business is a "can do" attitude. Turcotte, who described her position as a Continuing Education Entrepreneur, is owner of Professional Learning Services (PLS). PLS offers quality continuing education seminars, dental hygiene refresher courses, clinical workshops and private instruction.

"When I presented my company to others and talked about presenting programs or hiring speakers to present for PLS, I did it with confidence and a positive attitude," she explained. "I clearly have a vision of success and will make whatever needs to happen occur so that I will achieve the success I envision."

Judith Dember-Paige, RDH, turned her dental hygiene experience into storybooks. Dember-Paige's first book, *Smile Wide Look Inside, Nicole's Trip to the Dental Office,* told of a child's visit to a dental office from a dental hygienist's perspective.

"The idea was to educate children about what they may experience while at a dental office, facts about their teeth, and how to prevent tooth decay from a very early age," said Dember-Paige, who has been a dental hygienist since 1982, and practices part-time dental hygiene with Dr. Robert Amsterdam.

"I love my job," said Pamela J. Myers, RDH, who has been licensed since 1974, and has worked in the Texas Department of Criminal Justice (TDCJ) since 1985. While she was the first to say that dental hygiene practice in a state prison is not for everyone, she added: "I get to practice dental hygiene like I was taught. The patient is important, not the dollar. I am not tied to a rigid schedule. If one patient requires more time than another than that is what is done. I don't have to be concerned about insurance or other 'business' aspects of private practice."

Is a career role outside the norm for everyone?

"It is incredible to look back and realize where you started and what you have learned along the way," Dellanina concluded. "You have experiences that most Americans only dream about. One thing I have learned is that you don't have time to think, 'I can't.' You just do what you have to do."

A Day in the Life

It can be hard to imagine work life outside the operatory. However, many of the same skills are used regardless of the environment in which dental hygienists practice.

A typical day for Myers begins at 5:00 a.m. in the clinic at the state prison. She schedules patients in groups of two or three "as I may not receive one every 45 minutes to an hour due to security."

She explained that a count of all offenders is done every couple of hours throughout the day and at night to ensure that no escapes have occurred. During the count process, no offenders may move from their current location; offenders already in the infirmary, where Myers practices, must stay and no others may enter.

"I don't provide care to more than one at a time, but I must have multiple patients waiting in order to have a steady flow," Myers continued. She provides patient care for four different facilities. She also oversees the preventive program for the University of Texas Medical Branch – Correctional Managed Care (UTMB-CMC) in more than 100 different clinics scattered in the eastern two-thirds of the state of Texas.

"My practice has over 125,000 patients – it's the size of a city!" she stated. Myers coordinates all of the dental staff continuing education programs and designs online courses for staff. She has written statewide policy for dental services.

In forensic work, the scenario may be different each time. It has become standard procedure to get training in formal courses in forensic dentistry before applying for a position on a team. Furnari observes it more in urban areas where many more people want to do forensic dentistry.

"Volunteer dental hygienists should be available at any time of day. They should expect no compensation. There will be times when a medical examiner's budget will allow compensation for the work the dental identification team performs. This is welcomed but should not be expected," Furnari continued.

Furnari observed that in addition to local and state societies that serve a medical examiner in times of disaster, the United States Government has a federally funded organization that offers a formal team position. A dental hygienist may apply to become a member of a Disaster Mortuary Response Team (D-Mort). Professionals can apply to the region of the country in which they reside. There are many pages of the application and thorough background checks are made.

"Members of D-Mort may be dispatched to any area within the U.S. and to other countries where U.S. assistance is requested. Members are usually dispatched or activated for two weeks at a time and are paid a small stipend along with travel reimbursement. During this activation they are temporary Federal employees but work under the guidance of the local authorities. Members of D-Mort can be activated according to the skills, education and training they possess. They would be utilized according to people's needs after the disaster and their expertise. Dental hygienists would be called upon to assist in all aspects of identification, comparable to and recording antemortem and postmortem records, exposing radiographs, accurate documentation and other administrative duties."

"This involves formal training each year," she explained.

"I have become acquainted with many dentists and dental hygienists who practice Forensic Dentistry via the D-Mort program, and they find this is a pathway for them," said Furnari.

The U.S. Public Health Service (USPHS) is one of the uniformed services and a part of the Department of Health and Human Services, Furnari explained. In peacetime disasters the USPHS augments the nation's response capability, and it assists state and local authorities in dealing with disaster impacts.

Panico, a dental hygienist since 2000, has been an affiliated practice school-based dental hygienist since 2006, working with Head Start, Dignity Health and elementary schools. Her current position is as a contract employee for Dignity Health Chandler Regional Medical Center working at San Marcos Elementary School and Galveston Elementary Schools in Chandler, Arizona.

When dental hygienists determine their personal strengths, passions and preferred patient population, Panico explained about this type of work, they should demonstrate how oral health is important for the population and how their work to improve oral health would benefit partner organizations.

"For example, in the population (school children) and organizations (elementary school and a local hospital) I work with, the children with improved oral health have better general health, less distraction of pain, improved ability to eat, less visits to the hospital emergency room for oral concerns, fewer missed days of school and higher performance in school. The result is higher student test scores, more funding for the school, and less cost for the hospital as they treat fewer dental infections in the emergency room," Panico stated.

She said it also can be helpful to network through other professional associations. Becoming a member of other professional associations such as a teacher, nurse, public health or school-based clinic associations can open opportunities and an understanding of the needs of those professional groups that the dental hygienist could address.

For Shaughnessy, as a business owner, the day is consumed with a mix of dental hygiene and business operations. As mentioned before, she occasionally sees patients, but primarily manages all aspects of the business, from human resources to treatment follow up, the implementation of new policies and ideas, staff meetings and accounting, payroll and marketing.

Shaughnessy also oversees the recall system and patient relations maintenance, while she also functions as a peace keeper, manages the website with a web designer and works with the dentist to meet his needs and help him in any way to carry out his work. She manages the purchase and repair of new and existing dental equipment and computers.

The work day is not that different in a veterinary practice than in a human practice, observes Linda K. Bohacek, RDH, MA, CDHC, FAADH, who works as a clinical dental hygienist at Oakwood Hills Animal Hospital in Eau Claire, Wisconsin. She is quick to point out the differences, too.

"Beyond clinical hygiene, my responsibilities include the development of educational materials for patients, designing dental charts and dental instruments, maintaining dental equipment and inventory of dental supplies, providing dental education for staff, consulting on dental hygiene protocols and overseeing patient recare," Bohacek reported.

As one might expect, Panico, in her position as an affiliated practice elementary school dental hygienist, provides full preventive dental services (radiographs, oral evaluations, prophylaxis, dental sealants and fluoride treatment) to uninsured, underinsured and underserved children from birth through 18 years of age living in Phoenix's East Valley suburban communities.

Dellanina shared that those who invent products frequently attend conventions to market the product, make calls to businesses or dental supply companies to sell the product and need to develop a user-friendly website to support online sales. Inventors answer calls, take orders, visit local hygiene schools and send out information to local dentists and dental hygienists about the invention.

"If you are a hygienist looking at becoming an inventor," Dellanina commented, "you must believe in what you are creating or it will never sell."

This might also be said of creating and selling yourself in a new career position!

As an editorial director, Rethman's day involves several aspects of the publication for which she works. Collaborating with other editors, she plans the editorial calendar each year.

"We develop concepts for each issue, determine topics of interest for our readers and identify qualified authors," Rethman stated. "I also review articles when they are submitted to see if they are a good fit for our scope and mission, and then recommend if they should undergo peer-review. Since all of our feature and continuing education articles are peer-reviewed, this is a process that is very important to us. We have an excellent editorial advisory board and group of reviewers who ensure our articles are accurate and top-notch."

Rethman also has an opportunity to write for Dimensions® of Dental Hygiene.

"In each issue, I write either an 'Editor's Memo' or a column called 'Tips on Technique,'" she explained. In addition to the writing and article reviews, she travels to many of the major dental conventions to work with the publication's editorial and sales teams.

Turcotte also gathers trends and needs in the profession. As the decision maker for all programs selected, advertised and promoted for Professional Learning Services (PLS), Turcotte described it as her passion and responsibility to keep abreast of the professional needs of dental hygienists.

PLS offers dental offices and healthcare facilities training in CPR, infection control, medical emergencies and clinical remediation and advanced techniques to meet the facility's needs. PLS also offers training in professional presentation skills to dental professionals, corporations for sales training and educators for faculty workshops.

"These areas have been developed due to the unique specialties that I have and therefore offer," said Turcotte. "I do this through examining trends, consulting with the PLS professional advisory board, connecting and communicating with key opinion leaders, academic and corporate affiliations and reviewing all audience evaluations on a regular basis. I also review articles and website for ideas and information."

Professional Characteristics that Equal Success

In the first few chapters, the characteristics needed for success as a dental hygienist were carefully described. In Chapter 2, "Professional Roles," experts in the profession explained the characteristics needed to succeed in other, more traditional areas of the dental hygiene field. Chapter 5 will explore what is necessary for working outside the operatory in less traditional areas of oral health.

Dember-Paige cited some of her own characteristics that have helped her and would help others pursuing something not found in traditional dental hygiene textbooks, including:

- A genuine care for others;
- A positive attitude even when the current situations is not;
- Maintaining that perfectionist style of personality without being obsessive; and
- A high attention to detail.

In this section of Chapter 5, we will explore four over-arching professional characteristics that employ these personal traits to work toward career success and satisfaction. These characteristics are:

1. **Passion and Problem Solving:** Developing a typical career path into a passionate cause and problem-solving the way to achievement.
2. **Fortitude:** Withstanding the tests delivered by those who either don't see a purpose for a new position, challenge the dental hygienist to defend it or openly oppose it. Fortitude also encompasses the daily grind of doing something that no one else – or few others – has undertaken.
3. **Creating and Maintaining a Long-Term Plan:** No career plan can survive on passion alone. Creative planning is required to ensure that goals are met and a vision for work is established.
4. **A Love for Life-Long Learning:** To support what professionals do in any field, they must be a constant student of the literature.

1. Passion & Problem-Solving

Becoming an inventor, according to Dellanina, required passion and problem solving skills.

"I love working with people and helping them improve their health. I want to make a positive difference in others' lives. I have a strong desire to do things efficiently and tend to get frustrated with inefficiencies," she continued, describing herself as driven, persistent, self-motivated and self-reliant.

The business world is a natural area for problem solvers, according to Shaughnessy.

"In order for dental hygienists to open a practice, they must do a lot of problem solving/research at first," she explained. First, clinicians must determine if the state in which they practice will allow them to own a dental practice.

"I went in as a business owner; not a dental hygienist. California posed too much red tape to achieve this, hence, I moved to Arizona to get my practice," Shaughnessy continued.

Myers, a self-described eternal optimist, is also very analytical. In addition, she is a born leader, quiet and reserved. Above all, she said, if anyone had asked her about practicing dental hygiene in a prison setting, she would have said "no."

"I don't think any RDH has a burning desire to work with convicted felons upon graduation, but I would encourage students to consider the rewarding career path my life has taken," she commented, describing corrections work as a career in which "you can truly make a difference." She further described correctional dental hygiene as a career with stability, regular hours and great benefits.

2. Fortitude

"It takes years to establish a label/name brand, and patience and perseverance is required to go forward," Turcotte said. "There will always be setbacks, but you know if you're cut out for this if you develop tough skin, don't let obstacles be barriers but have them be inspiration and allow opportunities for creative thinking and problem solving. Sometimes your competition could be your allies and be mutually beneficial, depending on what services are offered and in what territory."

Much as with corporate time schedules, discussed in Chapter 2, Dellanina shared that the inventor's work day is far different from the clinician's regulated timetable. She described a schedule that includes starting earlier in the morning for businesses located on the East Coast and staying up later to find time to write emails, stuff envelopes with brochures and samples or just fill orders. She added that this is a departure from clinical hygienist work that is done when the professional leaves the office.

"Not so when you are an inventor. An inventor has to have a 'Just Do It' attitude. Honestly, the hard work and long hours an inventor puts in will eventually pay off. You have to take risks if you want the rewards," she related. "There isn't any guarantee of steady income like you have in dental hygiene, but the reward and possibilities are exhilarating," Dellanina said.

The business of inventors and entrepreneurs is not for the weak or shy. People suited for this business are typically confident, passionate, persistent, do not take "no" for an answer and like to problem solve, according to Dellanina.

"A few things to realize if choosing this road: You need thick skin," Shaughnessy said. "You cannot let all the little details weigh you down. You cannot be prone to taking things personally and you need to have a good business sense. You always need to be caring and compassionate at the same time, because the patient is always No. 1."

Next, Shaughnessy said to consider the stress. "It is very stressful at first. Many people will tell you it cannot be done. You have to ignore them, but of course you need a good solid business plan that makes sense financially as well. Then you can ignore all the naysayers. One also needs good solid financial backing," she said.

Turcotte noted that the person who is best suited for the entrepreneurial life is one who is a self-starter and motivator. In her own business, Turcotte determines each day what she needs to do to move the business forward.

"I consult with members of my advisory board as needed, but each day, I am in charge of my schedule ... sometimes that means a 60-hour work week, and sometimes that means a 20-hour work week. It offers a high degree of flexibility," she said, adding that her husband's job offers their family a steady income and health benefits that give her position a higher degree of flexibility and savings.

"I also had good support for childcare when I traveled on overnight trips. If I were single, I still would have made the choice of owning my own business because of my independent personality; however, I would have had to make compromises that I may not have had under my circumstances," Turcotte stated.

Gurenlian listed her personal strengths of persistence, honesty, hard work, fair balance and a sense of humor as good characteristics for public speakers.

"I doubt very much that we could live life well without a sense of humor. So, even while speaking, I will find myself laughing at myself. I try not to make too many mistakes during a presentation, but it does happen," she said.

Gurenlian shared a story about a struggle she had with a remote device during one of her presentations.

"I kept either advancing the slides too fast or somehow going backwards. It was very frustrating, but I handled it by making a joke. If you can poke fun at yourself, the audience is usually forgiving of your blunders," Gurenlian explained. She added that honesty is the best policy.

"Invariably, someone will ask a question, and I don't know the answer," she said. "Rather than make something up to try to sound good, I simply say that I don't know and will research the answer. People know when you are faking it and that destroys credibility."

Rethman explained that if a dental hygienist has an interest in a similar career path, he or she should keep an open mind.

"Don't be afraid to step out of your comfort zone," she advised. "Take small steps toward a direction that might be interesting to you (such as writing, speaking, working in the dental industry) and build a foundation. We don't know what the future holds and the next opportunity may present itself in ways you never imagined."

Myers echoed this sentiment. While she has never felt unsafe, threatened or insecure, she noted that the professional setting in the prison's dental operatory is not for everyone.

"If you are 'faint of heart,' it probably is not for you. I work with convicted felons. That means murderers, rapists, robbers and pretty much all of those human beings that society would like to forget. However, it is never boring and every day is a new adventure."

3. Creating and Maintaining a Long-Term Plan

Gurenlian stated that if dental hygienists are seeking a position that is not typical for the profession, look for a course on owning a small business and learn about managing finances, creating contracts for their work, setting goals and a fee schedule and obtaining equipment that will enable them to do their job. It is also important to identify specialists to help entrepreneurial professionals succeed. These specialists might include audiovisual experts, financial planners or accountants.

Turcotte said that in order to become a continuing education entrepreneur, professionals must first establish credibility within their target marketplace. It is also important, she added, to have a professional connection with the state and local dental hygiene association.

"The first place to start is to do a feasibility study to determine if there is a need for this business locally, regionally or nationally," Turcotte said. "Find out who already offers courses in your area, what are the loyalties (i.e., alumni, membership, etc.), what are strategic locations, what is the interest in topics and speakers and what price will the market pay." It is also important to determine who the market is and what the competition looks like. Turcotte advised aspiring entrepreneurs to explore their strengths and talents to determine their uniqueness in the marketplace.

It is important, too, for the potential business owners and dental hygienists with a lot of autonomy in their practice to have a long-term plan.

"How will you get the dentist to stay and work hard?" Shaughnessy questioned. "After all you need the dentist there! In order to overcome this, currently, I am moving into a possible partnership for the dentist to eventually be part owner. This is an inevitable step in my case if I want to have security with the dentist. We also are planning to purchase the real estate involved in order to make this a wise, long-term investment as well. I eventually would like to use this model to open more practices in the near future, with my dentist partner."

Myers developed the preventive program for the UTMB-CMC in 1986. At that time, she explained, the TDCJ was under federal court monitorship, and her program had to be reviewed by the deans of the three dental schools in the state of Texas.

"The deans agreed that my plan was an ideal program, but commented that it would never work. The words 'never' and 'can't' are simply not in my vocabulary," Myers said. "Our periodontal program not only has been successful, but has been recognized by the American Dental Association (ADA) and the departments of corrections in other states."

4. A Love for Life-Long Learning

Continuing education is an important factor for Bohacek. She explained that many states allow veterinary assistants with on-the-job training to provide basic dental hygiene services in the field of veterinary medicine. In addition, certified veterinary technicians are allowed to provide enhanced dental hygiene services and in some cases, tooth extractions.

"Personally, although I was overqualified as a dental hygienist, I was under-qualified as a veterinary assistant or veterinary technician," Bohacek observed. Building on her education as a dental hygienist, she "enrolled in animal behavior courses, then attended veterinary conferences and signed up for every continuing education course possible in the area of veterinary dentistry."

Dember-Paige loves to attend continuing education seminars to meet other dental hygienists, explore networking opportunities and develop mentoring relationships. "Talking to other dental hygienists helped me to discover outlets to some of the inner frustrations I had," she related. "Many of my progressive ideas came out of hearing a presentation or having an encouraging conversation with someone who could relate to my experiences."

Gurenlian's planned career path includes learning and teaching for the rest of her life.

"I truly enjoy dental hygiene and health-related topics," she concluded. "It is natural for me to keep reading and learning. I regularly purchase new text books and subscribe to scientific journals. They are as interesting to me as a mystery or romance novel."

Further Advice for the Adventurous

The wonderful aspect of practicing dental hygiene today is that many pioneers already have taken "the road less traveled" as Rethman quoted from the Robert Frost poem. Those trail-blazers are more than willing to share advice that has helped them to succeed.

One aspect that all of the contributors in this chapter agreed on is that although dental hygiene professionals might get into an allied position without an advanced degree (such as a bachelor's, master's, doctorate), those credentials do help ensure one thing necessary to success: credibility. As each succeeding generation moves into the work force, more often than not a four-year college degree, advance training or graduate work does offer a stamp of approval on pursuits and ambitions in the healthcare profession.

Rethman stated that while there was not a specific degree requirement for the various positions she has held, most recently in dental hygiene editorial, she knows that her education at Ohio State University was a necessary and fundamental foundation.

"I also know that a bachelor's or master's degree can give someone that extra level of credibility to have certain opportunities within dental hygiene," Rethman added. At minimum, she continued, a bachelor's degree can provide the educational level to follow a career path similar to her own. "The combination of experience and education, however, are unbeatable," Rethman said.

Another position that may not require an advanced degree would be an education entrepreneur. Turcotte noted, however, her academic background, experience and credibility to evaluate educational programs made this course a good fit for her.

"As an educator, I designed and implemented educational seminars and retraining programs. These unique topics and niches in the market place drew attention to the business and services offered," Turcotte said. For example, for 15 years, PLS offered education-vacation packages that increased its national exposure with a focus on dental hygiene audiences.

"What also had a significant impact on being a leader in continuing education are the years of volunteer service, including president of the state dental hygiene association and a national academy. These experiences led to recognition and awards by my peers further enhancing my credibility," Turcotte continued. When considering lecturers to speak on various topics, Turcotte takes into account: credentials, experience, research and teaching qualifications, special skills that all play a role in the selection process.

While professional speakers may not need an advanced degree, Gurenlian said, "I believe that an advanced degree lends additional credibility as a speaker, which is why my company requires a minimum of a baccalaureate degree to be an associate," Gurenlian commented. She added that it is imperative that the public speaker has excellent presentation and research skills. In addition, it is important to develop an area of expertise.

"Pick something that interests you and study the information that is available," she advised. "You must develop a command of the topic and update it regularly. Test the design of the program by volunteering to speak at a local component or study club. That gives you the opportunity to refine your content and speaking techniques. Once the topic is well developed, you can market it to other associations and organizations."

Gurenlian suggested that if dental hygienists like a challenge, travel and giving all their energy and expertise to an audience, public speaking is a great career choice.

"However, it does tend to sound more glamorous than it is," she cautioned. "Think of the travel to all those wonderful places. The reality is that I often fly to a site, spending more hours in the airport than the time it takes to get to the meeting location, sleep in a room that is foreign to me, and fly home either the same or next day. It sounds impressive to travel, but I never really get to see anything other than a hotel room and the airport! I could take a few extra days to experience my surroundings, but that would mean giving up time with my family. So there are trade offs. Of course, when going to certain places, like Australia, my husband and/or children will join me and that is delightful."

Gurenlian advised those who are considering a career as a professional speaker to think carefully about how to approach this choice:

- Will this become full-time work or a part-time initiative? How should aspiring public speakers market their presentations?
- Are they willing to make changes based on audience feedback and not take things personally?
- Are they willing to take on the work challenge involved in thoroughly knowing the subject matter?

"If you just want to present fluff, you may find that your career is somewhat short," Gurenlian observed. "If you are willing to provide substance, you will have longevity in this career."

While an advanced degree was not required for Myers position with the department of criminal justice, she believed that a higher educational level would be required in the future. She anticipated that along with the degree will be a need for a minimum of five years full-time experience in correctional dental hygiene.

"I strongly believe that the proposed Advanced Dental Hygiene Practitioner (ADHP) will become reality in the future and would work so well in a correctional setting," said Myers, encouraging others to pursue advanced educational opportunities.

Furnari recommended a formally recognized course of study for those interested in forensics, whether the dental hygienist lives in an urban or rural area.

"This usually involves five – to seven-day intensive training that includes lectures and laboratory exercises. At this time, forensic dentistry is not a viable option for a 9-to-5 position. It may be some day, and I sincerely hope it will," Furnari said, explaining that those who choose to serve, serve mainly as volunteers.

Being an inventor and launching a new product requires networking, according to Dellanina.

She advised aspiring inventors to become more involved with dental hygiene associations to give their name and product more recognition. Dellanina also recommended that aspiring inventors work for a dental supply company to see how they sell dental products, or even consider hiring someone to market the product.

"The best advice I can give to those interested in becoming an inventor is to have some marketing skills or have someone you know that could help you with a marketing plan. Marketing your invention correctly improves your chances for success," said Dellanina. "Take advantage of your strengths and possibly hire out your weaknesses. Hire a bookkeeper if you are not good with numbers," she continued.

Making wise choices when it comes to money is extremely important to those new in business. Dellanina recommended some savvy business negotiations and exchanges between business people. Work with attorneys, manufacturers, magazines advertisers and others to find compromises that benefit both professionals.

"Remember, everything in life is negotiable," said Dellanina. "Give and take is OK. Be creative when it comes to having someone do work for you. Possibly offer to advertise them on your website in exchange for a reduced fee." In positions such as Panico's affiliated practice position, it is required to have not only a solid dental hygiene education, but also to practice and be accredited in a state that permits dental hygienists to expand their practice without direct supervision by a dentist. Her position requires an Associate of Applied Science degree, Arizona Registered Dental Hygiene license and an Affiliation Agreement.

"While this position does not require an advanced degree, the Arizona state law and Arizona Board of Dental Examiners' requires an Affiliation Agreement be completed by the affiliated dentist and dental hygienist," explained Panico. "Though an advanced degree is not required, the knowledge I gained from completing my master's degree has allowed me to be a significant contributor in the planning and assessment of the school-based affiliated practice dental clinic, CHW East Valley Children's Dental Clinic."

Panico recommended Affiliated Practice or other alternative practice positions to those interested in a career change, but not to those new to dental hygiene.

"In my opinion, it is best to obtain experience in a traditional setting first to hone your clinical skills in efficiency and patient management," she concluded. "Then you can apply these mastered skills in non-traditional settings."

Shaughnessy stated that her work as a business owner does require a degree.

"One would not technically need a degree to own a practice, but I do not see how any one person could run a business with no experience in dentistry or college. In my opinion, earning a degree, any degree, is basically a test of person's stamina and critical thinking skills. The path to a degree prepares the person to solve problems. If you do not have problem-solving abilities, whether it is a degree that prepares you for it or just plain old life experience, then that person could never run a dental practice or be a dental hygienist for that matter," Shaughnessy said.

Dember-Paige also commented that authorship does not require many degree credentials, "although it doesn't hurt," she added. What she does recommend is that dental hygienists and aspiring authors alike discover a passion in the field.

"I have had the opportunity to work in most specialties in dentistry. It is how I discovered that pediatric dentistry is my favorite. If there is an area that you want to know more about, consider spending some time working in that area of specialty. For example, observing during an implant surgery or assisting during a root canal. Find an area that you love and keep building on your learning," Dember-Paige stated. She also recommended that dental hygienists balance professional and personal life. "Working hard and playing hard will bring years of personal satisfaction and happiness," she concluded.

"It's important to keep positive people around you," Dellanina said. "There is no problem hearing the truth and being open to constructive criticism. With that said, occasionally you will come in contact with people who may not be fans of your success or efforts. Therefore, go around individuals who can be negative road blocks!"

The Importance of Mentors in Career Opportunities

Mentors, as was discussed in Chapter 3, provide that important reference point in any career. However, when a dental hygienist expands the career horizon and moves into an area where few are practicing, having a mentor is critical for a number of reasons.

To expand practice, dental hygienists may need the mentorship of policy makers in the profession. To create a new role outside the traditional diagram, they may need the mentorship of others in the healthcare profession. To build a business that is allied to the dental hygiene profession, career planners may need the mentorship of someone from the corporate or business arena. There are a variety of reasons that seeking outside help is essential. Another reason is validation: The aspiring professional may need the morale boost to overcome naysayers.

Turcotte credited her mentor as the inspiration for starting her own business – her mentor was the one to actually propose the idea.

"She provided her dental knowledge, wisdom, market sensitivity, business and political connections and unlimited guidance," Turcotte explained. "We started out in a student-teacher relationship in the 1970s and became teaching colleagues from 1981 to 2003 when she passed away. She was the one person I could call for advice anytime, and I could trust her intuition. I also have several other friends in dental hygiene that provided unlimited support and guidance from their professional experiences. Ultimately, you make your own decisions, but it is important to surround yourself with trusting and loyal friends and colleagues within and outside of dentistry to help maintain balance and perspective."

Rethman commented that other dental hygienists who have roles outside of clinical practice can be very helpful.

"I had several mentors early on who gave me guidance," she said. "Without their help I would not have achieved what I have today."

Dember-Paige said that she has enjoyed the privilege of having many mentors, not just one.

"When attending professional conferences, locally as well as nationally, I would go there with the mindset to meet other dental hygienists," she explained. Virtually everyone she approached to ask for help was willing to lend assistance without taking credit for Dember-Paige's work.

"I would look for people who had accomplished what I was looking to do, and exchange business cards with them to keep in touch. Many times I was at a crossroads not knowing what direction to take when after having a good conversation with a mentor, the path became clearer," Dember-Paige described. "Venturing outside your comfort zone may be scary, but it is the first step toward opening the door to many new opportunities."

During an all-day continuing education course on forensic dentistry, Furnari learned of a local forensics group. Driven by the desire to make a difference in a place that most people would go out of their way to avoid, Furnari joined the group.

"The dentists in the local group welcomed me and saw that month after month I attended every meeting and course they offered. Each of these dentists became my mentor and continue to this day to be both mentors and friends," she commented.

"My display of interest and commitment prompted them to call me in to help with a plane crash in 1992. My participation in this disaster secured my appointment to the NYC Chief Medical Examiner's Forensic Dental Identification Team," Furnari continued.

Bohacek took a similar approach in building mentors and contacts in her unique field. A flyer from the annual Veterinary Dental Forum, a conference devoted solely to issues related to veterinary dentistry, led her to many researchers and board certified veterinary dentists from all over the world.

"I met three other dental hygienists at this conference," Bohacek shared. One dental hygienist was employed at a university in the research department where she provided dental hygiene services to beagle dogs participating in research studies. Another dental hygienist worked with a veterinary supply company and was developing dental instruments and oral health products for pets. The third dental hygienist also went through schooling to become a certified veterinary technician and was practicing in a veterinary practice.

"As there were so few of us in veterinary medicine, we three dental hygienists became colleagues and mentors," Bohacek continued. Her most valued mentoring came from the veterinarians and the certified veterinary technicians with whom she practiced.

"Thank goodness for their patience and devotion to caring for those who cannot speak for themselves," she observed.

Panico found a similar situation when she began affiliated practice. At first, there were only three affiliated dental hygienists working in Arizona when she began practicing.

"Since my colleague, Lynnette Martin, RDH, and I were the second and third Affiliated Practice Dental Hygienists in Arizona, we had to be intentional about establishing mentors," she explained. The mentors they sought out included Sharon Heuer, MS, MEd, RDH, RD, and Micki Banks, RDH, developers of the first Arizona affiliated practice dental clinic in an elementary school, and Cindy Klienman, CDA, RDH, BS, developer of a hospital-based intensive care unit oral health program.

"We also sought mentorship with Kneka Smith, RDH, MPH, the past Chief Officer of the Arizona Office of Oral Health and a contributor to the development of the Affiliated Practice Relationship law, and Marge Reveal, RDH, MBA, who encouraged me to continue my advanced education," Panico continued.

"I have been lucky enough to have many mentors that have guided me down the path of becoming an inventor. My dad was my first, encouraging and supporting me with words of wisdom from his 50 years of entrepreneurship," said Dellanina.

Dellanina appreciated the help of her friend, employer and mentor, Dr. Rena Vakay, a dentist in Alexandria, VA. Working with her has been an education in itself.

"I became more articulate; she pushed me to grow professionally and personally. She took the time to show me my potential and took me outside my comfort zone. She encouraged creativity which helped build my confidence as an inventor. She taught me to trust myself, my judgment and that there are more ways than one to do things. That experience helped me years later as an inventor," shared Dellanina, who also appreciated the help of mentor Jackie Fried, RDH, MS, her thesis advisor at the University of Maryland, at Baltimore.

"She too took the time and effort to support my creative efforts and brought out my persistent and tough side," Dellanina said. She also named Vonda Manley, RDH, MS, as one of her most recent mentors and inspirations. Manley was the original patent holder for the Edge-Ease X-Ray cushion product line.

"She is a brilliant, humble, down-to-earth woman with a huge success story behind her company, Strong Dental Products, Inc., which was acquired by Crosstex International in 2007," said Dellanina. "As an inventor, there is nothing she hasn't done. She has taken me under her wing and supported my efforts by sharing her knowledge and experience, which has been invaluable! My mentors have been an inspiration to me in so many different aspects that I hope I can help others in the same way."

While Gurenlian did not have one particular mentor to help her develop her business, she did have plenty of encouragement and friends who used a word-of-mouth approach to help her market her courses.

"To this date, my preference is to use word-of-mouth versus a refined business plan, as it helps me maintain a balance between work and family. If I did not pay attention to this aspect, I would be working constantly and never having time with my family," Gurenlian commented.

Career Satisfaction

Is it easy to achieve career satisfaction in an unusual area of the profession? Absolutely, said those who have the experience. The passion to create a path for others is one of the most satisfying aspects of working in a new area.

"I have achieved career satisfaction as an inventor because I know my product, the Prophy Aid, has helped thousands of dental professional inside and outside the U.S.," said Dellanina. "By taking the time to problem solve, I not only solved my own problem, I solved a problem for thousands of others like me. The internal reward is wonderful and will eventually be financially rewarding."

As a forensic hygienist, Furnari observed that she has achieved yet another level of satisfaction with her career choices. Ten of her more than 23 years as a dental hygienist have been as a dental hygiene educator. She also has some experience as administrator and researcher in her career. These professional roles lie in the parameters of the traditional dental hygiene professional.

"Forensic hygienist is a unique avenue that is truly outside the traditional paths and has brought further advancement to my dental hygiene career. It has offered me an opportunity for both professional and personal growth. It allows me to take on new challenges wherein the success is most rewarding," said Furnari.

Panico valued that her career option in affiliated practice dental hygiene offered her autonomy, deep appreciation from patients, a sense of fulfillment from integration in the community, and challenge and change that develops the mind to "think outside of the box." She added that a dental hygienist who has passion for public health, community dentistry and primary prevention is best suited for this career option.

Admitting to the emotional ups and downs of her own unique role in dental hygiene, Bohacek immediately stated that those pale in comparison to the gratification received through helping pets lead healthy lives.

"As only 1% of pet owners provide daily mouth care, dental disease is the most common disease in pets. To be an integral part in providing such a valued service to pets is very rewarding," Bohacek concluded.

Dember-Paige highly endorsed authorship. "Being an author of a book is a great compliment to what you are already doing. It gives you credibility as an expert in your area. Anyone can write a book based on his or her own experience," she commented. She concluded: "Writing a book automatically puts you in a position to be a mentor. Most people will look to you with admiration. It is up to you to show humility and choose to help them reach their goals as well."

Career satisfaction for Gurenlian comes every time she stands in front of a room and delivers a great presentation.

"I can see the light bulbs go off in participants' minds," she said, "and if I have made one person think about adding another dimension to their professional practice that will improve the health of the public, I have done my job."

"Little did I know when I graduated from Ohio State I would be doing what I'm doing today," remarked Rethman. "I never conceived that I would have the opportunity to write, speak, travel and meet such wonderful colleagues around the world. But the important point is that while I never imagined such things were attainable as a new dental hygiene graduate, I never closed my mind to the possibilities."

"The main satisfaction I have achieved with this area of dentistry is all the aspects of success that have followed," Shaughnessy concluded. She explained that she is very happy now.

"I do not stress about the future and wonder if I will ever make it through another day of dental hygiene. I know I have an investment for my retirement. I make more money now. I have an opportunity for new and exciting ventures in the near future. Every day is different, but I will always be a dental hygienist, no matter how I use it."

Critical Thinking Exercises

1. Use the in-depth information from this chapter to develop a list of potential opportunities you may be interested in pursuing in the dental hygiene profession.

2. Prioritize the list of opportunities and determine if further education, training, continuing education courses, communication, time management, management, presentation or other skills will need to be developed to pursue the top two priority career opportunities.

3. Identify key networking contacts who could be identified to speak to in order to pursue this avenue in dental hygiene.

Key Concepts

1. Pursuing positions that are not immediately listed in the professional roles diagram also will require the dental hygienist to expand his or her comfort zone.

2. It is important to recognize which dental hygiene skills translate well into new positions and utilize those skills to the best of one's ability to support the new role.

3. Some positions outside the professional roles diagram are not easy for most people and may require other skills and additional education beyond what is acquired in dental hygiene school.

4. Autonomy and problem-solving skills are important factors in moving outside the professional roles grid.

5. Capturing unique ideas and packaging those ideas in a marketable way are key to success in roles that fall outside the typical dental hygiene positions.

6. Knowing when to partner with other professionals in and outside the oral healthcare field is another important part of succeeding in unusual career opportunities.

7. When a dental hygienist determines what his or her personal strengths, passions and preferred patient population are, he or she should demonstrate how oral health is important for the population and how improved oral health would benefit partner organizations.

8. Networking through other professional associations or becoming a member of other professional associations such as a teacher, nurse, public health or school-based clinic associations can open opportunities and an understanding of the needs of those professional groups that the dental hygienist could address.

9. Four over-arching professional characteristics that ensure the success of the dental hygienist who moves into another career path include: passion and problem-solving; fortitude; creating and maintaining a long-term plan; and possessing a love for life-long learning.

10. Advanced degrees will be required for moving into a position in education, research or a corporate environment to assist in providing the necessary knowledge and skills for success.

11. Mentors provide an important reference point for a dental hygienist who is expanding his or her career plan and moving into an area where few are practicing.

12. To expand into other areas of the profession, a dental hygienist may need the mentorship of policy makers in the profession, professionals outside of the dental profession, but still in health care, or someone from the corporate or business arena.

Chapter 5: Personal Perspectives

"Why not ME?"
My Career as an Inventor
Gina Dellanina, RDH, BS, MS

Founder of Bubble Gum Smiles and owner of the Prophy Aid

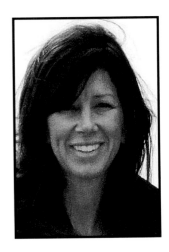

Figure 5.1. Gina Dellanina

I did not have any experience in product development prior to creating the Prophy Aid®. I have always been a problem solver and love to work with my hands. Years ago, I read a wonderful book given to me by my dad, an entrepreneur himself, about how an entrepreneur's mind works. It basically said any time you get frustrated with something and a problem arises, you have to see that as an opportunity to problem solve. That is the difference between inventor minds and those that are not inventors. The entrepreneur or inventor sees a problem as an opportunity, not a problem.

The idea of the Prophy Aid® came to me after about 10 years of practicing dental hygiene. I became very frustrated with the polishing part of the dental hygiene appointment. My time was limited at the end of the appointments, my patient's were pooling with saliva and would need to rinse. I would have to stop polishing to suction. Reaching for the small suction during the polishing process took time away from polishing and caused continual fatigue in my back. The prophy paste was constantly popping out of the metal ring and there was splatter occurring. I knew there had to be a better way to polish.

Eventually I was holding the prophy paste in the blue prophy paste holder and the suction at the same time so I could polish, suction and retract at the same time. That is when I thought there has to be a better way. Then I thought, "Why not ME?" Why can't I develop something to solve my problem? If I have a problem with polishing, I bet other dental hygienists probably get just as frustrated as I do. Maybe the patients will be happier with a new method, too. That is how the Prophy Aid® started.

Some experiences truly helped me achieve success as an inventor. For example, I received my Master in Dental Hygiene degree at the University of Maryland, in Baltimore, in 2000. While an advanced degree was not required for my work as a clinical dental hygienist or inventor, the experience of developing my thesis for my master's degree helped me grow personally and professionally. I worked extremely hard on something I believed in. I was out of my comfort zone. Therefore, defending my thesis was a moment I will never forget.

I now know I can do anything I set my mind to. That did not come easily. I understand now that taking dental hygiene boards in several different states, getting a master's degree, etc., pushed me to develop personally and do things I never thought I could accomplish. Now looking back, I can see my career as an inventor slowly developing, but it was never my intention.

Some steps dental hygienists should think about if they would like to become an inventor include paying attention to what frustrates them and following a plan something such as this:

1. Identify a problem.
2. Find a solution to the problem.
3. Sketch out what the invention might look like.
4. Make a rough working model to see if it works (called a "prototype").
5. Start taking notes in pen and document dates as you develop your invention (i.e., the date you came up the idea, the date you sketched it, etc).
6. Go the U.S. Patent and Trademark Office (USPTO) on the Internet. Decide if you want to file a provisional patent or a utility patent. A provisional patent *protects your idea with patent pending status for a minimal cost for one year before you have to file a utility patent. The cost is roughly $100 (in 2009) if you do it yourself. This is an extremely important step to take to protect your intellectual property before showing the product to others, who might be inclined to replicate it without compensating you.
7. Once you have patent pending status and your idea is protected, have some colleagues try out your invention. Get feedback and make adjustments as needed.
8. Find non-disclosure agreements (NDA) on the Internet, bookstores or your local library. Have anyone you want to show your invention to sign it. An NDA states that whoever you share information about your product with will not and cannot talk to anyone about it. The NDA also states that the idea and product is yours alone.
9. Go to the USPTO website and do your own search on your product topic to see if anyone has had your idea.
10. Research what type of materials your product will require. Talk to several companies in your area or do a Google search for those companies that might be willing to manufacturer it for you.
11. Once you know you have a patentable invention, and you want to start a business. File a business name with your local newspaper, register with the Board of Equalization, then apply for a business license and tax ID number.
12. Keep positive people around you to keep your progress going.

My advice to anyone in the profession of dental hygiene would be to consider being an inventor. Dental hygienists, new or experienced, are constantly problem solving, therefore, the next step to becoming an inventor is developing those skills even more.

Being an inventor is invigorating, exciting, challenging and personally rewarding. It doesn't seem like work when the project is your own. It's a learning experience while providing you with a new appreciation for business owners!

Chapter 5: Personal Perspectives

"Be Prepared to Serve"
My Career as a Forensic Dental Hygienist

Winnie Furnari, RDH, MS, FAADH

Forensic Dental Hygienist

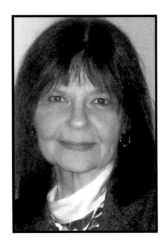

Figure 5.2. Winnie Furnari

My searches for ways to further help the public while using my skills and experience steered me towards forensic dentistry.

Mortuary Science has always interested me as I became aware in my youth that I was not uncomfortable in the presence of death. I also realized at a young age that tragedies befall us daily and that I would have the presence of mind to be able to work well under pressure, help others during a tragedy and still maintain an ability to perform tasks with strength to share. I planned that one day I would be contributing to mankind on a larger scale than in a one-chair operatory.

During my dental hygiene education, I came across an all-day continuing education course in New York City on Forensic Dentistry. I attended, listened to the lectures and went to the morgue for hands-on experience. It solidified my intentions and confirmed that there would be a place for me in this field, but I would have to create it.

One can find several different yet similar definitions of Forensic Dentistry or Forensic Odontology. In just about all of them you find a common word, law. The work entails becoming involved in the legal aspects of dentistry. Forensic hygienists assist the law with our expertise. Forensic professionals skillfully apply their science to the law. This is applicable to all the disciplines of the Forensic Sciences.

My position has always been as a member of a team involved in human identification and also as a course presenter to share my knowledge and experiences.

I have participated in the identification efforts associated with several major disasters since then and have been sharing my story with other dental hygienists and dental professionals through course presentations. I have also created and taught a course for students in a Bachelor of Dental Hygiene program at New York University College of Dentistry in New York City.

Dental hygiene students participate in Forensic Dentistry lectures on expert testimony, human abuse, identification, anthropology, bite marks, organizations, ethics, post traumatic stress disorder and team participation. They participate in a hands-on oral autopsy at the Office of the Chief Medical Examiner in New York City. Each student is required to research an aspect of human abuse. The students also receive catastrophe preparedness training, Core Disaster Life Support Certification and participate in a Point of Dispensing Exercise.

These life-changing experiences have prompted me to further my education in catastrophe preparedness. I also share with the public and those in the dental field how to be ready for many types of catastrophic events. I have completed a Master in Bioterrorism and Catastrophe Preparedness degree. Here, too, there is a place for dental hygienists to participate in community preparedness, response and mitigation.

Current events and television programs have raised interest in Forensic Dentistry and the science of Forensics. Many more professionals are getting involved and raising their knowledge base with formal courses of training.

One of the missions of Forensic Dentistry, which is also one if its rewards, is to help the families of deceased persons. Some will find a closure knowing that a death is confirmed. Forensic Dentistry is not just about identification. Dentistry contributes expertise on the living also. Bite mark interpretations and Forensic testimony in courts of law for criminal and civil cases are integral in this field. An exceptional aspect of Forensic Dentistry, of which I am most passionate about, is human abuse. I will always tell my colleagues that even if you don't participate on an identification team, you are practicing forensic dentistry as you evaluate children, elders and partners for physical, emotional and neglectful abuse. In this way the forensic science can save a life or make the quality of life better. One other important aspect of Forensic Dentistry is documentation. When dental hygienists record and keep the utmost accurate records they contribute to what may be a life-saving event or a legal proceeding. This may be for a stranger, a colleague or his or her own protection.

Some would say it takes a special person to do this work, but I know that dental hygienists are more than willing to contribute skills for the benefit of others. I also know that if any of us had to do this work, the overwhelming majority of us would be there to help in yet another path to career satisfaction.

Chapter 5: Personal Perspectives

"Caring for Those Who Cannot Speak for Themselves"
My Career in Veterinary Dentistry
Linda K. Bohacek, RDH, MA, CDHC, FAADH

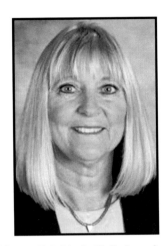

Figure 5.3. Linda K. Bohacek

I have been a practicing dental hygienist since 1971. During the past 41 years I have practiced in a variety of settings including nursing homes, hospital dental clinics, private solo and group practices, educational institutions and within the public health arena. My passion for the profession of dental hygiene, however, has been most heightened from my 22 years in the field of veterinary medicine.

My familiarity with the field of veterinary medicine came quite naturally as I married a veterinarian in 1975. I spent many hours on emergency calls with my husband, as well as, time at the animal hospital. In the mid-1980s, I became a mom and took a leave of absence from dental hygiene to raise my two children. It didn't take long for me to realize that I missed dental hygiene practice. So, when my husband asked for my help in developing preventive dental services in his practice, I jumped at the challenge. Fortunately, I did not have to write a resume and interview!

My journey into the field of veterinary dental hygiene was, as I recall, uncharted territory. My dental hygiene education provided a strong foundation, but I also needed knowledge of animal dental anatomy and the ramifications of treating animals undergoing general anesthesia. I gained a lot of knowledge through on-the-job experience. I recognized early that I needed small feline dental instruments so I worked with a dental instrument company to design them for me. I learned that healthy pocket depths vary from breed to breed and species to species and that animals have a much better immune system to fight off dental infections. The composition of their teeth, however, lends itself to fracturing easily. As animals age five to seven times faster than humans, oral cancer is more prevalent.

As a result of my years of practice in a veterinary setting, I have insight as to the attributes and skills that I feel are important for being successful as a dental hygienist in veterinary medicine:

- _Compensation_ – Expect monetary compensation to be a third to half of the current hourly wage in private dental practice.
- _Flexibility_ – A typical day of work varies depending on scheduled surgeries and unexpected emergencies, however, 9 am – 6 pm is typical. Typically procedures are performed in the morning followed by record keeping and call backs into the early afternoon. Discharge appointments are usually scheduled in the later afternoon.
- _Multi-tasking_ – While performing dental hygiene procedures, additional tasks are required, such as, cleaning ears, trimming nails, combing out mats, collecting laboratory samples and monitoring cardiac output, respiration, blood pressure and blood oxygen levels.
- _Teamwork_ – A veterinarian, vet assistant and certified veterinary technician are always close by and may be performing other procedures or minor surgeries on your patient while dental hygiene procedures are performed. Practicing without supervision in a separate room is not an option as all pets are under general anesthesia.
- _Adaptability_ – Often equipment and instruments with which dental hygienists are accustomed may not be available. Operator positioning for treatment can be a real challenge and physically demanding. Endotracheal tubes and oral monitors may hinder view of the oral cavity so adjustments to instrumentation and positioning are required.
- _Animal Handling_ – Attendance at animal behavior continuing education courses are required as bites and scratches are the number one injury in veterinary hospitals. Understanding body language is important for recognizing aggressive, submissive and fearful behavior. Cat and dog scratches and bites are potential occupational hazards. Therefore, it is recommended to be vaccinated against Rabies and maintain recommended Tetanus immunization intervals. Be prepared with a back up set of scrubs as one never knows when a pet will voluntarily or involuntarily urinate, express anal glands or pass stool on your clothes or your body.
- _Physical Fitness_ – Expect to lift up to 50-pound animals and use stretchers or gurneys for larger animals. Bending and twisting of the back is a normal day occurrence. Expect pulling and tugging from leashed animals of all sizes.
- _Veterinary Assistant Skills_ – It is recommended that dental hygienists become proficient in veterinary assistant/ technology skills. Veterinarians will be more likely to hire a dental hygienist who has more to offer than only a dental hygiene degree.
- _Job Shadow_ – One of the quickest ways to know if you are suited for veterinary dental hygiene is to observe at an animal hospital. Ask specifically to observe dental hygiene procedures. In the past, many dental hygiene colleagues have asked to observe as I practice. I make sure to inform them that it is important to NOT observe their own pet as the emotional bond becomes a distraction.

For those who seek practicing in a veterinary hospital as a way to be close to animals, be warned. There is more to working in a veterinary hospital than being close to animals. The daily encounters with animals and owners bring a variety of emotions and insights.

Many pet owners love their pets just as their children and would do anything to keep them healthy. There are also pet owners who believe that animals are just that – animals. They chose to do the bare minimum for their pet and sometimes chose euthanasia over treatment.

Death and illness are a constant part of the practice of veterinary medicine. It is important to understand and respect varying pet owner viewpoints so that you can determine whether you wish to handle the emotional aspect of working in this field.

Chapter 5: Personal Perspectives

"Looking to the Future"
My Work as a Dental Practice Owner
By Jammie Shaughnessy, RDH

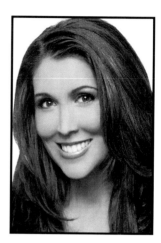

Figure 5.4. Jammie Shaughnessy

I love dental hygiene. In fact I miss having the rapport with the patients I had as a clinical dental hygienist day in and day out. I do not miss the physical aspect of dental hygiene: it can be mentally and physically exhausting at times. What I do now is tiring, but only mentally, not both. The mind and body can only handle so much before it burns out, and that is what was happening with me. I did not want to throw all of my education down the tube, after all the money and time I spent at University of Southern California School of Dentistry. So I thought, "How can I use my knowledge, but not actually physically work on patients all day?" I knew I wanted to work well into my 50s and even 60s, and I was in my mid 30s at the time. It was already hard on my body to do dental hygiene four full days a week. How could I ever last?

The light bulb that went off in my head that prompted me to own a practice was when I worked for a dentist who owned a large, 20-operatory practice, but did not actually practice any dentistry. I saw his success and his failures and thought, "I bet I could do what he is doing. I mean he is not even 'doing' dentistry." And of course as a dental hygienist I cannot do dentistry either. But I could "run" a dental office.

As I mentioned before, one also needs good solid financial backing. A non-dentist cannot qualify for a loan to purchase an office on their own. You either need a co-signer or a partner, or have some decent capital that you are willing to risk. You should assess whether you want to open a practice from the ground up or buy an already established office. I wanted to go into a practice with some goodwill in order to have instant cash flow. I did not want to sit and wait for patients without even having hired a dentist yet! So I bought a practice that was four years old; the selling dentist worked on for nine months until I found my own lead dentist to take over. The transition was difficult, and the practice lost some money at first. However, I chose a very good dentist, and after our rocky transition was ironed out we instantly saw our numbers soar. We changed the practice into a full-service practice, everything from professional cleanings to dental implants and everything in between.

The irony of this situation is that when I first had the idea to open up a practice, none of the dentists I knew or approached would partner with me. They were all too wary. But I knew I would always have this monkey on my back. My dentist is asking me to partner with him, now he sees that I mean serious business and get things done.

Chapter 5: Personal Perspectives

"Operatory On the Go"
My Work as an Affiliated Practice Dental Hygienist
By Michelle Panico, RDH, MA
Affiliated Practice Elementary School Dental Hygienist

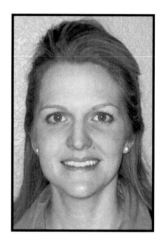

Figure 5.5. Michelle Panico

I learned about being an Affiliated Practice Dental Hygienist (APDH) in 2004 through the Arizona State Dental Hygienists' Association (ASDHA) newsletters and journals. My passion for public health and desire to serve the underserved drew me to this area of the profession. This opportunity opened up to me because I actively pursued and developed it. Once I had completed the Affiliated Practice requirements, I completed a business plan with my colleague, Lynnette Martin, RDH. Together we then made a list of possible community partners (Head Start, WIC, YMCA, Boys & Girls Club, Community Health Centers, elementary schools and non-profit hospitals) and began making contacts to share our business plan and vision.

The steps that dental hygienists would need to go through to be considered as an elementary school dental hygienist include:

- *Creating a business plan to clearly communicate your ideas;*
- *Contacting organizations that would be interested in partnership for developing and funding the program; and*
- *Assembling a team to implement the strategies and achieve the program objectives.*

To make the transition to this career option smoother, it is advantageous to have experience in administration, public health concepts and pediatric dentistry, strong written and verbal communication skills, cultural competence and sensitivity and a self motivated, assertive and kind personality.

The major difference between my position and other dental hygiene roles is that I am able to play an active role in designing a public health program, have greater autonomy, work without a dentist present and provide services for a poor population, which requires understanding the culture of poverty. This position would work for others who enjoy public health and want to grow personally and professionally.

I am able to achieve satisfaction in my position as an Affiliated Practice Dental Hygienist because I experience a sense of purpose, unlimited possibilities, and a potential for growth professionally and personally. Since our clinic continues to change and expand to reach more community members efficiently and with more services, it feeds my professional desire to be challenged at the same time as fulfilling my personal need for purpose and serving the community.

Chapter 5: Personal Perspectives

"Testing the Waters"
My Career as a Professional Speaker
By JoAnn R. Gurenlian, RDH, PhD

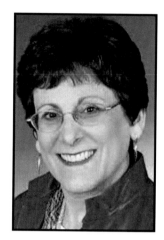

Figure 5.6. JoAnn R. Gurenlian

Technically, I have been a dental hygienist for 36 years. However, I always considered myself a dental hygienist from the moment I started dental hygiene school. I truly was invested in this career from the beginning, and feel very proud to say that I have been part of this profession for so long.

I started in dental hygiene school in 1974, graduated with an Associate in Arts degree from Fairleigh Dickinson University in 1976, and then obtained a Bachelor of Science degree from that same school in 1978. In 1979, I graduated from Columbia University with a Master of Science degree in dental hygiene. Since there was not a doctoral program in dental hygiene, I continued my education at the University of Pennsylvania, and received a Doctorate in Education specializing in Educational Leadership in 1991.

I started teaching at Thomas Jefferson University in Philadelphia in 1979. The program had just started, and I became the instructor who taught education-related courses. As I developed my own skills, the department decided to begin to offer continuing education courses, and I became the coordinator of those courses. In developing event planning skills, I also carefully evaluated the presentation styles of the various speakers we hired for programs.

Over the years, I developed my own presentation style and began to teach continuing education courses. One of my first courses was for the Southern New Jersey Dental Hygienists' Association (SNJDHA). Remarkably, this organization gave me many first starts: as a speaker, leader for the New Jersey Dental Hygienists' Association (NJDHA) and as president of the ADHA. The members of this group have been an invaluable resource for my learning, as they allow me to present new courses I develop to them as a way of "testing the waters." Without them, I don't know that I would have been nearly as successful in my career.

Presently, I am an entrepreneur. I started my own company, Gurenlian & Associates in April of 1993. My company provides consulting services and continuing education to healthcare providers. I design continuing education programs that are meant to be informative and practical to provide healthcare providers a means to implement what is taught. My goal is to promote best practices to improve the health of the public.

In 1993, when I began this venture, I was the Director of the Department of Dental Hygiene at Thomas Jefferson University. During that time period, finances in the state of Pennsylvania were tenuous at best and universities and colleges had to make cuts. The handwriting was on the wall, and the department was in jeopardy. After working for months on trying to save the program, it was clear that it was going to be closed. I happened to be a speaker at a meeting in Boston with Irene Woodall. We had dinner together the night before the presentation, and I shared with her my concerns about the program and my need to move on to something else. Irene had created her own business and was working as a professional speaker. She encouraged me to consider doing the same. The next week, I went home, looked into the prospects of starting my own business and decided that was the right move for me. My brother assisted me by teaching me how to start a company and putting me on the path of learning about small business practices. Sixteen years ago I formed my company and the rest is history as they say.

In addition, timing was a part of my success. I had just completed tenure as President of the American Dental Hygienists' Association in 1991. I had the good fortune of name recognition and used that to market my business. I could easily talk about professional status and recognition issues, independent practice and dental hygiene diagnosis. It did not bother me to speak about controversial topics and these were of great interest. When organizations found out I also had experience teaching pathology and oral medicine topics, it allowed me the chance to broaden my speaking opportunities.

I have lectured locally, regionally, nationally and internationally. I will lecture anywhere except a war zone! Some of my favorite places to speak have been in Southern New Jersey, Canada, Switzerland, Italy and Denmark.

As a speaker, my role is to research content that is evidence-based and relevant, and present it in a manner that is understandable and usable. I have learned over the years that a program that does not include the "how to use this information," does not have the same impact. I want the participants to think about going back to work the next day and implementing and evaluating what they just learned.

My most exciting experience as a speaker was talking about independent dental hygiene practice at a dental educators' meeting in New Orleans. It was my first national presentation and the topic was so controversial, I was not sure that I would live to see the next day. There was standing room only when I gave the presentation. It was scary and exhilarating at the same time.

Another truly thrilling experience was when I was undergoing breast cancer therapy and was asked to speak in Calgary. I had not taught for six months because I had been ill from the chemotherapy. Arrangements for me to speak had been made before I was diagnosed with cancer, and the organization invited me to speak even though I was still undergoing treatment. I was slated to deliver three presentations in one day, and the association had made arrangements for a dear friend to fill in for me should I not feel well enough to complete the courses. I taught all of the programs scheduled and received a standing ovation, something the hosts said had not occurred before. I don't know if they were being kind, but it was very empowering for me to present that day. It made me feel that I could do something productive other than worry about cancer, and got me back on track with my business. I felt whole again.

I would recommend becoming a professional speaker to those interested in this career path because I am always learning something new. Also, there is the added benefit of making connections with colleagues from around the world. It is amazing how similar our professional concerns are around the globe.

The major difference between my position as an entrepreneur and professional speaker and other dental hygiene roles is that I am independent and responsible solely to myself. In other dental hygiene roles, you are likely working within a center or setting in which you are an employee. I am responsible for myself and to myself, no one else. There is great freedom and great responsibility that come with those terms.

I started out wanting to be an educator, and I plan to continue in that arena with my business for as long as possible. I do have other interests as well, one of which is politics. I have ventured into running for political office and working with political candidates. It is something that allows me to address other topics of local and national importance.

Chapter 5: Personal Perspectives

"Trying My Hand at Writing"
My Career as an Editor and Editorial Director
Jill Rethman, RDH, BA

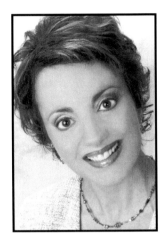

Figure 5.7. Jill Rethman

I graduated from the Ohio State University School of Dental Hygiene in 1974. The time has gone by so quickly, especially because I thoroughly enjoy my chosen profession.

I didn't plan to become a dental hygienist – it was a career I luckily "fell into." As I was approaching my sophomore year at Ohio State, I had not yet declared a major. I had a part-time evening job at a local department store, and it just so happened that several of my co-workers were in the dental hygiene program. I had no idea what I wanted to do, but their stories of what they were learning and how they were beginning to treat patients in the clinic intrigued me.

After numerous conversations with them, I decided to go for it – I made up my mind that I wanted to be a dental hygienist! I went through the interview process with the program director, Dr. Nancy Reynolds Goorey. She was a true inspiration – at the time there were very few women dentists. I painstakingly wrote a long, heartfelt essay on why I wanted to be a dental hygienist and what inspired me to choose the profession. Lo and behold, I was accepted to the program!

There were 86 people in my class, a very large group compared to today's dental hygiene classes. It was only after I was admitted that I realized how fortunate I was – nearly 500 people had applied for those coveted 86 spots. My classmates were highly intelligent, talented young women (no men in my class), many of whom had fathers, brothers and other relatives who were dentists or dental hygienists. I also came to realize that a large number of them had wanted to be dental hygienists their entire lives. It was then that I understood how fortunate I was to be in this profession and to be chosen by Dr. Goorey. She gave me the chance to spread my wings in ways I would have never dreamed possible.

For most of my career, I worked in clinical practice. I was able to treat all kinds of patients, including general, pediatric and periodontal practices. (As an aside, the most difficult clinical position I have ever had was working in that pediatric practice! I substituted for a dental hygienist who was on vacation for a week. It was non-stop action, and it sure gave me a great appreciation for those who work with children full time).

In the mid-1980s while living in New Jersey, I drove to Manhattan one day to attend the Greater New York Dental Meeting. I had never seen such a large dental exhibition and was impressed by the scope of educational programs and exhibits. I was hoping to find a position where I could supplement my clinical work with travel to dental meetings – I thought it would be a great experience to work with a dental products company and broaden my horizons in dental hygiene.

I approached the Johnson & Johnson booth, since I heard they utilized dental hygienists to provide product samples at conventions and to answer product-related questions. I was in luck. The individual in charge, Ada Beth (Benton) Harris was there. We chatted, I handed her my scant resume, and by some miracle she called me. This started a wonderful adventure of travel with other dental hygienists from across the country – many of whom are still very dear friends. I attended all the major dental meetings while working in clinical practice. It truly opened my eyes to the "industry" side of dentistry and gave me a wider range of experience within the dental hygiene field.

After several years, the Johnson & Johnson role was phased out. But luck was on my side once again. I found a similar position with Pfizer. My role with Pfizer was as a convention representative, and after a few years that, too, ended. But before it did, I met some wonderful fellow dental hygienists who had managerial roles with Teledyne Waterpik. Candy Ross and Carol Janz managed the Waterpik professional educational program. This program utilized dental hygienists to not only work at dental conventions but to provide educational lectures at dental and dental hygiene schools. I applied for a position as the northeast educator, and was more nervous than I have ever been in my life at that interview. I was required to give a ten-minute lecture on a topic in dental hygiene; I had never done public speaking. I remembered all those times during speech class when I was scared beyond belief. I would lie awake at night thinking of my presentation, and when it was over, it was as if a huge weight had been lifted off my shoulders. So here I was, applying for a position where I would be speaking in front of groups of people on a regular basis. I remember thinking at the time that I must be out of my mind! Candy and Carol were wonderful, and in spite of my nerves, they hired me. This propelled me to yet another phase in my dental hygiene career.

I held the position at Waterpik for several years and then a new opportunity came along – one in which I would not only give educational programs myself, but I would also manage a group of dental hygienists to speak across the country. I became the director of educational programs for Sultan Healthcare in the early 1990s. Another door opened as another part of my dental hygiene career began. I was still in clinical practice part time, living in Maryland now. The position with Sultan was extremely rewarding, but that, too, came to an end. Yet somehow in 1995, I was in the right place at the right time. A publication called the Journal of Practical Hygiene had started. I decided to try my hand at writing and had several articles published within JPH. They liked my work and named me to their editorial board. In the fall of 1995, the publisher approached me to be the Editor-in-Chief. Needless to say, I was amazed and honored – I jumped at the chance to start another wonderful phase of my dental hygiene career. I remained as the Editor-in-Chief of JPH for seven years.

I continued to present CE programs and was starting to get more and more requests to speak. The major dental and dental hygiene associations were calling me, and I had to pinch myself, realizing that my career had taken an interesting turn. I kept wondering where the next "fork in the road" would take me, and it wasn't long before I had my answer. During my time at JPH, I definitely caught the writing bug. I heard about Dimensions® of Dental Hygiene, a new publication for dental hygiene professionals. I was impressed with the quality of the articles and the individuals involved. Anna Pattison was the Editor-in-Chief and Lorene Kent was the Publisher – both dental hygienists. This made Dimensions® unique since it was the only dental hygiene journal with dental hygienists at the helm. I knew Anna for quite some time and was aware of her excellent reputation and high standards. I met Lorene at a dental meeting and we realized we shared a common mission – to provide quality information to dental hygienists in a practical format. In 2004, at the ADHA meeting in Dallas, I was introduced as the Editorial Director for Dimensions®.

As I look back on the various steps I've taken and roles I've had in dental hygiene, I realize that each one has been a building block. One opportunity has given me the experience that has led to another opportunity. Each one has built upon the other and no position or experience has been wasted.

Speaking, writing and working in publishing are perfect avenues for someone who wants to work independently and craves flexibility. With each issue of Dimensions®, new topics present themselves that keep my mind working and my knowledge up-to-date. This also enables me to stay current for the educational programs I present at various dental and dental hygiene meetings. It's a wonderful synergistic relationship that encourages me to be my best.

However, if you think "routine" and a "typical 9-to-5 job" are important, this career path won't work well for you. For many dental hygienists, knowing that the workday ends at a specific time is important due to family considerations and other activities. The major difference between what I do and clinical practice is just that – my workday never ends and various projects are always with me. I work all hours of the day (and night), including weekends. My computer and email are constant companions since deadlines don't take breaks or vacations. But I wouldn't trade the wonderful experiences I've had for anything.

One of my favorite quotes is by poet Robert Frost: "Two roads diverged in a wood, And I took the one less traveled by, And that has made all the difference." That "road less traveled" is a perfect description of my career path in dental hygiene!

Chapter 5: Personal Perspectives

"The Time to Take Action"
My Career as a Continuing Education Entrepreneur
By Joyce Turcotte, RDH, MEd, FAADH

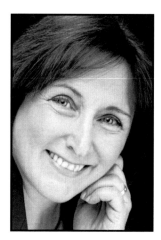

Figure 5.8. Joyce Turcotte

I graduated from dental hygiene school in 1973. I have held an active license and currently practice as my schedule permits.

Professional Learning Services, LLC, (PLS) began in 1987. I am the founder and have been the President and CEO since its inception.

I learned about this area of dental hygiene when I decided to leave full-time teaching. My colleague and mentor suggested I consider starting my own business. With my credentials and teaching experience, she inspired me to develop and present/conduct continuing education classes in Connecticut. A proposed Bill was submitted for review by the Connecticut State legislature and regulations would soon follow. This was the time to take action. The law was passed in 1988 and Professional Learning Services began in 1987. I had introduced the business name and service to the marketplace one year before the law became regulated and created a niche.

Thinking back over the past 25 years, I had a lot of weaknesses in business training. I reached out to associates, friends and family who had strengths in accounting, business planning, forecast, marketing and advertising, just to name a few. I also tapped into a free government service, the Small Business Administration (SBA) and the law that provided extensive assistance in all aspects of business and service. They also provided guidance in the legal arena. I took a lot of business related workshops and consulted with individuals with expertise in the business area.

I fortunately have an excellent network of close associates and friends who are experts in business, accounting, law, marketing and advertising, and a resource for specifically dental continuing education. I spent hours discussing ideas, strategies, concepts and plans. Technology was just coming into the mainstream and I needed the support for computer applications. Programs and systems that are considered out of date today were cutting edge in the 1980s, and I persevered to establish a reputable business.

I would recommend this area of the profession because it is important to provide quality education to your peers, a resource the market can trust. Over the years I have established great friendships, have had wonderful experiences, met thousands of dental hygienists, pushed my own levels of achievement and been able to balance raising a family with a home-based business. I have been in control of my travel and career path. My family has enjoyed traveling with me and I have been a positive influence on my children in being a business owner.

I also focused my business similar to an academic calendar and take more time off in the summer for family and traveling. The business operates 12 months a year, but the summer is a lighter schedule. With access to computers and cell phone, I can operate and manage business from different locations. With part-time office staff attending to the day-to-day operations, they help to keep up with phone calls, mail, advertising and other tasks and responsibilities delegated to them.

This is the type of business that you can operate part or full time. Depending on your educational expertise, you can offer a variety of topics or select speakers to provide seminars that meet your patient's needs and interests.

Anyone starting their own continuing education business should offer programs or services within their capabilities or within what services they could subcontract. As the owner, you have to determine where your priorities lie, what you can handle, what your passions are and what you can afford. My best recommendation is do what you love to do. Build in your area of interest and commit to what you can believe you can accomplish and always raise the bar.

Chapter 5: Personal Perspectives

"Putting It on Paper"
My Career as an Author
By Judith Dember-Paige, RDH

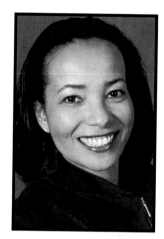

Figure 5.9. Judith Dember-Paige

While growing up, my dentist was the one who cleaned my teeth, I never heard of a dental hygienist. After having a conversation with the dental assistant at our local office, she explained she wanted to be a dental hygienist and what that would involve. I was intrigued and especially liked that I could have my own patients.

When I began to write my book I was already a dental hygienist for 22 years, and boredom for my profession had set in. I had begun to go crazy inside with the feeling of being closed in; there had to be more.

Writing my idea down on paper was the first step in the journey of developing my product.

Next, I had to transfer my hand written manuscript to a Microsoft Word program. It was amazing to see these words transforming into a book as I discovered how to take photos and download them into the pages. I shared the book's rough draft with about five colleagues for a critique and edit of my work. They would email me with corrective suggestions they thought I needed to make.

I only accepted the adjustments that were in line with my vision for the project. I was given the name of an excellent self-publisher, Jenkins Group Inc., which helped me pull my book together. They asked me three questions: Who is my target audience, who cares that I am writing this book and ultimately, who will buy my book? These questions helped me to define what the content of my book would be.

They offered me professional services like Critique, which asks critical questions, Editing, Illustration and Multiple Level Proofreading. They helped me with my cover and interior design, page layout and all the registrations necessary for its recognition. They coordinated and direct shipped the finished books to me; now I have become a book distributor. With the creation of each new book, it got easier. Book orders have come through my website, www.abcdepress.com, Practicon Dental Supply, Barnes and Nobles and other book stores ordered books directly through me. Dental hygienists are my biggest supporters; they have big hearts for their patients. Marketing my books has shown to be my biggest challenge. What I have found is, I am the one with the passion who knows my product best and I need to be the one behind the marketing.

After the completion of the first book, there was a strong request for a Spanish edition and in July 2008 *Sana Sonrisa, para toda la vida* was born. In addition, Carol Manocchi-Verrino, MAT, a teacher of middle school children in Westchester, NY helped me in creating a text for teacher's, *Smile Wide Teacher's Guide, Giving Educators the Tools to Teach Children's Dental Health.*

This guide serves to facilitate good dental habits through literacy-based learning experiences, for a classroom setting. With the insight children will gain from this program, my hope is that students can share with their parents and help end the downward cycle of young adults losing their teeth.

These lessons afford teachers the opportunity to cover more learning standards in less time with the inclusion of teachers' educational mandates. The goal is to help children take an active part in protecting their teeth now and in the future.

Becoming an author is an opportunity to write down your thoughts. They are unique to you and are not easily duplicated by someone else. I never saw myself as a writer. It was only when I was given the challenge to sit down and write an outline for my next book that it was discovered. I would have never thought of it by myself. It is never too late to develop your passion.

If you are someone who says "I can't write," this is simply not true. Writing gets better the more you do it, and the more you do it, the more opportunity you get to do it. Make the most of every opportunity that comes your way by showing you are interested in writing. Submit articles to our professional journals. They will not be shy about sending them back to you with needed corrections. Do not lose heart. Make the corrections and resubmit the articles.

This journey put me on a positive track toward writing and encouraging others. Finding groups of professional peers gave me a positive outlook with direction.

As I said, I never considered myself a writer but once I started writing, I never stopped. As a result, I have written many articles and three books. Practicing dental hygiene part time allows me the freedom to involve myself in other opportunities in which I may want to take part.

So take out a pen and paper and begin to write down some professional and personal goals that will help you to advance your career. Check out one of our professional journals and make plans to attend one of our next dental hygiene meetings. Take the next step toward fulfilling your dreams.

Chapter 5: Personal Perspectives

"Not for the Faint of Heart"
My Career as a Dental Hygienist in a Prison Setting
By Pamela J. Myers, RDH

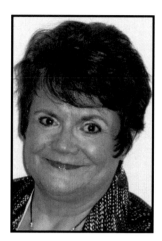

Figure 5.10. Pamela J. Myers

So what's it really like to work with prisoners every day? This story, which was published in *Chicken Soup for the Dental Soul* in 1999, is a good example.

One of my prison patients was a Vietnam veteran suffering from Delayed Shock Syndrome. He was brought to the operatory from solitary confinement. I was told he was having a bad day. He was in restraints and clearly agitated. As he came in, he told me, "They're coming over the hill."

"How far back are they?" I asked.

"A pretty good ways," he responded.

I told him that if I worked fast, and he stayed quiet, he would be out of the operatory before "they" got there. The patient remained quiet and immobile. I completed his treatment. As he left with two guards, he looked back at me with visible relief and said, "We made it, didn't we?"

I believe he was not aware of his surroundings that day; he was reliving a terrible memory of running for his life. God gave me the wisdom to manage the situation and allow this patient a few hours of peace. He remained calm the rest of that day, surprising the correctional officers.

Many of my patients have received very little if any dental care prior to incarceration. The average IQ is 92 and most have an average grade level of 7.9 upon entry to the Texas Department of Criminal Justice (TDCJ). They are a challenge to communicate with and definitely challenge any dental hygienist's clinical skills.

Patients are required to attain and maintain an acceptable level of oral hygiene to receive routine dental care. We instruct them in proper brushing and flossing technique and, on average, they show improvement in less than three appointments.

I learned about correctional dental hygiene opportunities from two of the dentists I worked with in private practice. They both worked part time for the prison system and advised me that TDCJ was hiring dental hygienists.

I know a little about the environment from their stories, wise counsel and mentoring. I was interested in the position because of the great state benefit package.

I applied for the opening and was offered the position. My husband literally talked me out of accepting the job as he was sure I would not like it. I talked to him for three years and convinced him I knew it was where I wanted to be. He relented, and I accepted.

Twenty-six years later, I am still practicing in corrections and am still married to the same wonderful man. We celebrated our 40th anniversary last year. He is the first one to tell others what a great job I have and how proud he is of me!

Professional Savvy, LLC, shares a warm and heartfelt thank you to Gina, Winnie, Linda, Jammie, Michelle, JoAnn, Jill, Joyce, Judith and Pamela for sharing their expertise in their professional roles in dental hygiene. Your valuable and meaningful words will provide so much learning and inspiration to students who are graduating as well as to practicing dental hygienists who need to make a change in their positions in dental hygiene in order to achieve a renewed success in their careers.

UNIT TWO:
Tools and Techniques for Career Development

Chapter 6: Career and Professional Development

By Christine A. Hovliaras, RDH, BS, MBA, CDE

Learning Objectives

The student dental hygienist and the dental hygiene professional will learn the following key objectives from this chapter:

1. Discuss the definitions and differences for personal vision and mission statements.
2. Identify goals and objectives for the future as well as assess your current career path.
3. Assess the satisfaction level in your dental hygiene career.
4. Preview and take the **Professional Savvy™ Career Development Assessment Test**.
5. Develop written vision and mission statements and information to direct your career planning annually and for regular intervals up to nine years.

Overview

Whether dental hygiene was the first step of a 10-step career plan, or if one gravitated toward the profession because of an interest in the healthcare field, career planners should develop a plan and seek outside counsel to review it. It is never too late to begin planning, and it is never too soon to consider options.

Maggie thought she had it all planned out: Two years in dental hygiene school while she continued in a four-year program to complete her bachelor's degree; two additional years working in a research laboratory while she finished her master's degree; and on to a teaching position at a dental hygiene program at a local university.

Julie created a plan for her career, too. Two years in dental hygiene school while she continued a four-year program to complete her bachelor's degree; two more while her husband, James, completed his bachelor's degree, during which time she would work full time in private practice. Then, when her first child came along, she could reduce her work hours to part time and continue with plans for the other two children the couple wanted. When the kids all reached school age, she planned to explore a corporate position with an oral health care products company to earn more money so James could work on his MBA program. They planned to have their family and education completed before they turned 40.

These two fictitious plans seem carefully thought-out; however, there should always be room for a change of direction or an unplanned situation in the career path. Both dental hygienists have taken a lot for granted if they have never considered the strengths and weaknesses of their personalities and work styles. Has each dental hygiene professional checked these plans with a mentor who is close enough to them to offer astute observations? It is likely that neither woman has considered a change of passion in her career path, let alone what might happen in their personal lives. What if Maggie discovers during her lab time that she has a greater passion for research than for teaching? What if Julie cannot bear to leave direct contact with patients for the corporate world?

The Personal Vision Statement

"Begin with the end in mind," wrote Stephen Covey in his book The Seven Habits of Highly Effective People.[1] Dental hygienists, or any healthcare professionals for that matter, should plot their career road map by first considering the destination.

There is no need to have an immediate elaborate plan, but instead to engage in a few self-defining exercises to guide decision making. A good starting point is to create a personal vision statement.

A **vision statement** is a one – or two-sentence description of what an individual hopes to become or achieve.[2] A good vision statement should include a motivation for developing meaning and purpose within a career path and selecting a direction that will enhance personal growth. It is wise to put this vision in writing and post it where it can be seen daily as a constant reminder of personal and professional goals. It will define how the professional's career advances for the future.

An established vision provides direction for the future, helps professionals set goals and objectives, and aids them in determining the quality of expertise and skills they have and may need in order to bring their career to the next level.

A personal vision statement should project where the dental hygienist would like to be in the next three to six years. As an example, consider the vision statement from Denise, a dental hygienist practicing in Raleigh, NC, which reads:

"I would like to work in the leading periodontal practice in my community and expand the patient base and dental technology within that practice."

More than words on paper, Denise will need an action plan to make her vision statement become reality. To succeed, she and other motivated professionals need to tap into three essential elements in her personality:

- **Confidence:** The belief that success is deserved and that she feels worthy of her vision.
- **Competence:** Her ability to be educated and utilize that knowledge and training to successfully complete tasks and solve problems.
- **Capability:** Her ability to create, define and control her life through structure, discipline and hard work. One must be capable in order to achieve success.

To further define her plan, Denise will need to create a personal mission statement.

The Personal Mission Statement

The next step is to write a mission statement. A **mission statement** captures the purposeful activities in which the professional wants to engage daily. While the vision statement encapsulates future plans, the mission statement reflects the here and now. For example, Denise's mission statement might be:

"To improve the oral health of my patients and to study current periodontal research to keep my dental team and our patients abreast of the latest findings in periodontology."

This mission gives her clear tasks for day-to-day practice and offers a bridge to help her grow into her vision statement.

Define Your Goals and Objectives

Together the vision and mission statements become guiding principles that help dental hygiene professionals plan, set goals and objectives and make decisions about their daily work life and future career goals.

Albert Einstein once said, "If you want to have a happy life, tie it to a goal. Not to people or things." Why? Because a **goal** is a personal benchmark; an individual achievement. Career planners won't have to rely on something or someone to assure their confidence and happiness when they have a goal to work toward!

Each dental hygienist should define at least two to three goals and objectives that he or she needs to accomplish in order to achieve their personal vision statement. Once each goal is defined then an objective should be developed to help secure that goal. An **objective** is defined as a strategy or step to attain an identified goal.[3]

For example, Denise has been working in a general dentist's office for five years. She wants to change her position and begin working in a periodontal practice to establish herself as a periodontal therapist. Her goal: Find a dental hygiene position in a state-of-the-art periodontal practice in Raleigh, NC.

With a defined goal, Denise can determine her objectives. One might be to make a list of state-of-the-art periodontal practices around Raleigh, the same area in which she currently works.

Her second objective: Determine which state-of-the-art periodontal practices in Raleigh have openings for her position. Denise may want to consult her fellow colleagues in Raleigh or contact a dental placement agency to determine which periodontal practices have technology and are in need of a dental hygienist.

Identifying Your Current Career Path

A good step for Denise, before she actually contacts any of these periodontal practices, is to identify her current career path. She will need to be clear about what she has to offer if she decides to apply for one of the available openings.

Dental hygienists in this position should evaluate the number of years spent as a practicing clinician and consider:

- Position currently held;
- Satisfaction with current career position;
- Dissatisfaction with current career position;
- What they can do to improve the current career position; and
- Willingness to improve the situation.

Are You Happy in Your Dental Hygiene Career?

Happiness is a relative term. Happiness does not have an accurate form of measurement. If we could pour it into a cup, lay a ruler next to it or place it on a scale, we might find that we actually have a large measure of happiness. Unfortunately, minor dissatisfactions frequently cloud feelings of satisfaction. Much of life's unhappiness results from boredom with the routine – whether that routine is good or bad.

Without an accurate measure, we are left to compare levels of happiness in relation to other times in our life or at other times in our career. For dental hygiene professionals to decide if they are happy in their present career paths, they should compare it to another point in their careers. To more accurately analyze it, the dental hygienist should pursue a self-assessment test.

Self assessment reviews values, interests, skills and expertise and personality. It provides a nice overview for dental hygienists to learn more about themselves and what motivates their actions. Students and professionals with years of experience should take a personality assessment exam, such as the Meyer-Briggs Type Indicator (MBTI). The MBTI is only one such exam, compiled by professional psychologists, that uses a field of more than 90 questions to reveal overall trends in one's personality type and preferences. I have recently taken the Forté Institute Communication Profile Survey and found it to be very accurate in assessing my personality and communication style skills. A quick search of a telephone directory should offer job counseling service centers where an interested party may find a qualified test administrator.

For an assessment test specific to the dental hygiene profession (students and practicing dental hygienists), consider the **Professional Savvy™ Career Development Assessment Test**, available at the end of this chapter and for purchase at www.professionalsavvychd.com. This test is administered to measure the aptitude specifically of dental hygienists for continuing growth in their careers. For student dental hygienists, see Figures 6.1 and 6.2 on pages 153-161 for the **Professional Savvy™ Student Dental Hygienist Career Development Assessment Test** and the **Professional Savvy™ Student Dental Hygienist Annual Career Development Plan.** For practicing dental hygienists, see Figures 6.3 and 6.4 on pages 162-170 for the **Professional Savvy™ Dental Hygienist Career Development Assessment Test** and the **Professional Savvy™ Dental Hygienist Annual Career Development Plan.**

Finding Career Satisfaction

The dental hygienist should always be sensitive to the signs of job dissatisfaction. This might include, but is not limited to, triggers such as unhappiness with salary increases, a stagnant level of responsibility in the practice, lack of appreciation for the dental hygienist's role in the practice by team members, and continuing team conflict. Dental hygienists need to quickly write down moments of job dissatisfaction, why it occurred, what can be done to change it and if they are willing to change it. They should also note how long the effects of these issues linger.

Several key studies conducted on dental hygiene career satisfaction reveal important points to keep in mind as professionals consider their situations. For example, one study showed that some of the most important elements required to keep dental hygienists in clinical practice for more than five years include:

- Quality and safety of a work environment;
- Time management for increased quality of dental hygiene services;
- Effective office policies and procedures;
- Employer support of professional career;
- Supportive work environment; and
- Variety in scope of practice.[4]

Additional factors that help professionals stay in a dental practice setting include: salary, benefits, decision-making capabilities, professional collaboration and family responsibilities. Those dental hygienists who left clinical practice cited family responsibilities as the number one reason for their departure; this was followed by boredom and lack of benefits.[5] Research shows that dental hygienists who are satisfied with their careers are more likely to promote dental hygiene as a desired profession,[6] while those who are not satisfied become bored, frustrated and burned out. These are critical concerns that need to be discussed for dental hygienists to consider if the current office they work in is right for them, or if they should pursue other career opportunities.

The ideal dental hygiene position is a combination of good work environment communication, trust and respect among the doctor and team members, understood responsibilities among the team members, time management flexibility based upon patient cases, and lifelong learning to continue to develop clinical and practical skills.

Dental hygienists should assess their satisfaction level with their current positions, and whether or not this would be their preferred position three years from now. They also should consider incorporating a timeline for goal planning.

Putting Professional Savvy™ Career Tools Goal Development Plans to Use

In the course of a busy life, it is easy to disconnect with goals. The complex act of juggling work schedules, school, leisure activities and family life can push career planning and goal tracking to the back of one's mind. This is why creating a goals development plan helps.

Professional Savvy, LLC, offers three **Career Tools Goal Development Plans** to keep the individual from drifting into dissatisfaction without knowing why his or her feelings have changed. These timetables help career planners and job seekers stay on track for making decisions. First, the **Professional Savvy™ Annual Career Development Plan** offers a measurement tool for rating the professional's position each year. Then, **Professional Savvy™ Three-**

Year Career Development Update takes the pulse on career goals over a three-year time period. The **Professional Savvy™ Six-Year Career Development Update** takes career goal planning from four to six years time. Finally, career planners can use the **Professional Savvy™ Nine-Year Career Development Update** to set out goals from a seven to nine-year period and identify further elements on which to focus that will bring goal attainment to a highly successful level. These tools help the busy professional track progress without allowing the task to become too overwhelming and help them to organize their career planning and development over time.

Professionals and students alike need to project a one – to three-year vision of their career. Many dental hygienists fall into the trap of not setting goals or objectives regarding their career. Professionals should carefully assess their satisfaction level in their current position and whether or not this would be their preferred position three years from now.

A proper career plan will help the dental hygienist evaluate opportunities and decide which are a good fit both personally and professionally. A dental hygienist can use Career Development Planning and the Three-, Six – and Nine – Year Career Development Updates to:

- Continue long-range career planning with established directed objectives to reach career goals in a timely fashion;
- Determine if additional training, certification or education is required;
- Establish the elements for success;
- Create a plan for achievement of career goals; and
- Utilize a mentor(s) to assist in career decisions and looking at future next steps.

Professional Savvy, LLC, has also developed these long-term Career Development Updates for dental assistants, dentists and dental specialists. Additionally, the Career Assessment Test and the Annual Career Development Plan is also available to student dental professionals (assistant, hygiene and dental), front office team, dental assistants, dentists and dental specialists. All of these Career Tool products can be purchased online at www. professionalsavvychd.com/career tools/.

Put Your Plan Together To Achieve Professional Career Goals

As the professional moves through the assessment process, career goals should begin to form. Dental hygienists and dental hygiene students should review the professional roles described in Chapter 2 to understand their current role in the dental hygiene profession and understand other roles for which they may have an interest or aptitude in the future. Consider: What roles sound appealing? Are there professionals in this role with whom to discuss if this position is a good fit? If so, the dental hygienist or dental hygiene student should set up a phone conversation with this person and identify questions they would be interested in asking this person.

Another aspect clinicians need to consider is how newly developed goals fit their current work environment. A wise career planner will identify at least two important goals to achieve in this position, and list those goals down on the **Professional Savvy™ Three-Year Career Development Update**.

Students can use the **Professional Savvy™ Dental Hygiene Student Career Development Assessment Test** and **Annual Career Development Plan** to assess their career plans in the same manner that a seasoned hygienist would do, but may rely on their mentors at school to assist in suggesting or helping to develop a few future goals.

Once career planners have listed a few important goals, it is important to develop the objectives that will need to be accomplished to achieve these goals. Developing these is an even more important area in which to gather help from a mentor. The objectives should also include a timeline of when they will be accomplished.

A mentor will provide career planners with the right direction and feedback to help them initiate this plan of action. A monthly meeting may need to be scheduled to help start the process and help the career planner to be accountable for his or her plan. A wise individual once said, "A failure to plan is a plan for failure." The better approach is to set achievable goals and objectives and make them happen!

References

1. Covey S. *The 7 Habits of Highly Effective People.* New York: Free Press; 1989, 145-150.
2. Mindtools website. Available at http://www.mindtools.com/pages/article/newLDR_90.htm. Accessed February 7, 2012.
3. America Heritage Dictionary website. Available at: http://ahdictionary.com. Accessed February 6, 2012.
4. Calley KH, Bowen DM, Darby ML, Miller DL. Factors influencing dental hygiene retention in private practice. *J Dent Hyg.* 1996;70(4):151-160.
5. Johns GH, et al. Career retention in the dental hygiene workforce in Texas. *J Dent Hyg.* 2001;77(2):135-48.
6. Dudian T. Dental hygiene career promotional behaviors and attitudes. *J Dent Hyg.* 1993;67(6):318-325.

Critical Thinking Exercises

1. Using the information gleaned from the text, write personal vision and mission statements that includes at least two to three professional goals. Write these out on paper or use a computer to create a Goals Evaluation for your own career pursuits.

2. Take the **Professional Savvy™ Career Development Assessment Test** to determine your relevant skills and expertise and career satisfaction in your current position(s) and determine future opportunities in your career. If you do not have a current opportunity to consider, use the table to evaluate a past job offer, internship or rotation in your clinical studies, a scholarship offer, a volunteer opportunity or a meeting that you have attended.

3. Review and take the **Professional Savvy™ Annual Career Development Plan** to determine your vision for the future, personal mission statement for the year, skills assessment and goals and objectives you want to achieve for the year.

Figure 6.1. Professional Savvy™ Dental Hygiene Student Career Development Assessment Test

PROFESSIONAL
Savvy

DENTAL HYGIENE STUDENT
CAREER DEVELOPMENT ASSESSMENT TEST

Date: _____

I. Personal Information

1. How long have you been a dental hygiene student? _____

2. Have you ever practiced as a dental assistant? _____

II. Personal Skills Assessment

1. What are your relevant skills in dental hygiene?

_____

_____

_____

2. What education have you received?

_____

_____

_____

3. What credentials do you hold?

_____

_____

_____

4. What experience and training have you developed as a dental hygiene student that make you unique?

_____

_____

_____

1 / 3

III. Career Assessment & Satisfaction

1. Are you currently employed in a position in dentistry?

Yes _____ No _____

If yes, what position are you currently in?

_____

If no, what type of position would you aspire to be in? [Please specify.]

_____

What are you looking for to be happy and/or satisfied in a future position?

_____
_____
_____

2. Does satisfaction in your work environment involve additional training or education?

Yes _____ [Please explain what is required.]

_____
_____
_____

No _____

IV. Next Steps

1. What next steps do I need to take place to achieve career happiness and success?

a. What additional education do I need?

_____
_____
_____

b. What additional training and certification do I need?

_____
_____
_____

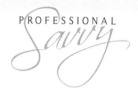

c. Are there any colleagues or mentors that I could work with to continue to achieve career happiness and success?

_____

_____

_____

d. Is there anything else I can do to achieve career success?

_____

_____

_____

e. Is there any opportunity you would be interested in pursuing in the next two years?

_____

_____

_____

3 / 3

Figure 6.2. Professional Savvy™ Dental Hygiene Student Annual Career Development Plan

PROFESSIONAL
Savvy

DENTAL HYGIENE STUDENT
ANNUAL CAREER DEVELOPMENT PLAN

Date: _____

I. Your Vision

1. What vision do you have in your dental hygiene career in the next year?

_____

_____

_____

II. Current Employment Position

1. Do you have a position in the dental profession?

   Yes _____ [Continue]   No _____ [Continue to Question 5]

_____

_____

_____

2. What led you to this current position?

_____

_____

_____

3. Is this current position the ideal position you would like to be working in the dental hygiene profession?   Yes _____   No _____

   If no, why isn't your current position your ideal position?

_____

_____

_____

4. What would your ideal position be in the dental hygiene profession?

_____

_____

_____

1 / 6

PROFESSIONAL
Savvy

5. If you currently do not have a position in the dental profession, what type of practice would you like to work in?

_____

_____

_____

III. Personal Skills Assessment

1. What are your relevant skills in dental hygiene?

_____

_____

_____

2. What is your educational background?

_____

_____

_____

3. What experience and training have you developed in your career as a dental hygiene student?

_____

_____

_____

4. What experience and training have you developed as a dental hygienist that makes you unique?

_____

_____

_____

2 / 6

PROFESSIONAL
Savvy

IV. Goals & Objectives for Current Position

1. What goals do I need to accomplish for my current position?

Goal: _____

_____

Goal: _____

_____

2. Prioritize the goals above.

Goal 1: _____

_____

Goal 2: _____

_____

3. What objectives need to be accomplished to help me achieve my goals?

Goal 1, Objective 1: _____

_____

Goal 1, Objective 2: _____

_____

Goal 2, Objective 1: _____

_____

Goal 2, Objective 2: _____

_____

4. What is the timeline for completion of each of the goals and objectives?

Goal 1, Objective 1: _____

_____

Goal 1, Objective 2: _____

_____

Goal 2, Objective 1: _____

_____

Goal 2, Objective 2: _____

_____

3 / 6

PROFESSIONAL
Savvy

V. Current Job Satisfaction

1. List the likes of your current position.

_____
_____
_____

2. List the dislikes of your current position.

_____
_____
_____

3. Identify how your dislikes may be enhanced to likes in your current position.

_____
_____
_____

4. Identify the time it will take to improve the dislikes to become likes.

_____
_____
_____

5. How will these likes and dislikes impact your future career vision?

_____
_____
_____

VI. Your Next Position

1. Do you have another position that you aspire to achieve in the next year of your dental hygiene career? [Please specify.]

_____
_____
_____

4 / 6

2. Is this position attainable in the next year?

Yes _____ No _____ [Continue]

If no, please explain why it isn't achievable in the next year.

_____

_____

_____

VII. Future Skills Assessment

1. What skills do I need to develop to achieve my future goals and objectives?

_____

_____

_____

2. Do I need further education or attend courses for my current position or to achieve my next position within dental hygiene?

Yes _____[List below.] No _____

_____

_____

_____

3. Do I need any additional training or certification for my current position or my next position within the dental hygiene profession?

Yes _____ [List below.] No _____

_____

_____

_____

VIII. Networking Strategies

1. Do I know someone who is in the position I am interested in pursuing for my next position in dental hygiene?

Yes _____ No _____

5 / 6

If yes, who is this person and how do I contact them?

_____

If no, how can I find the person who is in this position to contact?

_____

2. Are there any of my professional contacts who might assist me (i.e. past professors, associates, mentors or colleagues)? [Please list below.]

_____
_____
_____

3. If you are successful in finding the contact, determine how you will set up a meeting via phone or a personal interview.

_____
_____
_____

4. What professional organizations am I a member of or can I become a member of and learn about their Web sites? How they can help me network with other dental hygiene colleagues?

_____
_____
_____

6 / 6

Figure 6.3. Professional Savvy™ Dental Hygienist Career Development Assessment Test

PROFESSIONAL
Savvy

DENTAL HYGIENIST
CAREER DEVELOPMENT ASSESSMENT TEST

Date: _____

I. Personal Information

1. How long have you been a dental hygienist? _____

2. How many years have you practiced as a dental hygienist? _____

II. Personal Skills Assessment

1. What are your relevant skills in dental hygiene?

_____

_____

_____

2. What education have you received?

_____

_____

_____

3. What credentials do you hold?

_____

_____

_____

4. What experience and training have you developed as a dental hygienist that make you unique?

_____

_____

_____

PROFESSIONAL *Savvy*

III. Career Assessment & Satisfaction

1. In what position are you currently employed? [Please specify.]

_____

_____

_____

2. Are you happy and/or satisfied in your current position?

Yes _____ [Skip to Question 4]

No _____ [Continue]

If no, please explain why you are not happy or satisfied in your current position(s).

_____

_____

_____

3. What changes would you make to consider being happy and/or satisfied in your current position(s)? [Please explain in detail.]

_____

_____

_____

4. Does satisfaction in your work environment involve additional training or education?

Yes _____ [Please explain what is required.]

_____

_____

_____

No _____

5. Will you continue to work in this position for the next year?

Yes _____

No _____ [Please explain why.]

_____

_____

_____

IV. Next Steps

1. What next steps do I need to take place to achieve career happiness and success?

a. What additional education do I need?

_____
_____
_____

b. What additional training and certification do I need?

_____
_____
_____

c. Are there any colleagues or mentors that I could work with to continue to achieve career happiness and success?

_____
_____
_____

d. Is there anything else I can do to achieve career success?

_____
_____
_____

e. Is there any opportunity you would be interested in pursuing in the next two years?

_____
_____
_____

Figure 6.4. Professional Savvy™ Dental Hygienist Annual Career Development Plan

PROFESSIONAL
Savvy

DENTAL HYGIENIST
ANNUAL CAREER DEVELOPMENT PLAN

Date: _____

I. Your Vision

1. What is the vision for your dental hygiene career in the next year?

_____

_____

_____

II. Current Employment Position

1. What is your current position in the dental hygiene profession?

_____

_____

_____

2. What led you to this current position?

_____

_____

_____

3. Is this current position the ideal position you would like to be working in the dental hygiene profession?   Yes _____   No _____

If no, why isn't your current position your ideal position?

_____

_____

_____

4. What would your ideal position be in the dental hygiene profession?

_____

_____

_____

1 / 6

PROFESSIONAL

III. Personal Skills Assessment

1. What are your relevant skills in dental hygiene?

_____
_____
_____

2. What is your educational background?

_____
_____
_____

3. What experience and training have you developed in your career as a dental hygiene professional?

_____
_____
_____

4. What experience and training have you developed as a dental hygienist that makes you unique?

_____
_____
_____

IV. Goals & Objectives for Current Position

1. What goals do I need to accomplish for my current position?

Goal: _____
_____

Goal: _____
_____

2. Prioritize the goals above.

Goal 1: _____

_____

Goal 2: _____

_____

3. What objectives need to be accomplished to help me achieve my goals?

Goal 1, Objective 1: _____

_____

Goal 1, Objective 2: _____

_____

Goal 2, Objective 1: _____

_____

Goal 2, Objective 2: _____

_____

4. What is the timeline for completion of each of the goals and objectives?

Goal 1, Objective 1: _____

_____

Goal 1, Objective 2: _____

_____

Goal 2, Objective 1: _____

_____

Goal 2, Objective 2: _____

_____

V. Current Job Satisfaction

1. List the likes of your current position.

_____

_____

_____

PROFESSIONAL
Savvy

2. List the dislikes of your current position.

_____

_____

_____

3. Identify how your dislikes may be enhanced to likes in your current position.

_____

_____

_____

4. Identify the time it will take to improve the dislikes to become likes.

_____

_____

_____

5. How will these likes and dislikes impact your future career vision?

_____

_____

_____

VI. Your Next Position

1. Do you have another position that you aspire to achieve in the next year of your dental hygiene career? [Please specify.]

_____

_____

_____

2. Is this position attainable in the next year?

Yes _____   No _____ [Continue]

If no, please explain why it isn't achievable in the next year.

_____

_____

_____

4 / 6

VII. Future Skills Assessment

1. What skills do I need to develop to achieve my future goals and objectives?

_____
_____
_____

2. Do I need further education or attend courses for my current position or to achieve my next position within dental hygiene?

Yes _____[List below.]   No _____

_____
_____
_____

3. Do I need any additional training or certification for my current position or my next position within the dental hygiene profession?

Yes _____ [List below.]   No _____

_____
_____
_____

VIII. Networking Strategies

1. Do I know someone who is in the position I am interested in pursuing for my next position in dental hygiene?

Yes _____   No _____

If yes, who is this person and how do I contact them?

_____

If no, how can I find the person who is in this position to contact?

_____

5 / 6

2. Are there any of my professional contacts who might assist me (i.e. past professors, associates, mentors or colleagues)? [Please list below]

_____
_____
_____

3. If you are successful in finding the contact, determine how you will set up a meeting via phone or a personal interview.

_____
_____
_____

4. What professional organizations am I a member of or can I become a member of and learn about their Web sites? How can they help me network with other dental hygiene colleagues?

_____
_____
_____

Key Concepts

1. Dental hygiene professionals should create a one – or two-sentence personal vision statement that should include a motivation for developing meaning and purpose in their careers and a direction that will enhance personal growth.

2. Dental hygiene professionals should create a one – or two-sentence personal mission statement that should include goals and objectives to direct their daily activities.

3. Dental hygienists should define at least two to three goals and objectives that they need to accomplish in order to achieve their personal mission and vision statements.

4. Unhappiness with salary increases, a stagnant level of responsibility in the practice, lack of appreciation for the dental hygienist's expertise in the practice by team members and continuing team conflict are triggers for job dissatisfaction. Dental hygienists should record a moment of job dissatisfaction, why it occurred, what can be done to change it, and if they are willing to change it.

5. Minor job dissatisfactions frequently cloud feelings of career satisfaction. Professionals need to evaluate their current career path and key elements of it to determine their level of job satisfaction.

6. To achieve success in a dental hygiene career, a career goals development plan should be completed each year to determine short-, medium-, and long-term career goals and objectives.

7. A career goals development plan is achievable for professionals who take the time to analyze what their goals and objectives are in their professional careers.

Chapter 7: Searching for the Right Dental Hygiene Position

By Christine A. Hovliaras, RDH, BS, MBA, CDE

Learning Objectives

The student dental hygienist and the dental hygiene professional will learn the following key objectives from this chapter:

1. Distinguish resources and relationships they have through a continual process of research.
2. Identify elements of their personal life that shape their job search and career.
3. Determine if their current job is the right job for them at this time in their career.
4. Develop networking opportunities.
5. List the mentors who could assist them in the job search process to launch their professional career.

Overview

Searching for the right dental hygiene position begins with organization and preparation. Creating opportunity for oneself is a matter of identifying and continuing to develop the resources and relationships that meet the career goals and objectives already established.

Matt is a dental hygienist who has worked in the profession for six years in the same dental practice. He is pleased with his current position, yet he knows that with two other more experienced dental hygienists on staff, who are eight and ten years older than he, the possibility of promotion or expansion of his responsibilities is limited. His dental hygiene school contacts are not as current as they once were; he hasn't touched base with anyone for the past two years. He wonders how he can improve his career outlook. He considers a job search, but wonders how to begin one while working full time.

Many job searches end before they begin. If career planners are employed or do not face a financial burden, it is difficult to find time and motivation to search for a new position – even if their current position has multiple unpleasant elements in it. Beginning a job search is a monumental task whether the seeker is a new graduate, a seasoned professional, employed or unemployed.

The job applicant must be organized, readily prepared and optimistic throughout the duration of his or her entire job search. Career placement specialists project that job seekers can expect to add six months of searching for every $10,000 increment in their salary. While this outdated formula may seem overwhelming, know that some companies, dental practices and universities may create an opportunity when the right candidate becomes available. A job seeker with the right credentials may only send out one resume. However, if that seeker wants to create plenty of options from which to choose, it is a good idea to begin by contacting several well researched potential employers.

How Do You Start?

The best approach is to keep all resources, research and relationships in top form. These terms refer to the career planners' preparedness to act on new opportunities.

- **Resources** are the wide range of information about professions, companies and institutions and the job market in general.
- **Research** is necessary to help narrow down the possibilities to best fit the job seeker's talents, education and career goals.
- **Relationships** represent the human factor: the **networking** connections an individual has that might lead to an opportunity. Networking connections are the people the job seeker knows through others who might have needed information to make career-related decisions.

Resources and Research: Online and Off

The days of pounding the pavement and walking into dental or specialty practices to present a resume in person are in the past. Technological resources offer job seekers a wonderful tool for easily gathering information in one location. One click offers employment opportunities from the comfort of home, a local coffee shop or library.

Options in the dental hygiene field will lead the job seeker to a number of physical and virtual libraries, from the local public library to one located within a dental hygiene school or those found online through private entities.

Organizations such as American Dental Hygienists' Association (ADHA) Career Placement site at http://www.adha.org/careerinfo/dhcareers.htm and dental hygienists' state or local association, also offer job seekers information about job opportunities. Other online resources also are available through dental hygiene job posting sites such as Dental Workers at www.dentalworkers.com and Dental Jobs at http://www.dentaljobs.net, which connect job seekers with information about job opportunities available for potential employers. Professionals may want to contact their alma mater for job opportunities that may be offered.

To keep current with **contacts**, meaning the people who have first-hand knowledge of a professional, his or her work style, personality and work ethic, dental hygiene program graduates should return to their alma mater to look for a job first, and then seek out a few employment and other Internet sites next. Depending on the type of position (i.e., clinical, education, public health, research, administrative, advocate and corporation, etc.), dental hygienists may want to use online resources to locate a potential employer's website to learn more about the organization, its patients, staff and the typical procedures performed there. If dental hygienists are seeking positions in education, it is wise to visit educational institution websites, public health organizations within the job seeker's state and research facilities or educational institutions where research is being conducted.

While conducting research and compiling a list of resources, it is helpful to organize them into a simple reference table, such as Table 7.1, Resource Opportunities, found on pages 174-175. This gives job seekers an easy method of tracking their actions and progress. Such a table can be printed out for reference and can be stored in a personal or laptop computer for more convenient updating.

Table 7.1. Resource Opportunities

RESOURCE	CONTACTED
Professional Association Resources	
American Dental Hygienists' Association 444 North Michigan Avenue, Suite 3400 Chicago, IL 60611 Phone: 312-440-8900 Web site: www.adha.org	1/3/12: Emailed to register for annual session
Arizona State Dental Hygienists' Association 2415 E. Camelback, Suite 700 Phoenix, AZ 85016 Phone: 602-254-7210 Email: zrdh@msn.com	1/3/11: Called to register for CEU course 1/10/12: 1 p.m. CEU course at City University 2/10/12: Monthly networking session
Online Resources	
Job Placement Web sites for Dental Professionals **Dental Workers** www.dentalworkers.com **Dental Jobs** www.dentaljobs.net **RDH Jobs** www.rdhjobs.com **Dental Power** www.dentalpower.com	1/7/12: Reviewed resume with Jenny Collins
Job Placement Web Sites **Beyond** www.beyond.com **Career Builder** www.careerbuilder.com **Career City** www.careercity.com **Connect Careers** www.connectcareers.com **Headhunter** www.headhunter.com **Hot Jobs** www.hotjobs.com **Monster** www.monster.com **Job Hunt** www.job-hunt.com **Simply Hired** www.simplyhired.com **The Ladders** www.theladders.com	5/12/11: upload resume to site 5/16/11-5/18/11: answer three emails from auto response
Universities	
University of Missouri Kansas City Department of Alumni Affairs www.umkc.edu/advancement/Alumni_Association/aa_staff.asp **New York University** New York University School of Dental Medicine www.nyu.edu/dental	1/7/12: review job postings

Industry

Colgate Professional
www.colgateprofessional.com

GlaxoSmithKline
www.gsk.com

Johnson & Johnson
www.jjdentalprofessional.com

Procter & Gamble
www.dentalcare.com

WaterPik
www.professional.waterpik.com

Things to Consider in Looking for the Right Job

There are a number of considerations for career planners to keep in mind as they conduct employment research. While these could be regarded as limitations, it is better to think of them as guidelines for narrowing down a field ripe with opportunity.

These considerations include, but are not limited to:
- Goals for the next one to three years;
- Time and money investments needed to pursue a particular work area; and
- The type of schedule that suits one's life and personal career goals.

Goals should have been established at the end of Chapter 6. The career planner also should have assessed their time and money investment, as well as the schedule considerations, including the decision to work full or part time. Is the job candidate a part – time student? Are there childcare considerations that involve money and scheduling issues? These are aspects that need to factor into one's decision making.

If a job seeker's personal plan requires them to seek continued education, consider student loans or other educational funding such as grants and/or scholarships. This will help ease current financial obligations. Most educational institutions provide help in linking students with resources.

Next, career planners should consider what time they have available for taking classes. Those interested in continued education should speak with their employer about flexible schedules or part-time work during the time they will be going to school. Prospective students should also consider their personal motivation toward taking classes. Organizing work and school requires focused attention and strong organizational skills or knowing where to turn for help in strengthening these two areas. For those who require this type of help, contact the educational institution of choice for student counseling services. These programs frequently offer classes in how to become an effective student before one actually begins attending curriculum courses.

As career planners mull over potential openings or organizations of interest, they should consider if there is an area of the country in which they would want to work. If time and money investment are limited, consider local openings. Those with greater financial flexibility might have the luxury of choosing a location and beginning a job search there. However, do not forget to factor in relocation costs into the money investment part of planning.

Is Your Current Job The Right Job?

It might become apparent through completing assessment exercises, that the career planner already has the right job. The process of analyzing the position on paper may be all one needs to realize what its many advantages are. At this point consider:

- *Is my current job the right job for me?*
- *Am I content in this position?*
- *If yes, why is this the right position for me?*
- *If not, how can I achieve contentment in this position?*
- *Should I leave the job for another position?*
- *Do I feel I am receiving adequate benefits (medical/dental, vacation, sick leave, continuing education reimbursement, membership paid at ADHA, uniform allowance, meeting attendance, etc.) in this full-time position?*
- *Are there other opportunities I need to enhance my position?*

What a wonderful revelation career planners discover if they find they are already in the perfect position! If the planner knows this already, it is important to continue to develop professionally. It is at this point that the relationships the career planners form through networking among their professional peers can be an asset.

Relationships: Networking Opportunities

Whether the job candidate is a student or seasoned dental hygiene professional, the course of a single day offers numerous encounters with potential contacts. From patients to sales representatives to colleagues, everyone job seekers encounter represents a wide range of connection points for new opportunity. How does one prepare to act on something new? It depends on how much preparation that person has put into career planning.

To ensure preparedness for chance encounters, career planners should have an electronic version of their resumes on file at all times. It is important to update career information on an annual basis or any time that career facts are altered or added to the resume, which may include following:

- Completing a continuing education course;
- Completing a degree program;
- Changing jobs;
- Adding a part-time position to a work schedule; or
- Adding volunteer work to a work schedule that is germane to career plans.

Another idea is to have personal business cards printed and available in purse or wallet for easy distribution. Such cards are convenient tools when one attends educational seminars, association meetings or other gatherings where many colleagues will be present. These cards should include one's current address, telephone, email address and fax machine. Include daytime or work-hours telephone or cellular number only if the current employer does not mind if the occasional personal call.

Job seekers who do not want to rely on a chance encounter to advance their career options should seek out individuals who are in a position in which they have an interest. Contact these individuals for a brief informational telephone interview about their position, or suggest a lunch meeting to discuss it in person.

The best way to communicate job search intentions to a networking list is for career planners to describe what they are seeking. With preparation, dental hygienists can easily summarize their career goals and objectives for helpful networking contacts. Clinicians can seek out online career forums for employment ideas if they still need some guidance to refine goals.

Another good idea is to develop a simple table, such as Table 7.2, Networking Opportunities, below, that will place contacts into categories, while providing an easy method to record the latest contact date with that person.

Table 7.2. Networking Opportunities

RESOURCE	CONTACTED
Professional Contacts	
Professor Jones Phone: 123-555-7890	1/3/12
Dean Sturdivant Phone: 999-313-1234	1/3/12
Oral Health Care Sales Consultants	
Jane Smith Proctor & Gamble Phone: 234-555-8910	2/3/12
Joe Johnson Colgate Oral Pharmaceuticals Phone: 212-310-2007	2/2/12
Ron Jones Johnson & Johnson Phone: 973-385-7000	1/7/12
Community Contacts	
Tom Thompson City Chamber of Commerce Phone: 456-555-7890	2/10/12
ADHA Contacts	
Dawn Amaskane Manager of Meetings & Conventions Phone: 312-440-8903	2/9/12
Patient Contacts	
Dan James Citywide Hospital Phone: 678-555-9101	2/8/12

Utilizing a Mentor

A job search cannot be conducted alone. Because it is impossible to know everyone's connections in the profession, job seekers must employ everyone on their networking list, particularly mentors. Mentors offer perspective on dental hygiene positions and on the individual's personal work style that he or she might not see. Mentors may have connections beyond what their mentees have, resources they may not have considered and a point of view that the mentees need to launch and sustain a successful job search.

Mentors can introduce job seekers to networking contacts who hold positions in which they have interest and who may influence their job search. In addition, mentors can provide an educational assessment if further educational opportunities are needed to continue to develop lifelong learning. A mentor may also assist in further skill development such as writing, teaching, conducting research in the university or in the community.

Critical Thinking Exercises

1. Develop a resource table using the example from the chapter. Include organizations and websites you frequently consult with for career development. Track your progress over the course of a month

2. Develop a networking table using the example from the chapter. Include individuals you frequently consult for advice and career development. Also include anyone with whom you intend to build a relationship and track your progress in establishing that.

Key Concepts

1. Dental hygienists need to identify the key resources for career development to determine their next opportunity or position in the dental hygiene profession.

2. Job seekers need an organized method for logging resources and tracking the contact they make with that resource.

3. Dental hygienists should establish a diverse network of individuals with whom they can consult for assistance and advice in career planning.

4. Consider career goals, location and time and money resources during the research phase of the job search, using these elements to narrow the scope of the search.

5. Dental hygienists need an organized list of networking contacts and should track when and why they interact with those contacts.

6. Mentors offer perspective on job search opportunities that the job seeker might otherwise overlook.

Chapter 8: Career Tools

By Christine A. Hovliaras, RDH, BS, MBA, CDE

Learning Objectives

The student dental hygienist and the dental hygiene professional will learn the following key objectives from this chapter:

1. Examine the appropriate career tools to write, revise, maintain and update each year.
2. Develop a format for unique cover letters that introduce you to prospective employers.
3. Create a resume that best positions your expertise, qualifications and accomplishments.
4. Learn how to expand your resume as your career grows and your qualifications and accomplishments are developed and enhanced.
5. Understand when and why you should create curriculum vitae.
6. Create a professional portfolio to include any achievements, special qualifications, presentations and/or honors received while in school or during your career.
7. Build a list of references and seek recommendations to support your qualifications.
8. Develop follow up communication pieces to support your job search.
9. Track your accomplishments and update your career tools so that you are always prepared.
10. Create a professional electronic portfolio to put your accomplishments on display to show other dental professionals.

Overview

After assessing the research, resources and relationships to help support a job search, the job seeker must turn to the career tools that put qualifications, education and accomplishments in writing. These tools include the cover letter, resume or curriculum vitae, a typed list of references or letters of recommendation, follow up thank-you letters and potentially a professional portfolio. The key to maintaining the career planners' ability to advance as opportunities arise lies in an annual update of their career tools.

Building a career is similar to any other construction project: It requires a set of the appropriate tools. Whether job seekers are seeking their first job or tenth, they should be armed with the best precision tools available. In the age of computer technology, no one should lack a well designed cover letter, resume or curriculum vitae (CV).

Contemporary and traditional design templates for cover letters and resumes are available within most word-processing programs on today's computers. A quick browse on the Internet reveals even more elaborate designs, however, a black-and-white version printed on white or ivory bonded paper works well for job seekers of all levels of experience. Career-planning professionals observe that a too-clever design detracts from the applicant's qualifications. Unless a job seeker is searching in the graphic arts field, a standard style is a good choice.

The Cover Letter

Never send a resume by itself. The resume's faithful traveling companion is the perfectly edited, spell-checked and tailored-made cover letter, which introduces the job candidate and shares a bit of that applicant's philosophy about and qualifications for the position.

The cover letter is the applicant's first contact with a prospective employer. It provides the proper introduction for the resume and markets the job seeker's skills and qualifications to the prospective employer. Even in this age of technology where one might submit a resume electronically, the job candidate should do so with an email message that captures the formal introductory spirit of a cover letter.

Use the cover letter to establish a positive tone. It should not discuss salary information. While cover letters reflect the familiar format of a business letter and graphic design of the resume, the cover letter should be adapted when applying for different positions – even if those positions have the same title. For example, refer to Cover Letter 1, Seasoned Dental Hygiene Professional of Deborah Cole, RDH, BS, which is a letter to a Head Start Program.

DEBORAH COLE, RDH, BS
456 NEW PARK
HACKENSACK, NJ 07601

February 3, 2012

Ms. Dina Purcillo
Head Start of New Jersey
XYZ Lane
Anytown, New Jersey 60123

Dear Ms. Purcillo:

I am writing in regard to the position listed in the *Bergen Record* seeking a dental hygiene position in the Head Start Program in Teaneck, New Jersey.

My credentials would be an excellent fit for this position as I am a registered dental hygienist practicing for Dr. Jeff Miller of Gentle Smiles, and I love working with children. After receiving my bachelor's degree in early childhood development, I worked as a first grade teacher and later pursued dental hygiene as my next career. I am very interested in working in the public health setting with children to improve their oral health by preventing dental caries and offering preventive services.

I can be reached during the day at 275-567-1347 and I look forward to speaking with you soon.

Thank you for your time.

Sincerely,

Deborah Cole, RDH, BS

If the next lead in Deborah Cole's job search is an educator position at a university, she might highlight her bachelor's degree in education in that cover letter. See Cover Letter 2, Seasoned Dental Hygiene Professional.

DEBORAH COLE, RDH, BS
456 NEW PARK
HACKENSACK, NJ 07601

February 3, 2012

Jonathan Stone
New York University College of Dentistry
345 East 24th Street
New York, NY 10010

Dear Mr. Stone:

I am interested in the faculty position in the Department of Dental Hygiene at New York University that I saw in the fall edition of the *New York University Newsletter*. I have completed my Bachelor of Education degree and received my Bachelor of Science degree in Dental Hygiene. My passion is education, and I absolutely love teaching and working with dental hygiene students. I have enclosed my resume with this cover letter for your review.

I am currently practicing part time in an aesthetic dentistry office and am working part time in the dental hygiene clinic at Bergen Community College. I am very interested in pursuing a full- time position in dental hygiene education at New York University.

I can be reached during the day at 275-567-1347 and I look forward to speaking with you shortly.

Thank you for your time and assistance.

Sincerely,

Deborah Cole, RDH, BS

Deborah Cole shared that she has done some research regarding the institution, and indicated both past and present experience.

How fortunate for Deborah that her teaching career dovetails nicely with many aspects of dental hygiene. What if her previous career path had been as a florist? Then she should look for the career generalities that each career path must share: enjoy working with the public; help people find solutions tailored to their individual needs; act as educators in a subject most people do not understand; and direct the consumer's attention to new trends in the field. It might be a bit of a stretch, but Deborah's education in dental hygiene should make up the difference.

The chief marketing tool of any job search is the resume. It is the advertisement of who the applicant is, what his or her level of competence is and how the individual's accomplishments and experiences unfold. Resumes typically take one of three formats:

- **Chronological:** Listing the job seeker's primary work experience in order by date of employment (most recent to least recent).
- **Functional:** Listing the job seeker's primary skills sets and accomplishments.
- **Chronological/Functional Combined:** A combination of both strategies; by date and accomplishment.

For further information regarding what should be included in a resume, see Table 8.1.

Table 8.1.

A resume IS NOT:	A resume IS:
• A laundry list of responsibilities for the positions one has held	• A listing of accomplishments that are measurable examples of the job seeker's work experience
• A compilation of personal information	• A directory of career data
• A 10-page booklet detailing every job the applicant has held since high school	• Should not be more than two pages and should follow a classic format using a legible typeface
• To be sent out in a moment's notice after it has not been touched for 10 years	• Carefully proofread, spell-checked and distributed among the job seeker's most detail-oriented friends, associates and mentors before it is mailed, placed in the portfolio or posted on the Internet

Other key aspects of resume writing to remember:

- Job seekers should use keywords in their resume that reflect the areas of field in which they have interest, such as digital radiography or other new dental technology, community service work, evidence-based research, dental hygiene publications, dental diseases, oral health-systemic disease link, etc. Pick up these terms from the job opening resource. If an advertisement or other source mentions a need for proficiency in the latest dental hygiene technology and the job applicant has that skill, do not fail to mention it.
- Summarize education for those who have been out of school for a number of years, or for those who have been enrolled in several different educational institutions.

Resume Expansion with Career Growth

Certain aspects of the resume will appear on the document whether it is one for a dental hygiene student or a seasoned dental hygiene professional. These include basic contact information, a concise objective, professional experience, education received and awards or recognition. For students who lack a certain depth of work experience, it is easier to focus on academic achievement and then focus on any professional experience he or she may have received through clinical rotations or any type of community service activities in which he or she engaged to improve the oral health of their community (for reference, see Student Dental Hygienist Resume of Carl Rodriquez below).

Student Dental Hygienist Resume

CARL RODRIQUEZ, RDH
123 NEW WAY
LOS ANGELES, CA 90003
XXX-XXX-XXXX

Objective	To work in a state-of-the-art dental/cosmetic dental practice in Beverly Hills, California.
Education	Associate Degree in Dental Hygiene — June 2012 University of California San Francisco School of Dentistry San Francisco, CA
Professional Experience	Dental Assistant — 2006-Present Rhonda Mills, DMD, General Dentist, Berkeley, California Responsibilities included full mouth and bite wing radiographs, assist the dentist in dental procedures (i.e., restorations, aesthetics, prosthodontics), clean and sterilize instruments, provide infection control procedures between patients, set room up for patients being treated including tray set-up, and perform patient education when needed. Student Dental Hygienist — 2010-2012 Bright Horizons Preschool Program, Berkeley, California Student rotation - conducted intraoral and extraoral examinations, oral health education, application of fluoride varnish, and sealant placement when needed. Student Dental Hygienist — 2010-2012 University of California San Francisco School of Dentistry, Department of Dental Hygiene, San Francisco, CA Responsibilities included medical history assessment, intra/extra oral examination, vital signs, oral cancer screening, full mouth and bite wing radiographs, prophylaxis, fluoride application, and review of oral hygiene techniques.
Volunteer Experience	Give Kids a Smile Day, California — 2006-Present Worked with children in access-to-care populations and provided oral health education, fluoride varnish and sealant placement.
Professional Licensure	Dental Hygiene License in the State of: - California (Summer 2012)
Professional Organizations	American Dental Hygienists' Association, California Dental Hygienists' Association
References	Available upon request

More experienced dental hygiene professionals should categorize the type of dental/specialty offices in which they have worked and the type of job accomplishments they achieved. The professional should include the educational degrees received, state(s) in which he or she is licensed to practice, any type of community service activities in which he or she engaged to improve the oral health of their community (for reference, see Seasoned Dental Hygiene Professional Resume below).

Seasoned Dental Hygiene Professional Resume

DEBORAH COLE, RDH, BS
123 NEW PARK
HACKENSACK, NJ 07601
XXX-XXX-XXXX

Objective	To work as a dental hygiene educator in an astute and established university setting.
Professional Experience	Dental Hygienist 2003-Present Ira Green, DMD, General Dentist, Ridgewood, NJ Responsibilities included medical history assessment, intra/extra oral examination, vital signs, oral cancer screening, digital radiographies, oral prophylaxis, fluoride application, and review of oral hygiene techniques. Dental Hygiene Faculty Member 2004-Present Bergen Community College, Bergen, NJ Responsibilities include clinical education of first and second year students in clinic, teaching anatomy and physiology and preparing students for National Board Examinations. Kindergarten Teacher 1995-1999 Ridgewood Elementary School, Ridgewood, NJ Responsibilities included educating 20 kindergartens on vocabulary, spelling, reading, math for a 10-month period of time. Exercises included fun and exciting programs to gain the students interests.
Education	Bachelor of Science Degree in Dental Hygiene 2003 New York University, College of Dental Medicine, New York City, NY Associate Degree in Dental Hygiene 2001 New York University, College of Dental Medicine, New York City, NY Bachelor Degree in Education 1995 Fairleigh Dickinson University, Madison, NJ
Professional Licensure	Dental Hygiene License in the State of: - New Jersey, New York
Professional Organizations	American Dental Hygienists' Association, New Jersey Dental Hygienists' Association
Professional Honors	Honorary Member of Sigma Phi Alpha - 2007, Mentor of the Year Award - 2008
References	Available upon request

Curriculum Vitae

A curriculum vitae (CV) is a summation of an individual's educational and academic background as well as his or her teaching and research experience, publications, presentations, awards, honors, affiliations, continuing education information and other details. The CV is used mainly when applying for academic, education, scientific or research positions and also may be used to apply for fellowships or grants. A CV tends to be longer than a resume and includes more depth and detail. In Europe, the Middle East, Africa and Asia, the CV is the preferred tool for communicating a job candidate's background.[1]

Writing a CV requires a lot of attention. This is definitely a project in which to involve mentors – particularly those in teaching positions. Involve several mentors in reviewing the CV before sending it out. For further information regarding what should be included in a CV, see Table 8.2.

Table 8.2.

A Curriculum Vitae IS NOT:	A Curriculum Vitae IS:
• A single-version career tool	• Easily adaptable so the individual can have multiple versions that bring various elements of experience into focus depending on the type of position for which he or she is applying: research, education, grants, fellowships, etc
• Does not include personal information, a photo, salary history or references	• A summary of education, academic and work experience, as well as teaching and research experience, published articles, books and presentations, awards, honors and affiliations
• Full of abbreviations or slang	• Formal, with titles spelled out for easy identification
• Cluttered	• Clean and concise: It should painstakingly follow a consistent style (titles in bold, articles in quote marks, publications in italic, for example)

The CV is typically several pages long. The document follows a format that includes:
- Personal data
- Education
- Professional employment
- Teaching interests
- Teaching experience and development

- Professional experience and development
- Professional licensure
- Professional membership
- Professional courses attended
- Professional courses presented
- Community service
- University service (if applicable)
- Research and creative accomplishments
- Publications
- References (if applicable)

Professional Savvy, LLC, offers cover letter, resume and curriculum vitae writing services. Visit the Professional Savvy, LLC, website at www.professionalsavvychd.com.

References and Recommendations

Another important tool in the job hunting kit is the list of references and recommendations. Securing this can be a bit of a challenge in that sometimes the best resource for this information is someone whom the job seeker doesn't want to alert about a job search.

Rather than signaling one's current manager that her top employee is being considered for another position with a phone call from a prospective employer, it is better to use colleagues from past positions, or use a trusted friend within the current work place who is discreet and won't share pending plans around the office. The student has a distinct advantage in this area as everyone knows he or she will be moving into full-time employment!

Student dental hygienists however face the unique challenge of compiling references without actually having had a dental hygiene position. Students should utilize faculty as references for their clinical experiences and consider securing a letter of recommendation.

The letter of recommendation is a dated letter that may be mailed with the resume or presented during a job interview to a potential employer. An effective piece of communication for the new job seeker, the letter of recommendation should come from a recognizable authority figure (i.e., the dean of students, director of dental hygiene, or a professor from the student's college or university, or a supervisor from an internship or other position that relates to the one for which the applicant is applying). The letter should outline the applicant's general qualifications, reliable work ethic, excellent grades, awards, merits or other desirable characteristics.

The student may approach the intended writer of the letter in person or through some type of correspondence (i.e., email, business letter, etc.). When the student receives a letter of recommendation, he or she should write a letter, in turn, thanking the person for taking on the task of introducing the student. The student also needs to make certain that the contacts who provided the recommendation letter know that he or she is interviewing and may be contacted by a potential employer.

Likewise, when considering anyone to be a reference, job seekers should contact references, let them know of the seeker's intention to use them as a reference and, as a courtesy, ask their permission to do so. Those with many years of experience will want to touch base with anyone listed on their reference list before distributing it. It is a good idea to keep in touch with individuals on the reference list (see Chapter 7: Searching for the Right Dental Hygiene Position). A friendly phone call once a year keeps the connection current, offers a networking opportunity, and may be a source of job leads.

With a secured list of references, career planners should print those contacts on a separate sheet of matching paper stock that also coordinates with the design and typeface of the other job search pieces. On the resume itself, the list need only be referred to with a short sentence, "References available upon request." New and experienced job hunters should go to interviews with the list and present it when the potential employer asks for it.

A Professional Portfolio

A portfolio is a collection of the job seeker's experiences, presentations, writing samples (if applicable), certificates, listings of educational honors, merits, credentials, continuing education classes attended and the dates which the candidate attended them, letters of recommendation, and photos of professional activities. For both the student and the dental hygiene professional, the portfolio should also contain the resume. For the student, the portfolio can include pictures of the student working clinically, a list of patients treated during various educational rotations, a list of internships served and other student-oriented activities.

The information should be presented on matching or complementary stationery and can be contained in a plain, professional-looking binder or in a traditional artist's portfolio. The portfolio is an excellent method to present one's career experiences and qualifications, according to Hope-Claire Holbeck, RDH, MS, Chairperson of the Dental Auxiliaries Education Department at Middlesex Community College in Edison, NJ.

"From a professional health care point of view, we look at the portfolio as a collection of work or experiences that you have had," Holbeck said, adding that the portfolio gives a job seeker an opportunity to present greater detail than one could put into a resume.

"For me cover letters and resumes are very two-dimensional. The purpose of a cover letter is to pique the hiring manager's interest to get them to look at the resume. The purpose of the resume is to get you to the interview. These pieces show that you are qualified and that the hiring manager needs to investigate your qualifications. The use of the portfolio is to take it a step further," Holbeck continued. "It gives the potential employer more information about you that rounds you out and fleshes out this two-dimensional picture of your professional work. Resumes can have a sterile feeling."

Follow-up Communications

Like a firm handshake, making eye contact or waiting until another speaker is finished before talking, the follow-up letter and post-interview thank-you letter exhibit a professional's knowledge of common courtesy. It is part of sharing one's business etiquette and communication skills. Too many job seekers – both new and seasoned professionals – forget the important impression the follow up or post-interview thank-you letter leave. These both represent opportunities to re-state the mission of the job search, the key points established in early communication (particularly the job interview), and to input new information learned during the job interview. It is important to not be repetitive in either closing communication, but is a chance for the job applicant to creatively communicate another area of strength he or she would bring to the position. For example, job seekers may want to send follow-up letters regarding positions for which they have applied, but have not received either an invitation to interview or a rejection letter. For reference to this type of communication, see Follow-Up Letter – Seasoned Dental Hygiene Professional below.

Follow-Up Letter – Seasoned Dental Hygiene Professional

DIANE SMITH, RDH, BS
123 JANICE PLACE
HOBOKEN, NJ 07030

February 7, 2012

Dr. Larry Rosenfarb
Smile Experts
XYZ Lane
Anytown, NY 60123

Dear Dr. Rosenfarb:

I saw the dental hygiene position posted in the *New York Times* for the cosmetic practice in New York City highlighting this technology driven practice. I recently sent out my cover letter and resume for your review.

My experience working in an aesthetic dentistry office and at a university with assisting patients in whitening/bleaching techniques will be of importance for this position in your practice. I have worked with digital radiography, computerized charting and state-of-the-art appointment confirmation via email and texting and keep abreast of the latest technology in bleaching options and services.

I look forward to hearing from you and can be reached at 201-567-1347.

Thank you for your assistance.

Sincerely,

Diane Smith, RDH , BS

The post-interview thank-you letter might read like the Thank-you Note below.

Thank You Letter – Seasoned Dental Hygiene Professional

DEBORAH COLE, RDH, BS
123 NEW PARK
HACKENSACK, NJ 07601

February 8, 2012

Mr. Jonathan Stone
New York University College of Dental Medicine
XYZ Lane
Anytown, NY 60123

Dear Mr. Stone:

Thank you for the opportunity to interview for the position of Assistant Professor in the Department of Dental Hygiene at New York University College of Dental Medicine. I was very impressed with both the two- and four-year programs and the curriculum that has been established for these dental hygiene students.

My experience in education and working with a multitude of patients from young children through older clients has enabled me to work in many different capacities to diagnose oral diseases, assess restorative needs and periodontal treatment in order to keep these clients in a level of oral health and wellness.

It was a pleasure to meet you and I look forward to hearing from you shortly. I can be reached at 275-567-1347.

Thank you for your assistance.

Sincerely,

Deborah Cole, RDH, BS

This letter thanks the hiring manager, ties the position to the job seeker's experience, expresses enthusiasm for the position, and shares availability information. It answers the all-important questions:

- Why would the hiring manager consider this applicant?
- What would the applicant bring to the position?
- When is the applicant available to begin work?

Utilizing Career Tools to Get the Job

Timing is the important consideration in how these elements work together to secure a desired position. The cover letter and resume need to be presented as soon as the position is posted or as soon as the job applicant is made aware of the position. The follow-up letter should come at least a week after the resume and cover letter are received at the employer's location, if the job applicant has not received a call or other communication from the hiring manager for an interview. References and recommendations should be presented during the job interview, and the post-interview thank-you letter should be mailed the day after the interview. Delivery delays make the job applicant seem less interested, less motivate or less organized than other job applicants.

The Yearly Update and Tracking Accomplishments

A good end-of-the-year exercise, perhaps one to be scheduled for an hour or two during holiday time out of office, is to review existing career tools.

Consider the following:
- What responsibilities need to be updated?
- Did responsibilities expand this year?
- Was there a change in position altogether?
- What continuing education courses were taken?
- What other accomplishments, awards or recognition need to be added?

This task also could be scheduled before the time of an annual review. The point is to not let it become a five-year update. It is easy to forget key transitions in one's career or become overwhelmed and fail to update it all together. Career planners do not let an immediate opportunity find them with outdated career tools.

Career Tools in the Technological Age

Are any of the career tools relevant in the age of technology? Does a cover letter carry the same impact when it becomes an email message with a resume attached in an electronic file?

Many job postings currently offer an email address instead of a physical address or a telephone number. Job posting also frequently offer either generalized job responsibilities or highly specific tasks that might only apply to handful applicants. In spite of this, the traditional tools, a cover letter, resume and follow up communications, are still valid pieces of the job search. It's simply a matter that now job seekers need to have an electronic version of all the tools.

Taking that a step further, is what used to be the traditional portfolio.

Holbeck, at the suggestion of her college's information technology manager, took the traditional portfolio into the virtual world when she helped launch an electronic portfolio project that occurs in the final year of the dental hygiene students' education at Middlesex Community College. Through this program, students compile accomplishments and create a type of personal Internet page that is stored in a private, password-protected website hosted by the college.

Holbeck noted that students, in particular, have a difficult time with newspaper advertisements in the dental hygiene field. Many feature email addresses and few descriptions making it hard for students to know how to tailor their cover letters to suit the position. The e-portfolio allows students to present the full spectrum of their educational and volunteer experiences for this more vague inquiry for positions in dental hygiene.

Holbeck decided this was a great opportunity for students for a few reasons. When students graduate into entry level positions, they often feel they do not have enough experience to go with confidence into an interview.

"My first purpose was to make students realize the actual sum of the experiences they had in their dental hygiene education," said Holbeck. She commented that a student's accomplishment may include the variety of patient types whom the student may have attended, internships and extracurricular activities in which they participated, events the student attended, accolades, awards and scholarships.

"It helps them realize how qualified they are for interviews and positions in dental hygiene," Holbeck continued. "It gives them another tool to help them land a job."

She shared that the e-portfolio falls into a nice niche. "The way jobs are advertised today, the advertisement might read, 'send your CV'. You are usually emailing or mailing a CV, and they never really get to talk with you. What the e-portfolio does is let you put a link to your online e-portfolio into your cover letter," Holbeck noted. This link offers 24-7 access to the job seeker's qualifications.

"The student or professional can constantly upgrade it. It becomes a reservoir of the job seeker's accomplishments and experiences," Holbeck continued.

It also allows the dentist to review the full list of continuing education courses and the date attended. "That's normally a list you wouldn't give to an employer," Holbeck noted. The e-portfolio also shows the candidate as being more technologically savvy.

The e-portfolio's key elements are organized onto tabs – just as a typical web page might feature. These might include: an introductory page, academic samples, achievements, scholarships, professional goals the student is hoping to achieve, resume, work and internship experience, CPR certification, first aid qualifications or a radiology license. Another tab may include co-curricular activities: those things that don't relate to dental hygiene. Volunteer projects such as helping out at a homeless shelter or interesting aspects of the individual life – such as holding a black belt in Tae Kwon Do or being bi-lingual – could be organized here. Holbeck cautions job seekers to not include aspects of their life that are too far from easily recognized accomplishments, particularly any aspect of personal life which might be regarded as a work-place liability.

She enthusiastically endorses the e-portfolio program for her students and for seasoned professionals. "I think you will see more and more e-portfolios because we are working toward an all-electronic format," she commented. Given the time limitations of the average interview, and the possibility the candidate may not be invited to interview, an on-line link is highly preferable and gives the candidate a distinct advantage.

"It's a way to get into the technological age," Holbeck said. The rise of portable electronic devices give everyone continual access to the Internet and email. It is important to meet the potential employer in the time and space they have available.

"People are not tied to desks. If you have an e-portfolio online, you offer 24-hour access to your experience and credentials," she said, adding that dentistry no longer lags behind in the technology field anymore and hasn't for years.

"Graduates are so technologically savvy. There is a changing of the guard as the younger generation comes into the dental practice – this includes younger dentists hiring dental hygienists," Holbeck continued.

On a cautionary note, Holbeck advised students that an e-portfolio is not a Facebook or Twitter. It is a professional medium. She also advised students to be cautious of what other presence is attached to their name on the web.

"If you think potential employers are not 'Google-ing' your name, you are wrong. They are to see what comes up. You must be careful of what you have out there about you. An e-portfolio is private and tells the employer about your professional capabilities."

References

1. Doyle A. How to Write a Curriculum Vitae website page. Available at: http://jobsearch.about.com. Accessed: August 2008.

Critical Thinking Exercises

1. Using the text and the examples given, create a cover letter, resume and follow-up communication letter(s) for your job search. Create a curriculum vitae if it applies. You may design something for yourself, have a friend with a creative eye do it for you, or use a computer template.

2. Select two classmates to proofread and critique your completed cover letter, resume and follow-up communication letter(s) for your job search.

3. If you are a seasoned dental hygiene professional, update your resume at least once a year and include further education, training, certification and accomplishments you have achieved in it.

4. Select a mentor to proofread and critique your completed cover letter, resume and follow-up communication letter(s) for your job search. Evaluate these critiques and make necessary adjustments to your tools.

5. Compile all the elements you would want to include in a professional portfolio. Review both traditional and electronic portfolio formats and create a portfolio after deciding which will work best for your purposes.

Key Concepts

1. The cover letter is a unique communication piece used to introduce the job candidate and share that applicant's philosophy about and qualifications for the position and should be altered to suit each position for which the job seeker applies.

2. Resumes reveal who the job applicant is, what his or her level of competence is and how the individual's accomplishments and experiences unfold. Resumes may be formatted in chronological or functional order, or may be a combination of the two styles. Resumes need to expand as the individual's qualifications and accomplishments continue to grow.

3. A curriculum vitae (CV) is a summation of an individual's educational, academic or scientific background as well as his or her teaching and research experience, publications, presentations, awards, honors, affiliations and other significant contributions, and is used mainly when applying for academic, education, scientific or research positions and also may be used to apply for fellowships or grants.

4. A list of references for an experienced dental hygiene professional should include discreet co-workers, previous job managers and other professionals familiar with that person's work style.

5. A list of references for a student applying for a first job should include professors, internship and part-time position managers and any professionals familiar with the student's academic performance and work style. Students may want to have a reference write a formal letter of recommendation to introduce the student and his or her accomplishments.

6. A professional portfolio reveals the depth and breadth of a professional's or a student's experience. It should not include details that are too personal, but should be career-related and list co-curricular activities that make the job applicant appealing to the potential employer.

7. Follow-up communications should include thank-you letters to individuals with whom you have interviewed with for a position.

8. Professionals in dental hygiene should update resumes and/or curriculum vitae each year and know how to write an effective cover letter in order to secure an interview and then get the job.

Chapter 9: The Job Interview – Keys to a Win-Win Deal

By Christine A. Hovliaras, RDH, BS, MBA, CDE

Learning Objectives

The student dental hygienist and the dental hygiene professional will learn the following key objectives from this chapter:

1. Understand the significance of careful research when preparing for job interviews within dental/specialty practices, educational institutions, corporations and other organizations.

2. Identify and prepare for the six primary interview styles: screening interviews, traditional interviews, behavioral interviews, telephone interviews, panel interviews and working interviews.

3. Create a list of questions to ask of potential employers that suit the professional environment, whether it be private practice, a group dental practice, an educational institution, public health department or a corporate environment.

4. Develop an interview style that highlights your professional acumen and reveals aspects of your personality that suit the position for which you are interviewing.

5. Identify appropriate dress and behavior for the job interview that compliment your skills, achievements, talents and expertise.

Overview

A job interview is a stage production: It requires hours of preparation and rehearsals; it sometimes requires special costuming; it should be presented to an audience of helpful critics before it "opens" before a real crowd. If job seekers are not prepared, a job interview is like an opera singer taking the stage without having memorized the musical score or accompanying lyrics. This is the opportunity for the professional to "sing" his or her own praises in an orchestrated performance.

A single job posting opens a business' door for hundreds of applicants. The hiring manager must sort through these applicants to reduce the playing field to 20 to 30 face-to-face interviews. While many equally qualified candidates may interview for this single job opening, the one who secures the position is the competitor prepared to show that he or she has more to offer the employer than other applicants. While this may sound theatrical and intimidating, it is important to realize that the job interview is also a forum to examine the prospective employer and make certain the position is a good fit for both parties. Both the job interviewer and job applicant will try to seek the honest truth about each other. And both will present a positive image. How does one get to the truth?

The job applicant must complete some prior homework to ensure a successful interview. First, one needs to locate important information regarding the company, practice or organization with which he or she will be interviewing.

For the **dental practice**, the job seeker might want to determine:

- Number of years the practice has existed.
- Number of people employed by the practice, as well as what those individual's titles are and how many years each has been employed in the practice.
- Job responsibilities of the dental hygienist.
- Number of patients the dental hygienist treats per day (recare and periodontal therapy).
- Range of salary and benefits.
- How often regular staff meetings are held in order to communicate and discuss key office topics.

For a position in a **corporate setting**, find out:

- The philosophy, mission and goals of the company.
- Products manufactured by the company.
- New developments within the company.
- Sales and revenue.
- Number of employees.
- Dental professionals who work in the company.
- The nature of the position: is it new, existing, or has it been modified for this search from what it was before.

For any job, regardless of the setting, the job seeker will need to determine:

- In which department the position is.
- What are the roles and responsibilities of the position.
- To whom the position reports.
- If travel is required, what percentage of the new hire's time will be devoted to travel salary (type of).
- Sign-on bonus (if required).
- Benefits (vacation, sick days, holidays, medical/dental insurance, stock options, retirement plan).
- The average number of years other employees have been with the organization.

It is a good idea for job seekers to find someone who has or is working for the potential employer in which they have an interest to get an idea of the internal practices of the organization. Belonging to a professional association offers the notable advantage of providing dental hygiene professionals with networking exposure to other dental hygiene colleagues across the country. Networking at meetings and events ensures an expanded and diverse calling list when the job seeker needs information about other businesses. To get access to a similar network, the job seeker might also call a placement agency in the dental hygiene field to find someone who has worked for a particular organization or an employee who has left the position or is currently working in the same department.

For dental practice interviews, the job applicant may want to conduct an Internet search on the employer to gain a better understanding of the credentials and expertise he/she may have. An employee or former employee of the practice could share about their experience working in that office.

Preparation for the actual interview may begin with a visit to the library or book retailer, or might include a search of the Internet for sample interview questions. Anticipating what might be asked during job interviews has become an art form. Many books and websites offer lengthy lists of job interview questions and how to shape an answer to avoid giving the wrong impression.

The types of questions the job seeker will encounter depend on the style of interview being used.

The basic list of interview types include: screening, traditional, behavioral, telephone, case, working and panel, and may include any combination of these types.

Screening interviews are typically the first phase of interviewing. Conducted by hiring managers or even outside human resources counselors, screening interviews are designed to save time for the final decision maker. These interviews are shorter, cover broader aspects of the applicant's background and may be conducted by someone farther down the chain of command than the eventual direct supervisor. A screening interview may be conducted over the telephone. Typically, a second interview is arranged on a different date. In some instances, a screening interview will be conducted by the human resource manager and another interviewer on the same day.

Questions used during a screening interview might include:
1. Tell me about your past experience.
2. I see you work at Company XYZ or for a doctor. Are you still employed there? How does your background suit the requirements for this position?
3. Tell me why you are looking for other employment.
4. What are your future educational goals?
5. Are you willing to relocate?

Traditional interviews also rely on general, **open-ended questions** that require more than a "yes" or "no" answer. These interviews gauge the job applicant's overall presentation and ability to communicate, as well as if the applicant has the skill set and enthusiasm for the position. The questions asked during a traditional interview help the manager measure how well this person will fit into their organization.
In a traditional interview, the hiring manager may ask questions such as:
1. Tell me something about yourself.
2. Tell me why you are right for this position.
3. What are your strengths that you bring to this position? How could this benefit the position for which you are applying?
4. Are there any challenges that you have faced in a previous position? If so, how did you handle this challenge(s)?
5. Tell me where you see yourself in 10 years.
6. If you had a conflict with a co-worker, what would you do about it?

In some cases, when the job applicant and the prospective business are separated by many miles, a **telephone interview** makes the best use of everyone's time. The same preparation is required for this type of interview as for a face-to-face encounter. For the actual telephone call, one should conduct the interview in a quiet room, where he or she can concentrate and take notes without interruption. Applicants should be cautious not to fill in the silences in conversation, but allow space in the dialogue for thoughtful pauses. Sometimes an interviewer will use these pauses to test the interviewee's reaction. Instead of a rambling response, give one that is concise and follow it up with a related question.

Other interview types require even more careful preparation. **Behavioral interviews,** for example, gauge what the applicant's future performance might be by comparing that with his or her past performance in certain situations. The interviewer may pose questions such as, "Share a time when you faced an unexpected problem," or "Describe how you manage several patient visits that begin to overlap."

In advance of the behavioral interview, applicants should prepare scenarios regarding their job experiences that reveal their strengths. The stories should be well prepared and concise. The applicant needs to share the situation faced, the action taken and the results achieved. Also, the job applicant should prepare answers for questions that arise during the course of the story, as the interviewer will be probing for truthfulness, lessons learned, adaptability, flexibility and team relations. Interviewers frequently ask situational questions that probe hypothetical situations versus an applicant's actual experience.

During a **case interview**, the interviewer will present a specific case for the job applicant to analyze. Within this case, the job seeker will need to identify key business issues and discuss how to address the problems involved. For example, if an organization such as an assisted living home for the elderly frequently has trouble communicating oral health needs to the families of their patients, that will be the case the organization will want job applicants to analyze in the interview process. The dental hygienist will do well in such an interview by studying what types of cases might arise in the organization in which they will be interviewing. Reading case studies in dental hygiene publications will expand his or her knowledge beyond experience and enhance the answer he or she is able to deliver during a job interview.

Another more intense interview situation is the **panel interview,** which is one that involves more than one interviewer at one time. The job applicant may be required to discuss a position with three or more interviewers who represent various areas of the job. This can be a popular approach in working environments such as the dental operatory, where work is truly a team effort. While challenging, the panel interview creates an opportunity for the dental hygienist to experience how the team interacts. If it is too uncomfortable, that may be a warning sign that this job would not be a good fit.

A **working interview** may also be scheduled to provide candidates the opportunity to do at least a three – to four-hour work day within the office in which they may be interviewing. During a working interview, job seekers will be able to observe the team dynamics, how they communicate with each other and with their patients as well as the team collaboration in the work setting.

Regardless of the type of interview or the combination of interview types the dental hygienist may encounter, he or she must remain calm and consider each answer carefully. It is even advisable to pause before answering or restate the question to clarify what one has heard, even if the job candidate has a ready answer to the question. A thoughtful pause is particularly useful during interviews that have been specifically crafted to test the job applicant's coping skills. These interviews might purposefully not begin at the appointed time. The interviewer may engage in an aggressive or even sarcastic manner or conduct the interview in a loud, busy area of the company. These are the hallmark symbols of the **stress interview** and are devised to test how the job applicant handles pressure. The applicant should quickly assess the interview environment and adjust his or her attitude accordingly. It is important to avoid getting tense or angry, and counter the interviewer's demeanor with a professional approach. In these situations, the interviewer may ask questions such as: "Were you challenged with a difficult situation and how did you handle it?" In answering, the applicant should admit reasonable failures and how they learned from those situations.

In a hypothetical example, consider "Joyce." While Joyce was interviewing with Dr. Rogers, his office manager, Madeline, came into the office no less than 10 times to ask Dr. Rogers patient questions. Joyce was annoyed by the constant interruption and found it hard to maintain her concentration in sharing her qualifications. However, she continued to interview like a professional and well spoken woman. Joyce informed Dr. Rogers that her experience with digital radiography and computer software programs would provide a wonderful advantage to his patients and the dental team.

In another example, Dr. Rogers shared with job applicant Joyce that he allots 30 minutes of dental hygiene care time for a child patient and 45 minutes for an adult patient. He made it clear that this is the bottom line – no more time is needed, and the dental hygienist needs to be on a set schedule.

Joyce remained calm and explained to Dr. Rogers that there may be times when 30 minutes may not be appropriate for a child, as in the case of placing sealants on the first molars of a six-year-old patient in addition to a professional prophylaxis and bitewings. Joyce explained that it can depend on the child's behavior in that situation. She recommended that 45 minutes would be adequate pending everything goes smoothly. Dr. Rogers hesitated, clearly considering this, and agreed with Joyce. She then went on to discuss risk factors of dental diseases with adults. Joyce explained that a healthy adult patient could be seen in a 45-minute appointment, however, a new patient who has not been to a dentist and/or dental hygienist for a professional prophylaxis in seven years will require more time. This time would include the dental hygienist gathering a complete medical and dental history, bitewing or a full mouth series of radiographs, periodontal assessment , oral cancer screening examination, determining the treatment plan and then eliciting several appointments for ultrasonic therapy and scaling and root planning. Joyce suggested an hour-and-a-half appointment for this patient over the course of a few weeks. Dr. Rogers appeared frustrated, but understood her rationale for categorizing patient disease with patient care.

Both parties need to make a decision: Will Dr. Rogers accept a professional into his practice who may not agree with his every directive, yet will make every patient's care top priority, or will Joyce accept a position in a practice where she will continually need to crusade for the patient's right to treatment whether or not it fits a stringent time schedule? One can see that interviews benefit both the employer and the applicant. Both have the opportunity to assess the other's behavior and adaptability to the work place culture.

Working Attire

As mentioned before, a job interview requires preparation on many levels. While research and rehearsing prepare dental hygienists mentally for the job interview, they must also have a sharp outer appearance to satisfy that "first impression moment" as the interview begins.

Consider that a patient assesses a physician's competence as she enters an examination room. Students size up a teacher walking to the lectern. A busy office manager evaluates a sales person as he walks into her office. In any of these situations, advice will be taken, information will be absorbed or products will be sold based, in all likelihood, on a first impression. Like it or not, from the moment job candidates enter a room, their appearance begins telling a story before they begin to speak.

In the healthcare field, it is important to note that a tailored professional image underscores the competency of the job applicant. Short groomed nails with clear or neutral polish, a tidy hairstyle – pulled back if it is worn long – and a clean, pressed business suit (pants or skirt) let the candidate's qualifications shine without the unnecessary distractions of an unkempt or overdone appearance. Job candidates should avoid excessive jewelry, make-up, hair styles or clothing choices.

At the other end of the spectrum, if a job applicant has been in the field for awhile and has not updated his or her look in five or six years, he or she might ask a friend for guidance or a professional appearance consultant in choosing interview clothing that reflects current, professional styles and even newer eye wear if the job candidate uses prescription glasses. These are the safe areas of dress that show the job applicant as one who is current and up-to-date, without the event of becoming a fashion statement.

Making the Interview Work

The dental hygienist should be prepared for anything from road construction to a flat tire when traveling to an interview. It is important for job candidates to know the location of the office ahead of time to make certain that they get there on time. They should bring at least two to three copies of their resume in the event that they need to provide it to the potential employer or other parties with whom they may meet or interview. A copy of references should also be available so that the potential employer may contact previous employers. As stated in Chapter 8, job seekers should let the people listed on their references sheet know that they may be contacted regarding the applicant's work style and behavior.

It is important for job candidates to remain calm and be professional from the time they walk into the office. All eyes are on the job candidates from the moment they walk through the door and introduces themselves to the receptionist. This is a formal appointment and appearance and body language will be assessed whether or not the candidate is speaking.

"Relax" is the key word for any interview. Projecting an image of intensity and focus does not also have to include tension. Remember to smile during the interview.

When an applicant enters a room, he or she should reach out a hand to shake the interviewer's hand or the hands of each person on the interview panel. The job candidate should sit comfortably and avoid crossing arms and legs; a non-verbal stance which can be construed as aggressive or angry. The applicant should be certain to make eye contact with the potential employer.

Communication is key to conducting an effective interview. As stated before, the applicant should listen to each question thoroughly to understand what the interviewer is asking and provide open and honest answers that impart a sense of integrity and self esteem during the interview. If the applicant encounters a question for which he or she does not have a ready answer, he or she should take a moment to think about other ways to answer it. If an idea does not begin to form, the applicant should ask the interviewer if the question can be addressed later during the appointment. This is where a notebook becomes an important tool. The job candidate should jot down any questions in it that have been deferred until later in the interview so that he or she will not forget to answer them.

An applicant needs to be conscious of his or her movements and avoid touching his or her hair, unnecessary leg movements or any distracting, repetitive motions such as clicking pens, adjusting jewelry or tapping fingers.

Whether job candidates are new or seasoned dental hygienists, they need to be prepared to develop a list of questions to ask potential employers in the interview. These might include (if the following information was not secured in previous discussions with the hiring manager):
- What are the job responsibilities for the dental hygiene position?
- What is the time schedule to treat a new child or adult patient and a recare child or adult patient?
- How much time is scheduled for a patient with mild to moderate periodontitis?
- Does the team help each other during the day?
- Is there a dental hygiene assistant to work with the dental hygienist?

Use the helpful portfolio notepad during the interview to write down notes about the employer, colleagues and practice. It is also helpful to do some background research on the potential employers and their office. This can be done by talking with people who know of the practice or by reading the company website prior to going into the interview. Job seekers can read the dentist's biography, his or her philosophy, the types of services the office provides and key questions that the job seeker would like to have addressed. It is also a good idea to bring a professional portfolio to the interview to share accomplishments with the potential employer.

It is important to remember to share professional information during the interview and avoid over-communicating or sharing too much personal information in the course of the conversation. Some career experts advise that sharing a bit about hobbies and personal interests, when asked, can cement a lasting impression during the job interview, however, be as brief as possible in these answers. These revelations should tie back to the position for which the professional is interviewing. For example, a dental hygienist who is interviewing for a position in a pediatric practice might mention volunteer work he or she does with youth in the community. In yet another situation, the interviewer might mention that the weather that day is good for some type of activity that the job seeker also enjoys. It would be acceptable to mention it under those circumstances as it would create a connection with the interviewer; one that might help the interviewer to remember the candidate in a favorable light. Job candidates should be alert for natural conversation cues and should not bring up such things simply because the interviewer says, "Tell me about yourself." A job interview is not a good time to discuss anything of a highly personal nature.

At the conclusion of the interview, the job candidate should thank the interviewer for his or her time and state what a pleasure it was to meet. The successful job candidate always takes time to do his or her best in the interview to provide a professional appearance and personal conduct.

Students Preparing for Interviews

Students should consult with faculty members to help them develop a well written cover letter and resume and document their school experiences within these documents. The student and his or her faculty mentor should discuss the fundamentals of interviewing, including engaging in role playing to build the student's interviewing confidence. These steps ensure that the first-time job seeker will secure a fair salary and benefits package that reflects his or her expertise for the position.

It should be noted that a dental hygienist who has not engaged in an interview for a number of years also could benefit from a bit of role playing with a trusted mentor or colleague. Nothing offers the job candidate more confidence than preparation.

Critical Thinking Exercises

1. Develop answers to the interview questions in this chapter based on your resume and professional experience.

2. Using the interview styles described in this chapter, team up with a mentor, colleague or classmate and use role playing and your actual resume and career experience to act out an interview. The person acting as interviewer should try all of the interview types described in the chapter. The person acting as the job applicant should vary responses based on these interview types. If in a classroom setting, have the class offer helpful critiques of the role playing.

Key Concepts

1. Many qualified candidates interview for a single job opening; the one who secures the position is the competitor prepared to show that he or she has more to offer the employer than other applicants.

2. The job applicant must complete some prior homework to ensure a successful interview, the first of which is to locate important information regarding the company, practice or organization with which he or she will be interviewing. The next step is to prepare for the questions that might be asked during the interview.

3. Belonging to a professional association will give job seekers a notable advantage in connecting to someone who has or is working for the company in which they have an interest to get an idea of the internal practices and working environment of the organization.

4. The basic list of interview types include: screening, traditional, behavioral, telephone, case, working and panel, and may include any combination of these types. Regardless of the type of interview or the combination of interview types the dental hygienist may encounter, he or she must remain calm, listen to each question and consider responding to each answer carefully.

5. In the healthcare field, it is important to note that a tailored professional image underscores the competency of the job applicant. Make appropriate clothing, accessory and grooming choices to present the best possible image.

6. Do not over-communicate during any type of interview. Pause thoughtfully before answering each question, even if an answer has been prepared, and offer a succinct response that has a distinct conclusion. Do not let responses ramble to a close.

7. Job applicants in the interview must be careful of their non-verbal communication. Sit comfortably and avoid crossing arms and legs – a non-verbal stance which can be construed as aggressive or angry – and avoid touching hair, unnecessary leg movements or any distracting, repetitive motions such as clicking pens, adjusting jewelry or tapping fingers.

8. The new or seasoned dental hygienist needs to develop a list of questions to ask the potential employer in the interview.

9. At the conclusion of the interview, the job candidate should thank the interviewer for their time and state what a pleasure it was to meet them and shake their hand.

10. Students should consult with faculty members or seek out a dental hygiene consultant who can help them develop a well written cover letter and resume and document their school experiences in the resume. Students also need to discuss different interview approaches and engage in role playing to develop interview confidence.

Chapter 10: Career Business Savvy – Protecting Yourself

By Christine A. Hovliaras, RDH, BS, MBA, CDE

Learning Objectives

The student dental hygienist and the dental hygiene professional will learn the following key objectives from this chapter:

1. Understand the elements of employment arrangements, such as salary or other compensation, benefits, disability and liability.
2. Identify the importance of getting the employment agreement in writing.
3. Assess employment arrangements and negotiate those not to your benefit.
4. Analyze the practice structure and your role within it.
5. Create measurement tools, such as daily and weekly productivity sheets, to track your progress and prove your worth in the practice for your yearly review and bonus.

Overview

Part of protecting one's newly acquired position is developing an employment agreement. This written document should clearly define everything the employer and employee have agreed upon for a particular position to eliminate confusion and emphasize agreed upon goals. Using measurement tools ensures that the employee continues to adhere to the responsibilities outlined in the employment agreement, and helps the employee track the frequency of those duties not captured in the employment agreement.

Latoya was on top of the world as a dental hygienist of 10 years. She completed two successful interviews for a position within an exciting, state-of-the-art dental/cosmetic practice in California, and the hiring manager called to tell her the job was hers. She scheduled a time to go to the office to fill out paperwork and discuss the details. The salary offer was not quite what she hoped, however, nothing was going to dim the joy of this moment.

Does Latoya have time to negotiate an increase in the salary? When is the appropriate time to negotiate the terms of hiring for this position?

In Latoya's case, her opportunity to negotiate these items occurred during the phone call in which she was offered her the job. To create a negotiating opportunity, she may have wanted to direct the conversation in this manner:

Hiring Manager: "Latoya, we would be so pleased to have you as a part of our team. Dr. Johnston would like you to begin on Monday, May 22, and the salary for your position will be $60,000 annually plus medical benefits. We would like for you to come in next Thursday to sign the appropriate papers and meet the rest of our team. Do you have any questions at this time?"

Latoya: "Yes, actually, I do. During our two interviews, I did not feel that we had ample time to discuss salary and benefits. I would like to consider this offer and discuss the salary next Thursday."

Hiring Manager: "We did clearly explain that the salary was dictated by our budget. If it does not meet your personal requirements, we don't have any room to increase it."

Latoya: "I understand and appreciate that completely. What I may have are a few other compensation ideas I would like for you and Dr. Johnston to consider. If you have a moment now, I would be happy to explain it, or we can discuss it next Thursday."

Hiring Manager: "Sure. Let me know what your thoughts are now."

At this point, Latoya knows two things: First, the office is firm on their budgeting and will not consider negotiating the salary, and second, they might consider compensation that is not tied to a salary increase. What Latoya needs to have completed beforehand is her homework on compensation ideas. She should research what dental hygienists in her market are paid on average, know what she brings to the practice that is unique enough to earn her some extra salary or compensation considerations and, finally, understand what would be a reasonable compensation request.

As with every phase of the job search, negotiating a salary and other compensation and comprehending the terms of employment begin with research.

Determining Salary and Examining Dental Hygiene as a Business Opportunity

Knowing one's worth in the marketplace is critical and job seekers and those about to close on a position will want to determine the range of salaries in a given market.

A **salary**, or the money paid for the fulfillment of job responsibilities, is the wage the prospective employer is offering. Job candidates will want to compare that to the average rate of pay for the same job in his or her state and region. Pay can be offered on an hourly, per diem (daily) or on annual salary basis, or may be offered in the form of commission, salary-plus-commission or commission with guaranteed minimum salary. The dental hygienist also may become an independent contractor pending state practice regulations, meaning that he or she develops a contract with the dental practice and then sets and collects all fees associated with the services he or she provides and pays overhead costs with the profit fluctuation based on production, collection and expenses.

To determine the going rate for salary in a particular state or specific market area, the dental hygienist may contact other dental hygienists working in the area, contact the component dental hygienists' association employment chairperson, or contact a local employment agency specializing in dental office employment.

To find general statistics on dental hygiene pay, the job seeker may visit a few helpful websites, including the United States Department of Labor, Bureau of Labor Statistics (http://www.bls.gov) and search the title "dental hygienist" to obtain statistics on the profession. Sites such as www.payscale.com offer comparison between the prospective employer's salary and national standards. Both of the sites mentioned offer hourly and annual wages. In addition to this, RDH magazine conducts an annual dental hygiene wages and benefits survey and typically publishes this data in September. For more information, please visit www.rdhmag.com.

Occasionally, the job seeker encounters a job offer in which the salary does not meet his or her needs. This is the time to consider compensation that would make it acceptable to take a lower-paying position. **Compensation** is additional money, advantages or benefits that are not necessarily a part of the employee's standard salary or hourly wage that are given to pay for work done. Compensation may include reduced or flexible work hours or additional vacation time that may ease the salary burden for the employer and make a lower-paying position more attractive to a highly qualified candidate. A creative dental hygienist might even consider asking for a per-hour fee and additional commission for promoting and completing specific services or by fulfilling an over-and-above per-patient quota each day. This is the area in which the dental hygienist may make a business-within-a-business of the dental hygiene department. For more information on this approach, see Chapter 15: Dental Hygiene Is a Business of Dentistry.

Identifying Job Benefits, Disability and Liability

Another area to research is the value and exact cost of benefits and how those fit into the salary total. **Benefits** are non-monetary remuneration that enriches a position by offering a job candidate medical and dental insurance, retirement and any paid leave such as vacation time, sick time, continuing education time, uniform allowance, membership in professional organizations, paid holidays, additional education regarding expansion of professional responsibilities in the office, etc. In addition, some organizations also offer a monthly or annual bonus. To make an informed decision about the quality of the position he or she has been offered, the job candidate may want to inquire as to the exact cost of their benefits package so as to include those costs in the total salary. The candidate may also want to discuss moving and relocation costs, if he or she is relocating, to see if that is something the employer may cover.

It is also a good idea to negotiate any time out of the office that is already a part of the job candidate's life before the first day of work. This might include a day out-of-office or early departure times from work for continuing education classes in which he or she is already enrolled, vacation time scheduled with a previous employer for which travel tickets may have been purchased or any time-off for pre-planned medical procedures.

The start date itself is another point to negotiate. The job candidate should begin with what the new employer's business needs are. Next, the job candidate needs to consider personal needs required by this life change, as well as the needs of his or her existing employer. It is important to make a positive and graceful exit from any position!

No benefits discussion is complete without also including information about insurance. Some dental practices offer health insurance coverage for employees, some don't. The American Dental Hygienists' Association (ADHA) offers its members a variety of insurance policies that cover disability and liability/malpractice insurance through Marsh Affinity Group Services (www.seaburychicago.com). There are also other insurance plans such as Principal Financial Group (www.principal.com) and Assurant (www.assurant.com), as well as many others that can be researched on the Internet. It is important that dental hygienists consider purchasing disability and liability/malpractice insurance in order to protect themselves from the challenging situations that may occur while practicing dental hygiene.

Yearly Review and Bonus Timeline

Just as yearly review dates are established, so should a bonus timeline and methodology. While many private dental practices may not have a formal organization for written annual reviews and bonus plans, it benefits all members of the practice when it is in writing. If such writing does not exist, the new dental hygiene hire should consider presenting such a proposal. In addition, the new hire might ask to see the practice's performance evaluation form. This ensures that the dental hygienist thoroughly understands how he or she will be evaluated during their first and subsequent years of employment.

Once new hires research and assemble information on salary, compensation and benefits, they can begin to negotiate suitable employment arrangements. Once the arrangements have been agreed upon by both parties, a written employment agreement can be drafted.

Written Employment Agreement

Everyone, from the new graduate with a first-time job to more experienced dental hygienists, should request an employment agreement. The employer is not required to draft an employment agreement, and many dental practices do not offer such a document. However, it is a convenient tool that the new hire might draft and submit, if he or she lets the employer know that he or she intends to do so.

The employment agreement protects everything the employer and employee have agreed upon so nothing goes unanswered. It identifies all the important details of the contract and puts dates in place for performance evaluation and salary evaluation. It ensures the dental hygienist will receive the items that were agreed to verbally in the office, and ensures that he or she knows exactly the duties to be fulfilled within the dental practice. To protect everyone involved, it is important to put everything into clear language that all parties understand and agree.

A written employment agreement may contain, but is not limited to:
- Job title, description and start date;
- Brief overview of responsibilities and expected outcomes;
- Exact salary and specify direct benefits;
- Days of the week and hours of the day the new hire is expected to work and may not exceed;
- Any employer approved time-out-of-office and/or sick leave;
- A schedule of paid time-off and vacation time and how the vacation time is accrued;
- Performance evaluation within six months of the hire date; and
- Date of first salary evaluation.

Also included in this list should be an agreement from the dental practice to cover time and compensation the dental hygienist expends for additional training in the profession that might include continuing education for new technology and/or courses available under the expansion of the practice act within the state. For example, in the state of New Jersey, dental hygiene professionals may provide local anesthesia, and in that state they can take classes to become certified to provide that service.

In addition, the job candidate may also want to include the final details for his or her next review time, from the exact first-review date and goals to be met by that date, to written progress reports throughout the review period to underscore how the new hire is tracking with these goals. All of these elements, once agreed upon, need to be captured in writing.

Members of ADHA may visit the organization's website to log in and view a sample of an employment agreement. The new hire may even go so far as to seek legal counsel when an employment agreement is put together for review prior to signing it.

Roles and Responsibilities Defined for Position

The dental hygienist should meet with the office manager/dentist/specialist to discuss job details. New hires will need to know to whom he or she reports at the office, as well as the team members with whom he or she will be working. In addition, he or she will need to find out if a dental hygiene assistant is available, and if not, who helps when assistance is needed. The dental hygienist will also need to determine who other subordinates are and what accountability he or she has for those employees' work.

The Typical Hierarchy in the Dental Office

Dental or specialty practices may be small, medium or large facilities with many employees. Regardless of where dental hygienists practice, some of the positions will be the same. This brief listing shows the breakdown of the hierarchy. For an idea of the organizational structure of a small dental practice might be, see Table 10.1 on page 210.

Diagram 10.1. Sample Organizational Chart for a Small Dental Practice

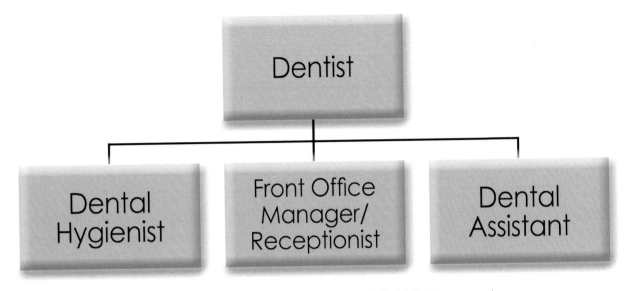

Moderate Size Practice

Dentist(s)

Specialist (Periodontist, Orthodontist, etc.)

Dental Hygienists (1-2)

Dental Assistants (2-4)

Dental Hygiene Assistant (1-2)

Receptionist

Front Office Manager

Insurance Coordinator

Large Practice

Dentists

Specialists (Periodontist, Orthodontist, etc.)

Dental Hygienists (2-4)

Dental Assistants (2-4)

Dental Hygiene Assistants (2-3)

Receptionist

Front Office Manager

Insurance Coordinator

Treatment/Patient Care Coordinator

Multicenter Practices (Within Each Practice)

Dentists

Specialists (Periodontist, Orthodontist, etc.)

Dental Hygiene Director
Dental Director
Dental Hygienists (2-4)
Dental Assistants (2-4)
Dental Hygiene Assistants (2-3)
Receptionist
Front Office Manager
Insurance Coordinator
Treatment/Patient Care Coordinator

The roles and responsibilities for each position should be defined within the practice and included in a practice management notebook within the office. Practices have their own ways of doing things and identifying what positions will be selected in conducting the responsibilities within the practice. Each year, goals and objectives would be defined for the doctors, specialists, dental hygienists, dental assistants and front office staff members. Depending upon the size of the practice, team colleagues would work effectively and collaboratively together to achieve both the dental hygiene and doctors' production goals for the year.

We know what the roles and responsibilities are of the **dentist, specialist, dental hygienist, and dental assistant**; however, roles may need to be reviewed regarding the dental hygiene assistant and what he or she will do versus the dental hygienist. The **receptionist** will be responsible for greeting all patients and alerting the appropriate team member as to the patient's arrival. The receptionist also will have the patient complete or update medical history forms and provide proof of insurance coverage.

The **insurance coordinator** would handle full responsibility of knowing all patients' insurance card information, submitting and documenting insurance programs and payments for patients within the practice. He or she would work collaboratively with the receptionist and the front office manager to ensure that insurance plans pay the doctor(s) in a timely fashion and that patients are charged for payments the insurance did not cover.

The **front desk manager** will coordinate all dental and dental hygiene services and make certain the adequate amount of time is being utilized effectively for maximizing productivity and profitability. He or she would collect information from several colleagues to produce the practice's quarterly profit-and-loss reports. This position would institute programs for inactive patients to return to the practice for dental and dental hygiene appointments and organize weekly or biweekly team meetings for enhancing effective communication and teamwork in the practice.

The **treatment coordinator/patient care coordinator** would get to know patients entering the practice to understand their specific dental needs and goals for working with the dental or specialty practice. This coordinator would conduct an initial appointment prior to the clinical examination and conduct dental radiographs (pending licensure). He or she would work directly with the doctor and dental hygienist to agree on the treatment plan for what the patient needs. The treatment coordinator would discuss the dental needs with the patients and define the treatment plan the doctor and dental hygienist agreed upon to optimize dental health. The treatment coordinator would also discuss the financial implications of treatment with each patient and payment options would be discussed.

In **multicenter practices** (such as Heartland and Midwest Dental) there may be a dental director and director of dental hygiene position who would work with each dental practice and is a member of a multifunctional team. The **dental director** will share the latest new technology and restorative, cosmetic, periodontal therapy and minimally invasive dentistry at each dental practice. The **director of hygiene** would develop guidelines for maximizing hygiene profitability in caries risk assessment, oral care screening, periodontal therapy, new technology and product recommendations based upon patient need assessment.

All too often, a position within this hierarchy will have loosely assigned duties that frequently cause trouble for the new hire before he or she settles into a routine with new co-workers. One would think that a small practice, for example, would have an easier task in defining each person's role. This is not the case. Small to medium-sized practices and companies require everyone within them to take on several roles. When dental hygienists hire into such a practice or company, they should be a willing observer but a cautious participant with duties not described in their written employment agreement. Review the activity the manager wants fulfilled before immediately saying "no." While it is important to be a team player, sometimes the clinician must also gently question an activity that is far beyond typical dental hygiene duties.

Also be prepared to consider the activity and how it may benefit future career goals. For example, dental hygienists also required to perform "front office" activities might get some much needed exposure to responsibilities that will guide them into administrative positions later in their career. Or dental hygienists required to occasionally fill in for the dental assistant may have an opportunity to observe new technology as well as a quality dental practice in action.

It is wise to make a list of any activities performed outside the scope of the employment agreement for discussion at the six-month review if the dental hygienist thinks those duties would require a salary adjustment. It is suggested that the dental hygienist speak to the employer prior to the one year review in regards to duties performed outside of the employment agreement. If these duties are not discussed, they may become absorbed into the position.

Position at Work

In establishing a new dental hygiene role, new hires can begin to shape their current job and future responsibilities by seeking answers to the following questions:

- **How much time is provided to evaluate and treat the following patient categories: a child, teenager, adult; new child or adult patient; child or adult recare; and an early periodontitis patient?** Keep in mind that new appointments should be longer, and that additional recare appointments are based on the oral care status of the patient; the greater the presence of disease, the more time the patient will require for treatment.

- **What are the goals and expected outcomes of the dental hygiene department?** The goals of the department should be aligned with the overall business goals of the dental and/or specialty practice. The practice should have estimated production guidelines for dental hygiene and set goals for each year thereafter depending not only on the dental hygiene goals, but also the dental hygienist's identifying further treatment necessary for the patient (e.g., redoing a restoration with a composite, placing a crown, a bridge or an implant, tooth whitening, etc.)

- **Who is responsible for the dental hygiene budget in the office for purchasing products, supplies, instruments, etc?** If it isn't the dental hygienist's responsibility, whose is it? What typically, if not ideally, occurs is that the office manager or dental assistant may do this on a regular basis. Ideally, this responsibility for the dental hygiene department should be given to the dental hygienist. A highly desirable dental hygiene position is one in which the dental hygienist is allowed to budget and purchase products with the approval of the dentist. This arrangement is a great indicator of expanding roles and responsibilities, as well as collaborative work situations for the dental hygienist.

  Purchasing is an important responsibility in practice. The dental hygienist should be responsible for the quarterly budget for purchasing the following items: instruments, equipment, materials for the dental hygiene practice such as cotton squares, bibs, infection control products and covers, suction tips, sterilization bags, film for radiographs, and dental hygiene products that include, but are not limited to floss, interdental cleaning devices, manual toothbrushes, electric or sonic brushes, toothpaste and mouthrinse. In addition, the practice team should have a professional products program in place to ensure optimal patient home care.

  It is important for the dental hygienist to know the quarterly budget and monitor the expenses generated. The best way to do this is by using a computer program that produces spreadsheets, such Excel, to determine what has been spent. Such a program also may be used as an inventory sheet so that the dental hygienist placing the orders knows how often a product needs to be reordered and how much of the budget remains. If another responsibility is to reduce supply costs, the exact percentage or range needs to be specified for that, and a worksheet is an easy way to line up and compare pricing and track savings.

- **Is the dental hygienist responsible for increasing the number of patients in the practice or reactivating inactive dental hygiene patients?** If so, the exact percentage should be specified. This may be a two-fold arrangement. First, it may require assessing the existing practice patient distribution by determining who has scheduled appointments in the past six months, who missed that six month appointment and why. What are the number of inactive patients from six months to a year ago? There may be a variety of reasons why a patient has not scheduled appointments that range from insurance coverage, to relocation, to a lack of motivation regarding oral health, etc. Second, the dental hygienist may be expected to bring in new patients. It is important to learn how the practice markets itself in the community. This is an area where business marketing strategies may need to be defined by a consultant. It is a task beyond a newly graduated dental hygienist.

- **What are those loosely assigned duties in the practice?** As mentioned before, every practice has a list of gray areas within the schedule for which the candidate might be expected to step in and offer service. This might include motivating former patients to return to the practice, offering a new service to existing patients to motivate them toward better oral health such as oral cancer screening assessment, cosmetic smile analysis for tooth whitening, replacing old mercury restorations with composite restorations, or any other new dental hygiene strategy to help patients achieve better oral health.

- **How is productivity tracked in the dental hygiene department?** While providing patient care is the concern of everyone in the healthcare profession, it is important to remember that dental hygiene is also a business. The easiest way to ensure that patients who need more care get the time and attention they deserve is to develop a schedule and be consistent with it. Even healthy patients appreciate a timely schedule that won't keep them waiting. If a new job does not have a productivity worksheet, offer to develop one. It is a good tool to prove the dental hygienist's worth during that yearly review.

The best way to begin to observe the needs of the patients in the practice is to document productivity each day. Tracking the day's appointments quickly reveals areas where the schedule can be adjusted. Identifying patient categories and time needed to conduct professional dental hygiene services will need to be determined. A Productivity Worksheet is beneficial to the employee and the employer. Used objectively, it helps both understand the schedule restrictions treatment time imposes. Review Tables 10.1, **Professional Savvy™ Dental Hygiene Weekly Productivity Worksheet**, and 10.2, **Professional Savvy™ Dental Hygiene Daily Schedule Worksheet** on this page and page 215 for further details.

Table 10.1. Professional Savvy™, LLC
Dental Hygiene Weekly Productivity Worksheet

Week of: _____

PROFESSIONAL SERVICES	MON	TUE	WED	THU	FRI	SAT
Total Adult Recare Appointments						
Total Periodontal Maintenance Appointments						
Total Debridement & Scaling and Root Planing Appointments						
Total for Placement of Local Delivery Agents (Arestin®, Periostat®, PerioChip®)						
Total New Patient Appointments						
Radiographs – Adults						
Radiographs – Child						
Mouthguards for Child						
Mouthguards for Adult						
Placement of Sealants for Child						
Placement of Sealants for Adult						
Total Dental Hygiene Service Fees						
Products Sold to Patients (Electric Toothbrushes, Battery/Electric Flossers, Dentist Sold Mouthrinses, Prescription Fluoride Treatments, Bleaching Kits, etc.)						
Total Product Fees						

Table 10.2. Professional Savvy™, LLC
Dental Hygiene Daily Productivity Worksheet

Date: Monday, 2/13/12

Dental Hygiene Services	Restorative/ Preventative Reco	Cosmetic	Implant/ Crown Bridge	Other Products
9:00 Adult Recare Mrs. Smith	Potential Composite #14	Maxillary Arch	None	Pulsar TB
9:45 New Child Patient Zach Jones (1 Hour)	Potential Fillings #2, 4, 8	None	None	Reco Listerine Smart Fl Rinse Restore Mouthrinse
11:00 Child Recare Donald Bucco (30 Minutes)	Sealants for first molars	None	None	Colgate Power TB
11:30 Child Recare with sealants (1 Hour)	Mouthguard for sports			Restore Mouthrinse
12:30 New Patient Mr. Don Jimmies (1 Hour)	Composite #3, 14 Crown #14	None	None	FMX Chlorhexidine Rinse, Mouthguard
1:30 - 2:15 p.m. LUNCH				
2:15 Adult Recare Mr. Jamison (45 Minutes)		In Office Tooth Whitening Maxilliary Arch		Prescription Fl Rinse
3:00 New Adult Patient Mr. Roberts (1 Hour, 15 Minutes)	Veneers on #6-11	In Office Tooth Whitening Mandibular Arch		FMX
4:15 Adult Recare Miss Johnson (1 Hour)	Bonding on #6, 11			Prescription Fl Rinse, MI Paste
5:15 Adult FMX Mr. Westin (30 Minutes)				
Total Dental Hygiene Service Fees $			**Total Product Fees** $	

Critical Thinking Exercises

1. Using the career goals you established in Chapter 6, write a sample employment agreement based on the material found in this chapter.

2. Research salary and compensation benefits for your position and area (city and state) on the websites described in this chapter and write a brief account of what you find.

Key Concepts

1. Negotiating a salary and other compensation, benefits and comprehending the terms of employment begin with research.

2. A job candidate will want to compare any salary and benefits offer he or she receives to the average rate of pay for the same job in his or her state and region.

3. Job seekers sometimes need to negotiate compensation to make lower-paying positions more desirable or to cover the cost of certain non-wage, yet job-related responsibilities.

4. To make an informed decision about the quality of the position he or she has been offered, job candidates may want to inquire as to the exact cost of their benefits package to understand how those costs fit into the total salary.

5. The employment agreement protects everything the employer and employee have agreed upon and identifies all the important details of the contract and puts dates in place for performance evaluation and salary evaluation so the dental hygienist will receive the items that were agreed to verbally in the office. The employment agreement ensures that he or she knows exactly the duties to be fulfilled within the dental practice.

6. New hires will need to know to whom he or she reports at the office, as well as the team members with whom he or she will be working, as well as who the subordinates are and what accountability he or she has for those employees' work.

7. In establishing a new dental hygiene role, new hires can begin to shape their current job and future responsibilities by determining such things as how much time is allotted to various types of patients; the goals and expected outcomes of the dental hygiene department; who is responsible for the dental hygiene budget in the office; who is responsible for increasing the number of patients in the practice; how loosely assigned duties are achieved; and how productivity is tracked.

UNIT THREE:
Practice Environment

Chapter 11: The Vision and Future for Dental Hygiene

By Harold A. Henson, RDH, MEd

Learning Objectives

The student dental hygienist and dental hygiene professional will learn the following key objectives from this chapter:

1. Identify the needs for different levels of dental hygiene education.
2. Understand the importance for creating a research infrastructure.
3. Understand the importance of self-regulation and the creation of an independent accrediting agency.
4. Identify the impact of the Advanced Dental Hygiene Practitioner (ADHP) and interdisciplinary collaboration on the profession.
5. Determine the future evolution of the dental hygiene profession.

Overview

This chapter will discuss the various trends and issues that affect and shape the dental hygiene profession. The topics discussed will have profound impacts on the further evolution of dental hygiene.

Education

According to the American Dental Association (ADA), there are currently over 300 dental hygiene programs in the United States with the majority of these programs being located in community colleges.[1] In 1986, the American Dental Hygienists' Association (ADHA) adopted policy to support the bachelor's degree for entry-level practice in the profession of dental hygiene.[2] The policy states that the association "*supports all aspects of formal dental hygiene education, which includes certificate, associate's, baccalaureate and graduate degree programs; however, the American Dental Hygienists' Association declares its intent to establish the baccalaureate degree as the minimum entry level for dental practice in the future and to develop the theoretical base for dental hygiene practice.*"[2] There are multiple reasons that the baccalaureate degree must become the entry-level degree. We now face a global population which is more culturally diverse in turn creating complex total and oral health needs.[3] Dental hygiene must be on the forefront in the areas of oral health promotion and prevention. There are many peer-reviewed research articles correlating oral health with systemic health. "*Dental hygiene treatment must move from a mechanical-based treatment to a wellness model of care*".[3] In order for the profession to continue to evolve, we must move forward to envision dental hygiene education into multiple education pathways. Associate-level programs need to establish articulation agreements with baccalaureate granting academic institutions. As this pathway continues to be established, we must continue to mentor our baccalaureate students to continue their education through graduate education. The American Dental Education Association (ADEA; formerly known as American Association of Dental Schools) published "*Report of the Task Force on Dental Hygiene Education.*" It states that "*the purpose of the Master of Science Degree Program in Dental Hygiene (MSDH) is to prepare professional dental hygienists with specialized skills in one or more of the functional roles: health promoter/ educator, manager/administrator, researcher, practitioner, change agent, and consumer advocate. To achieve specialization, the curriculum builds and expands upon theory and research skills gained in the baccalaureate dental hygiene curriculum.*" [4] The application of this degree is that the MSDH graduates will assume leadership roles within academia and various employment settings which will require advanced critical thinking skills.[4] Dental hygiene must evolve into the next educational level by creating a doctoral degree. Doctoral education creates the essential body of knowledge for a discipline to find answers to questions to advance practice and professional education as well as to explore and create new theories for the profession.[5] The four assumptions listed below clarify the need for the development of doctoral education in dental hygiene:[4]

1. *Dental hygiene is an important discipline of graduate study in which faculty and students search to verify dental hygiene knowledge regarding the science and modes of oral disease prevention and health maintenance, with focus on ways to apply this knowledge to promote, improve and sustain human health.*

2. *Doctoral programs will provide an intellectual climate and the necessary facilities to explicate, formulate and test knowledge and skills relevant to the scientific and humanistic dimensions of dental hygiene. Scholarship attainment and the promotion of scholars in dental hygiene should be the foremost goal.*

3. *No academic discipline has come into being without substantive research related to identifying, defining and refining its knowledge base and development of theory.*

4. *There is an implicit societal expectation that the dental hygiene profession will provide a sufficient number of dental hygienists who will be competent to care for and to help people with a variety of oral health concerns. This knowledge and skill, however, cannot be based in haphazard and intuitive guesses. Quality graduate programs for dental hygienists can help the profession achieve this goal and meet society's needs.*

Establishing doctoral programs would cultivate outstanding leaders, strengthen research capabilities, theoretical insights and overall scholarship.[4] Doctoral programs will also promote and align our profession within health care, educational pathways and advanced practice tracks.

Research

Research is the hallmark of any profession. Dental hygiene must be able to create new theories in order for the profession to evolve into advance practice. It is critical that we expand and strengthen our research infrastructure. In order to advance our research agenda, we must be able to integrate research into all aspects of the curricula. Dental hygiene theory and practice must be based on evidence-based research. All dental hygiene educational programs and continuing professional educational meetings need to emphasize the importance of research in clinical practice. All dental hygienists must utilize ADHA's National Dental Hygiene Research Agenda as the guide and collaborate with academic institutions in advancing the research agenda.[3] Dental hygienists must be able to integrate research regardless of their practice setting.[3] Research may seem like a daunting task, but all dental hygienists can play a significant role. For example, a clinical practice can become a clinical site for a research project. The dental hygienist can be the clinical research coordinator and collaborate with an academic institution on disseminating their clinical findings.

Our profession needs to have its distinct body of knowledge that furthers and deepens our philosophical understanding of the profession. As we begin to cultivate these new theories, we are able to explore collaborative research projects with other healthcare professions to provide interdisciplinary health care. Graduate dental hygiene programs must mentor their MSDH students to pursue research positions in the academic and private sectors. As these individuals become established researchers they can become future experts within the profession. For example, one institution can be known for systemic/oral health research while another would be known for dental hygiene educational research. It is the hope that with time these institutions would collaborate and begin to build a consortium of dental hygiene researchers with each group building upon the strengths of one another. This synergistic relationship can be developed with our international colleagues to create the research globalization for dental hygiene.

Another avenue that dental hygiene must explore is to collaborate with the National Institute of Dental and Craniofacial Research (NIDCR). We need to employ dental hygiene researchers within this institute so that we can generate and discover new theories. Once more dental hygiene researchers become established, the next goal would be the creation of the National Institute of Dental Hygiene Research. This institute's purpose would support clinical and basic research to establish a scientific basis for oral health promotion and prevention. Dental hygiene currently faces limited research funding and resources to advance the profession.[3] The institute would collaborate with ADHA's Council of Research and existing dental hygiene research centers such as the National Center for Dental Hygiene Research and Practice (NCDHRP) and Old Dominion University's Dental Hygiene Research Center. This dynamic synergism would allow us to further utilize ADHA's National Dental Hygiene Research Agenda.

The profession is currently facing a culturally diverse population, and new discoveries in the oral/systemic connection have begun to affect our clinical practice. The time has come for dental hygiene to become a major contributor to the nation's oral health research agenda and validate our role as the oral health prevention specialist.

The Advanced Dental Hygiene Practitioner (ADHP)

In June 2004, the ADHA House of Delegates adopted the policy to pursue the establishment of the Advanced Dental Hygiene Practitioner (ADHP).[6] The impetus for this policy came from the Surgeon General's 2000 landmark report, *Oral Health in America*. It identified oral health diseases as the "silent epidemic" in the U.S.[7] The ADHP was created to meet the need of the access to care crisis.[6] The ADHP's creation is of importance to the profession since it elevates dental hygiene to the level of other healthcare professions with advanced practice tracks. As this pathway becomes established within academic institutions it will provide new master-level tracks for dental hygiene graduate programs. However, the rewards of this pathway still lie ahead. The vision is that this particular track will create and generate new theories in oral health promotion and prevention. These mid-level practitioners will be able to develop new oral healthcare models that can be validated in their respective settings. Through the generation of new oral health theories, dental hygiene can begin to create mid-level oral health specialty tracks.

The ADHP has truly fulfilled several new pathways. The first pathway is the elevation of dental hygiene practice to a master's degree. This is also occurring within the fields of nursing, physical therapy and occupational therapy. The second pathway for the ADHP will be in oral health research due to that educational discipline's master's level education. The third pathway for the ADHP is in creating new theoretical and clinical models that can help to further develop the ADHA's National Dental Hygiene Research Agenda. Finally, the fourth pathway is to create interdisciplinary collaborations with other healthcare professions in order to further the national healthcare research agenda. Ultimately, the ADHP will disseminate research findings at national conferences resulting into advanced practice textbooks, peer-reviewed journals and various types of electronic media.

Independent Accrediting Agency

The ADHA explains that "*accreditation is a formal, voluntary non-governmental process that establishes a minimum set of national standards that promote and assure quality in educational institutions and programs and serves as a mechanism to protect the public.*" [8] The American Dental Association's Commission on Dental Accreditation (ADA CODA) currently oversees the dental hygiene profession. A critical issue that the profession faces is having organized dentistry regulating dental hygiene. Dental hygiene has a professional responsibility to be able to control its own destiny in order for professional evolution to occur. Organized dental hygiene must begin an open dialogue with the U.S. Department of Education in order to establish its own accrediting agency.[9] Research on dental hygiene outcome assessments and self-regulation must be conducted to support the importance of its creation.

Self-Regulation

Self-regulation "provides a profession with the autonomy to govern licensed professionals within the boundaries of patient safety, while maintaining the profession by encouraging expertise in professional practice." According to ADHA, self-regulation means that the state government turns to members of the regulated profession for advice and assistance in carrying out the practice act.[10]

According to ADHA, there are currently 17 states that either have dental hygiene advisory committees or varying degrees of self-regulation.[11] Currently, the dental hygiene profession is regulated under organized dentistry, which may limit the advancement, control and governance of the profession. Issues such as preceptorship will continue to arise and become a major challenge during legislative sessions. Dental hygiene is highly capable in developing its own destiny. Self-regulation would provide the profession with the means to make critical decisions in education, licensure and enforcement. In relation to the role of the dental hygienist and patient care, research has indicated that "*discourse can be effective in changing the public's perception and awareness of oral health care services and providers. As the oral care discourse is transformed through legislation and public awareness, the public will hopefully, be able to directly access dental hygiene services, and dental hygienists themselves may increasingly recognize their importance as contributors in the health care system.*" [12]

An historical event occurred in June 2008, with California being the first state to attain self-regulation. According to the California Dental Hygienists' Association (CDHA), "*The law is necessary because the profession of dental hygiene has evolved into a specialized area of oral healthcare that requires specialized skills and responsibilities warranting a separate regulatory body.*"[12] All dental hygienists must continue their legislative efforts to make self-regulation a reality in all 50 states.

Interdisciplinary Collaboration

Today's scientific literature now indicates the emerging link between systemic and oral health. Dental hygiene must continue its momentum to establish itself as an interdisciplinary team member. It is vital that the dental hygiene profession continues to educate and inform the public of the important role that dental hygienists' portray everyday in a patient's total health. Various healthcare settings and institutions should envision a healthcare team that is all inclusive to provide patient-centered health care. Academic healthcare institutions will need to develop curricula that can create synergistic bridges between all healthcare professions. This team of interdisciplinary experts will be able to provide comprehensive treatment. Other healthcare professions would recognize the importance that oral health plays in a patient's well-being. This would generate new opportunities such as collaborative research projects and new patient-centered care models all of which would highlight the importance of dental hygiene.

Future Timeline

So what will dental hygiene look like in 10 years, 20 years and beyond?

10 Years

In 10 years, it would be expected that all 50 states will have passed legislation that all RDHs are permitted to administer local anesthesia, nitrous oxide and minor restorative procedures. There would be at least 10 to 15 ADHP programs. A group of states would have self-regulation and independent practice. The baccalaureate degree will be established as entry-level practice. Online baccalaureate degree-completion educational programs will continue to increase in order to provide associate level graduates the opportunity to attain their Bachelor of Science degree in dental hygiene. Another important milestone is the establishment of various specialty tracks. Upon completing an entry-level program there would be concentrated tracks within the following specialties: periodontics, geriatrics, pedodontics, orthodontics, oral medicine/diagnostics, hospital dental hygiene, veterinary oral health, teledentistry and dental public health. These specialty tracks would give rise to the creation of specialized peer-reviewed dental hygiene journals.

20 Years

The master's degree will be the entry-level degree to practice. This would be comparable to other health professions such as physical therapy, occupational therapy and nursing. ADHPs would have evolved into specialty tracks of their own, just as the entry-level practice tracks have done. These ADHP advance tracks would specialize in research of rural public health, innovative pathways in oral health promotion and develop new theories in addressing the oral health needs of the global population. During this time doctoral level dental hygienists will emerge developing, testing and evaluating theory for the profession. The National Institutes of Health would have inaugurated a new institute named the National Institutes of Dental Hygiene Research. This section would further strengthen the dental hygiene research infrastructure by allowing dental hygiene researchers to delve into areas of research such as proteomics, genetics, diagnostics, informatics and translational research. The vision of the profession would be to create a consortium of dental hygiene researchers in which we could to continue to cultivate masters and doctoral level dental hygienists in their perspective research areas. In addition, we would see that independent practice is established in almost 50 states and the complete self-regulation of dental hygiene would occur.

21 Years and Beyond

The Doctor of Science in Dental Hygiene (DScDH) will be the entry-level degree to practice.[3] In addition, there will be academic programs offering PhD degrees in dental hygiene which will expand our current knowledge of health care. Dental hygiene will be involved in extensive teledentistry and there will be various centers of teledentistry. Dental hygiene education will involve the extensive use of clinic simulation centers. Technology will continue to evolve with hope of one day having holodecks, a room equipped with a hologrid containing omnidirectional holographic diodes that enable holographic projections, depicting simulated facilities for training dental hygiene students from all education levels. There will be multiple dental hygiene research centers. Each center will be known for their unique expertise in the scope of dental hygiene theory and practice.

At this time, the scope of dental hygiene practice nationally and internationally is equal. Internationally, we have strong collaboration with other countries. There would be numerous established foreign exchange programs not only for students and faculty, but for clinicians wishing to expand their professional knowledge base. Also, at this time we would be celebrating a milestone of the International College of Dental Hygienists. This would be an extension of the International Federation of Dental Hygienists' (IFDH). The college would confer international honors to dental hygienists who have contributed significantly to the profession of dental hygiene. There would be the creation of an International Dental Hygiene Research Institute in which a dental hygienist in any practice setting would be able to conduct research with international colleagues.

References

1. American Dental Association. Dental Assisting, Hygiene and Lab Technology Programs – U.S. Available at: http://www.ada.org/prof/ed/programs/search_dahlt_us.asp. Accessed December 5, 2008.
2. American Dental Hygienists' Association. ADHA Policies. Available at http://www.adha.org/downloads/ADHA_Policies.pdf. Accessed December 10, 2008.
3. American Dental Hygienists' Association. Dental Hygiene: Focus on advancing the profession. Available at http://www.adha.org/downloads/ADHA_Focus_Report.pdf. Accessed December 12, 2008.
4. American Association of Dental Schools. Report of the Task Force on Dental Hygiene Education 1992, Standing Committee of Dental Hygiene Directors 1988 – 1992, 23 – 25.
5. Somerville, JI. Report on the Council of Graduate Schools – Graduate Record Examinations Board 1976-77 Survey of Graduate Enrollment, Part II 1977, Graduate Record Examinations Board, N.J. 08540.
6. American Dental Hygienists' Association. Advanced Dental Hygiene Practitioner. Available at http://www.adha.org/downloads/ADHP_Fact_Sheet.pdf. Accessed December 2, 2008.
7. Oral Health in America: A Report of the Surgeon General, US Surgeon General, 2000.

8. American Dental Hygienists' Association. Dental Hygiene: Educational standards position paper 2001. Available at http://www.adha.org/profissues/education_standards.htm. Accessed December 12, 2008.

9. American Dental Association. The Site Visitor's Guide. Unit 1 The Accreditation Process. 2005, 1 – 28.

10. American Dental Hygienists' Association. Self-regulation of dental hygiene – state listing. Available at http://www.adha.org/governmental_affairs/practice_issues.htm. Accessed on February 13, 2011.

11. McKeown, L, Sunell, S, and Wickstrom P. The discourse of dental hygiene practice in Canada. Int J Dent Hyg. (2003), 1, 43-48.

12. California Dental Hygienists' Association. Self-regulation bill. Available at http://www.cdha.org/downloads/FINALSB853-6-13-08.pdf. Accessed December 15, 2008.

Critical Thinking Exercise – Part 1

Go to the American Dental Hygienists' Association (ADHA) website, www.adha.org.
Download the PDF document: *Dental Hygiene Focus on Advancing the Profession*. Divide the class into small groups, each taking a major topic heading. After reading the topics have the class critically reflect on the readings utilizing the following questions:

1. How will this affect your future?
2. How can you be the change agent?

Critical Thinking Exercise – Part 2

Assignment: Write a paper on the philosophy of dental hygiene. Incorporate ADHA's *Dental Hygiene Focus on Advancing the Profession* to support your philosophical views.

Key Concepts

EDUCATION

1. The entry level for a dental hygienist to practice must be a baccalaureate degree because *dental hygiene treatment must move from a mechanical-based treatment to a wellness model of care.*
2. The master's degree graduates will assume leadership roles within academia and various employment settings that will require advanced skills.
3. The doctoral pathway creates the essential body of knowledge for a discipline to find answers to questions to advance practice and professional education as well as to explore and create new theories for the profession.

RESEARCH

1. Research is the hallmark of any profession. Dental hygiene must be able to create new theories in order for the profession to evolve.
2. Dental hygiene theory must be based on evidence-based research.

ADHP

1. The ADHP will create and generate new theories in oral health promotion and prevention.
2. The ADHP will affect the evolution of the profession by elevating dental hygiene to the same level as other healthcare professions with advanced practice tracks.

INDEPENDENT ACCREDITING AGENCY

1. Dental hygiene has a professional responsibility to be able to control its own destiny in order for professional evolution to occur.

SELF-REGULATION

1. Self-regulation provides a profession with the autonomy to govern licensed professionals within the boundaries of patient safety, while maintaining the profession by encouraging expertise in professional practice. In relation to dental hygiene, self-regulation means that the state government turns to members of the regulated profession for advice and assistance in carrying out the practice act.

INTERDISCIPLINARY COLLABORATION

1. Dental hygiene must establish itself as an interdisciplinary team member in order to create new models of patient care and collaborative research theories/topics.

FUTURE TIMELINE

1. Dental hygiene must continue to evolve in order to compete in a global healthcare field. The profession must set timelines to elevate the profession with other health professions.

Chapter 12: Population Health Considerations for Improving Oral Health

By Ellen J. Rogo, RDH, PhD

Learning Objectives

The student dental hygienist and dental hygiene professional will learn the following key objectives from this chapter:

1. Understand a population health approach to health care.
2. Compare the health determinants and interventions in an ecological model of health at the micro, mesio and macro levels.
3. Value the ethical responsibility to promote change to improve access to oral health care.
4. Understand social action as a way to change the status quo, the personal commitment needed and the resulting empowerment and vulnerability.
5. Explain the educator and advocate role in social action.
6. Discuss strategies to employ focused communication and emotional intelligence to build relationships and gain support for social action.
7. Demonstrate the process for improving oral health during the assessment, planning, implementation and evaluation phase.
8. Understand the Synergy in Social Action Theory and the key elements for sustaining social action to improve access to care.

Overview

Dental hygienists are healthcare professionals whose mission is to improve the oral health of the population. Population health has a broader focus on health determinants within the community and systems that influence oral health. Practitioners have the ethical responsibility to improve population health through engagement in social action to enhance access to care. In social action, the professional roles of educator and advocate are essential to building relationships to gain support to change the status quo of systems that influence oral health. The process of improving oral health at the community and policy level involves four phases: assessment, planning, implementation and evaluation. The Synergy in Social Action Theory helps us understand the interaction of multiple factors that influence the sustainability of social action to improve access to care.

Population Health

Dental hygiene clinicians have traditionally viewed health as an individual condition influenced by daily self-care performed by the patient and services provided in the dominant delivery system, namely the private practice employee model. However, the current healthcare paradigm has shifted from a focus on individual health to population health. The goal of population health is to improve the health outcomes of a collective group who have common personal or environmental characteristics. Viewing health from a population perspective broadens the lens to focus on the health determinants in the environments in which an individual lives. Three approaches to population health exist: high risk population, targeted population and whole population approach. A high risk population approach targets groups of individuals who have the highest risk of developing a disease or condition, while a targeted approach focuses on groups who have a greater risk than the general population of developing a disease or condition. A whole population approach is concerned with an entire society's health and has the broadest focus.

The United States Department of Health and Human Services (USDHHS) is the governmental agency responsible for the health of the U.S. population. The department implemented the Healthy People initiative more than 20 years ago to set a comprehensive health agenda for the nation. The goals for the 2020 Healthy People framework were to increase the quality and longevity of healthy life, establish healthy environments conducive to health promotion and eliminate health inequities among population groups and promote collaboration between private and public entities to improve health.[1] The determinants of health addressed in the latest version of the Healthy People initiative were individual health, biology and genetics, health services, social environment and physical environment.[2] Health was divided into 42 focus areas, one of them being oral health.[1] Seventeen objectives outlined the prevention and control of oral and craniofacial diseases, conditions and injuries as well as improvement in access to oral health care.[3] In addition, the national health initiative discussed advancing the oral health in the children/adolescent and elderly population improving oral health interventions at the community level and within the current systems of delivery increasing the monitoring system of oral health and craniofacial disorders and lastly, improving the public health infrastructure of the nation.[3]

In 2000, the Surgeon General published a landmark report on oral health as a health issue in the U.S. population and the importance of oral health to general well-being throughout the lifespan.[4] The evidence presented in the report confirmed oral health disparities among various population groups based on the characteristics of age, gender, race and ethnicity and special needs.[4] Despite safe and effective prevention measures for oral diseases and craniofacial injuries, improvements in the interventions at the community level, including water fluoridation, and the systems level need to be implemented.[4]

A population health approach to interventions focuses on health determinants in the community and systems. The ecology of health is important to help understand population health interventions. An ecological approach views the relationship between individuals and their environments (for reference, see Diagram 12.1 Ecological Model of Health on page 228).

Diagram 12.1. Ecological Model of Health

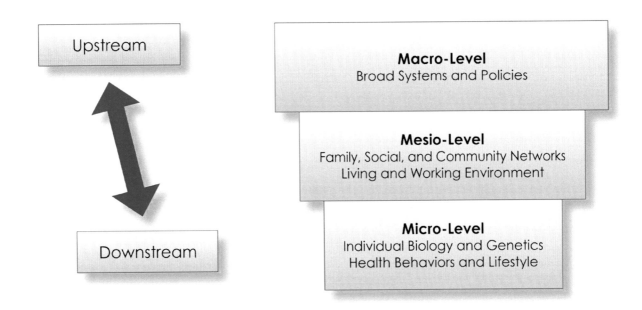

Within individuals and each of their environments are health determinants that interact and influence health.[5] At the center of the model is the individual, whose biological factors, behaviors and life style comprise the individual determinants of health at the micro level.[5] The next level, called the mesio level, reflects the family, social and community environment including health determinants in living and working surroundings.[5] The macro level is broadest level which represents systems and policies that are the determinants of health of a population.[5] Systems include economic, health, social, cultural and political determinants of health.[5] Policies made within the systems have the greatest influence on the population as a whole.[5] For example, within the Medicaid system, a policy to allow direct reimbursement to dental hygienists for oral health care influences the health of a large population.

Population health interventions focused on an upstream approach provide the greatest potential for improving the health of a whole population.[6] An upstream approach considers the broader determinants of health at the mesio and macro levels and the effects of these changes trickle down to the levels below.[6] A downstream approach focuses on the micro level and the individual determinants of biological and behavioral factors.[6] However, the Institute of Medicine recognized that interventions at all three levels provide the best solution for improving the health of the population.[5]

Professional Responsibility to Improve Oral Health and General Well-Being

The challenge of improving access to health services is one of the problems identified in the Healthy People initiative[3] and the Surgeon General's Report on Oral Health.[4] One way to improve oral health at the individual level is for dental hygienists to provide direct access to care. Direct access is defined by the American Dental Hygienists' Association (ADHA) as "the dental hygienist can initiate treatment based on his or her assessment of the patient's needs without the specific authorization from a dentist, treat the patient without the presence of a dentist, and can maintain a provider-patient relationship."[7] At the present time, more than 30 states have some form of direct access to dental hygiene care; however, many states restrict direct access to underserved populations or geographic areas.[7] Improving the oral health delivery system from the traditional practice model where dental hygienists are "tied" to a dental office,[8] to one that provides opportunities for care in alternative practice settings is needed.[9] Improving the oral health delivery system means changing laws governing the practice of dental hygiene at the state level. Dental hygienists need the ability to operate their own businesses to sustain a dental hygiene practice in alternative settings. To be successful as a business person and continue to provide access to direct care, fees for services rendered need to be reimbursed by public and private insurance companies. In order to be properly reimbursed for dental hygiene care, insurance codes need to be developed for every procedure dental hygienists can perform.[10] A change of this magnitude requires improvement of the dental insurance system at the macro level to impact the oral health of the population.

Macro level changes within the systems that influence oral health are very challenging since they require changing the status quo. Why should dental hygienists fight the "system" to change the status quo? As healthcare professionals, dental hygienists have the responsibility of adhering to high standards of conduct set forth in the ADHA Code of Ethics.[11] The standards of professional responsibility to the *community and society* include promoting "access to dental hygiene services for all, supporting justice and fairness in the distribution of healthcare resources."[11] This responsibility to society translates into *action* to improve access to care by challenging and changing systems, namely the dominant oral health delivery system and the dental insurance system. Action taken to resolve a social problem (e.g. access to care) is known as a *social action.*[10] Social action stems from an awareness of a problem and making a personal commitment to changing the status quo or challenging the system.[10] Personal commitment often times takes on the form of a vision or a mission to improve oral health, influenced by personal values.[10] Engaging in social action has a wide range of outcomes from empowerment to vulnerability.[10] Empowerment of the individual is influenced by the feeling of *making a difference* in the oral health of a population or improving laws that govern the practice of dental hygiene.[10] Social action can lead to a certain amount of vulnerability experienced as personal risks and financial risks.[10]

Social action also expands the professional roles of educator and advocate.[10] As an educator, the dental hygienist educates individuals and groups to enhance their awareness of oral health problems in underserved populations, the oral-systemic link, the dental hygiene profession and legislative initiatives.[10] Education is also important to developing a collective consciousness for the need to change the status quo to support justice and fairness in access to care.[10] In social action, an advocate is the *voice for the voiceless underserved populations* who lack access to health services. The advocate role encompasses being an initiator of change to systems that impact oral health. The educator role and advocate role are integral to social action efforts as dental hygienists change the status quo to improve the access to direct care problem.

Strategies that educators and advocates might find useful to influence change are *focused communication and emotional intelligence competencies.* When educating an individual or group, it is most effective to frame the social problem in a portrait and landscape view.[12] A portrait view of a problem puts a face to the name of a problem and portrays real individuals who are affected by the problem.[12] The landscape view frames the problem in a larger context.[12] For example, the access to care problem can be framed in the Healthy People initiative, the Surgeon

General Report on Oral Health and specific disease rates in one's state. When framing a health problem, credible resources are used to locate evidence supporting the notion that there is a problem (for reference, see Table 12.1 Resources for Evidence below).

Table 12.1. Resources for Evidence

WEBSITE	TYPE OF EVIDENCE
American Dental Hygienists' Association www.adha.org	Governmental Affairs (Practice Issues, Advocacy, Legislative Tracking) Professional Issues (Position Papers, Preceptorship Information) Members can access the document, Building an Effective Legislative Team
American Academy of Periodontology http://www.perio.org/resources-products/posppr2.html	Clinical and Scientific Papers (Parameters of Care, Position Papers, Academy Statements, Clinical Resources)
Centers for Disease Control and Prevention www.cdc.gov **CDC National Center for Health Statistics** http://www.cdc.gov/nchs **Oral Health Fast Stats** http://www.cdc.gov/nchs/FASTATS/dental.htm	Data and statistics on oral health Oral health resources Infection control in dental settings
Health Resources & Service Administration http://bhpr.hrsa.gov/shortage/	Health Professional Shortage Areas
Medicaid & Medicare www.cms.gov	Research, statistics, data, and systems
National Institute of Dental, Oral and Craniofacial Research Data Resource Center http://drc.hhs.gov/	Annual report with statistics on oral health Morbidity and Mortality Weekly Report (MMWR) Data tables and Data Query System (create a statistical analysis or oral health data)
Office of Minority Health http://www.omhrc.gov/templates/browse.aspx?lvl=3&lvlid=209	Oral health data on ethnic and racial groups

Table created by Dr. Ellen Rogo.

Focused communication strategies for education include:
- Assessing the audience's knowledge and values related to the social problem;
- Making the message relevant to their situation and needs;
- Engaging in an interactive dialogue between the audience members with a free exchange of ideas (do not preach).
- Having a clear and short message for solving the problem and expressing ideas in layman's words.

As an advocate responsible for initiating change in the status quo, it is imperative to build support for these changes. Building support means building relationships, strong relationships, where mutual trust and respect is experienced.[10] One strategy to build support incorporates the development of emotional intelligence competencies, which provide a foundation on which relationships are built. There are four emotional intelligence competencies (for reference, see Table 12.2 Emotional Intelligence Competencies below): Recognizing one's own emotions through *self-awareness*, controlling one's own emotions through *self-management*, recognizing other people's emotions through *social awareness*, and building relationships through *relationship management*.[13]

Table 12.2. Emotional Intelligence Competencies

EMOTIONAL INTELLIGENCE COMPETENCY	BEHAVIORAL COMPONENT
Self-Awareness	• Recognize one's own emotions and their effect on one's life • Develop an awareness of one's strengths and work towards improving weaknesses • Be self-confident that one can accomplish a task
Self-Management	• Control feelings and emotions • Exhibit integrity and responsibility for actions • Adapt to dynamic situations • View situations as opportunities and being optimistic • Adhere to high standards of excellence, and lastly • Take initiative and action
Social-Awareness	• Be empathetic and culturally sensitive • Aware of power in relationships • Commit to helping others
Relationship Management	• Mentor others • Inspire others through leadership • Communicate in an engaging manner • Influence change • Handle conflict in a positive manner • Build and maintain friendly relationships or networks • Work collaboratively and cooperatively with others

Table created by Dr. Ellen Rogo.

Dental hygienists who engage in social action need to use focused communication strategies during the education of others and emotional intelligence to gain support for their efforts to change systems that influence oral health. Building relationships and support is necessary within the dental hygiene profession and with individuals and groups outside of the profession.[10] There is strength in numbers when groups of individuals have a collective consciousness for change.[10] This consciousness is nurtured through educational strategies and emotional intelligence competencies that foster *collective action*. This action to solve a social problem has *collective power* and strength greater than individual action.[10]

Process for Improving Oral Health at the Community and System Level

The process of improving oral health as a social problem consists of four phases: assessment, planning, implementation and evaluation. Assessment is an examination of the social problem, partners, policy makers, opponents and resources to make the improvement become a reality. Planning is determining the methods to accomplish the targeted improvement. This phase involves procedures to develop a vision and mission, determine realistic outcomes and complete a Strengths, Weaknesses, Opportunities and Threats (SWOT) analysis before creating a strategic plan. The implementation phase is the individual and group action to achieve the improvement in oral health; whereas, in the evaluation phase the previous phases are examined retrospectively and the quality of the outcome is judged. The evaluation phase provides valuable feedback for future endeavors to improve oral health.

The initial phase, assessment, is a critical component of the process and one on which the rest of the phases are built. Substantial time and effort are required to thoroughly assess the problem, partners within the profession, partners outside of the profession, decision makers who make policy changes, potential opponents and resources.

The first step in assessment is the examination of the social problem. Define the problem in clear, concise language and decide what populations it affects. Identify what barriers and obstacles exist for solving the problem. Gather evidence in the form of statistics from local, state or federal agencies. Decide on a solution to the problem and alternatives and compute a dollar amount or an allocation of resources to institute the solution. Then investigate how other states have solved this problem to investigate alternative solutions.

The next step is determining support for the social action, which starts at home within the profession. Gaining the support of the executive board of a local or state component of ADHA is a first step. Most states have a Practice and Regulations Committee or a Governmental Relations Committee that is charged with initiating legislative changes. Committee members who have experience with changing legislation and the lobbyist employed by the state dental hygienists' association can provide valuable insight into the change process, especially when considering a change to state laws or statutes. Working with the membership of the designated committee, the leadership of the association and the lobbyist builds support through a collective consciousness and collective action. However, partnering with groups outside of the profession creates a stronger collective action. Many diverse groups have similar interests in improving health such as an oral health coalition or task force, nursing association, rural health association, public health association, senior advocacy group or children's health advocacy group. Through the use of an Internet search engine, one can locate a group's website and read the mission to determine if the organization is dedicated to the improvement of health.

The next step in the assessment phase is to identify the decision makers who have the power to make a policy change. For example, it is vital to identify the representatives and senators who are members of standing committees that deliberate on health bills in the state legislature when initiating a change in state laws that govern dental hygiene practice. A legislator is needed to sponsor the bill when it is introduced in the House and Senate. A clear understanding of the legislative process is needed to determine the process of introducing a bill, reading of a bill, referring it to committee, hearing testimony on the bill, etc., until it becomes a law. Most state legislatures' have information on the legislative process posted on their website. Before a legislator supports a health initiative, he or she wants to understand how this change is going to benefit their constituency and what financial resources are needed to institute this change.

It is also essential to the assessment phase to evaluate the opponents of the legislative change. Useful questions to answer are (1) who are the potential groups interested in blocking the change, (2) what are the groups' strengths and the weaknesses, (3) what power and influence do they hold on the decision makers, (4) how will they discount that the problem is not as bad as the evidence suggests, (5) what alternatives might they offer that are less effective to solve the problem, (6) what strategies might they use to discredit legislative efforts and (7) what type of vulnerability, personal and financial, does the dental hygiene professional's group have in relation to the opposition?[14] It is best to spend time understanding the opponent because the best offense is a good defense. Learning from past interaction with the opponent can help dental hygiene professionals plan a strategy to combat the opposition's negativity about the campaign.[14] Tactics to counter the opposition is to turn their attempts to discredit the dental hygienists' legislative initiative into an issue by itself and raise people's awareness of their strategy of passing the responsibility of solving the problem to others.[14]

The last consideration during the assessment phase relates to resources available to complete the initiative for improving oral health. Resources include manpower or volunteers willing to donate their time and talents to the effort. Financial resources are usually limited, and it is best to assess the dollars needed and the amount available to support the activities necessary to make changes.

The next phase in the process of improving oral health at the mesio and macro levels is the planning phase to develop a vision, mission and intended outcomes. A vision statement articulates the "dream" for the future, which is inspiring and simple to communicate.[15] Next, a mission statement is developed to describe, in broad terms, *what* improvement is going to be made and *how* it is going to be accomplished.[15] The outcomes for the change initiative are written as statements of achievement to accomplish the mission.[15] These outcomes must be measurable by clearly stating an action for achievement within a time frame. The vision, mission and outcomes must align very closely together (for reference, see Table 12.3 Vision, Mission and Outcomes on page 234) and be developed prior to the completing the SWOT analysis and strategic plan.

Table 12.3. Vision, Mission and Outcomes

EXAMPLE #1	EXAMPLE #2
Vision Statement Healthy Smiles, Healthy People **Mission Statement** To promote oral health through a statewide initiative to change legislation to improve access to dental hygiene care. **Outcomes** By September 2012, build support for the legislative change within the state dental hygienists' association and groups outside of dental hygiene. By October 2012, build a relationship with a legislator willing to sponsor the access to oral health care bill. By November 2012, write a bill to be considered by the 2013 state legislature to increase access to care by expanding the scope of dental hygiene practice by practice to include a mid-level provider.	**Vision Statement** Stop Abuse, Save a Life **Mission Statement** To create awareness of child, domestic and elder abuse through collaboration with professionals in oral health care, health care and the community. **Outcomes** By November 2014, build support for the implementation of a statewide continuing education program on the recognition of abuse and reporting mechanisms, within the dental hygiene community, other health care professions and community groups. By April 2015, launch a campaign for the statewide implementation of the continuing education program. By April 2016, see a 20% improvement in reporting suspected abuse to the authorities.

Table created by Dr. Ellen Rogo.

The planning phase also involves conducting a SWOT analysis and developing a strategic plan. The SWOT analysis identifies strengths and weaknesses *within* the organization and opportunities and threats *external* to the organization (for reference, see Diagram 12.2 SWOT Analysis on page 235).[15] Strengths within the organization include characteristics that have a positive impact on achieving the outcomes; whereas, weaknesses are the characteristics within the organization that have a negative effect.[15] Opportunities are external to the organization that might have a positive impact on achieving the outcomes and threats are conditions that might have a negative effect. A brainstorming session among group members can identify the components of the SWOT analysis. The components of the analysis are addressed in the strategic plan; strategies are planned to profit from the strengths, decrease the effects of the weaknesses, capitalize on the opportunities and protect against the threats.

Diagram 12.2. SWOT (Strengths, Weaknesses, Opportunities, Threats) Analysis

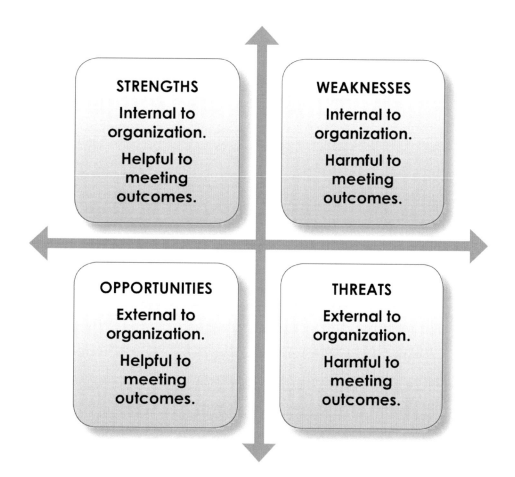

Diagram created by Dr. Ellen Rogo from cited information found in Nagy J, Fawcett SB, Berkowitz B, Schultz J, eds. The Community Toolbox. An Overview of Strategic Planning or "VMOSA" (Vision, Mission, Objectives, Strategies, and Action Plans).[15]

The strategic plan is a road map for achieving the outcomes. Components of the plan include the actions, person responsible, date for completion, resources needed, evaluation related to the action, and future planning considerations (for reference, see Table 12.4 Strategic Plan on page 236 for an example of a strategic plan). An initial strategic plan can be developed by leaders of the organization; however, the support of the membership is needed to get volunteers to complete the actions.

Table 12.4. Strategic Plan

Actions	Person Responsible	Date for Completion	Resources (People, time, talent, money)	Evaluation Related to Action	Future Planning Considerations
1. Discuss legislative change with the Executive Board	Sample Name: Mary Haas	October 1	Person needed to help design PowerPoint (2 hours)	Executive Board supportive	Include board members in all future communication
2. Gain support from the Practice & Regulations Committee	Sample Name: Linda Sardy	November 5		Committee members supportive	Attend all Committee meetings and include members in all future communications
3. Build support in the local components	Sample Name: Susan Tread, coordinator	December 1	People needed to educate North, SE, SW, Central components (3 hours)	Component members are supportive and some volunteered their time	Get contact information for those willing to help and include in all future communication

Table created by Dr. Ellen Rogo.

As implementation of the plan ensues, the strategic plan is considered a living document and evolves as actions are completed and new actions are added. One person should be responsible for ensuring the strategic plan is current at all times and incorporating information from all members working on the initiative.

One important aspect to the implementation phase is educating others to build support for the initiative. Building relationships, as previously discussed, is imperative to the success of the effort. Inspiring a shared vision can be promoted through the creation of a fact sheet that communicates the vision, problem and supporting evidence; a clear message of the solution to the problem; and contact information in a professional and attractive manner. Fact sheets can be distributed to decision makers via e-mail; however, building relationships means personal contact with the individual, on an ongoing basis, to build support for the change initiative. The ADHA developed a document, *Building an Effective Legislative Team*, as a resource for dental hygienists to assist in their legislative efforts, including a sample letter to a legislator and a fact sheet.

Another consideration is the manner and frequency in which communication will occur within the organization and with partners and decision makers. Keeping everyone apprised of completed actions, their effect on the outcomes and new actions that need volunteers, is vital to sustaining a forward movement of the initiative. A designated person needs to maintain current contact lists and write the updates in the form of a short newsletter that can be e-mailed monthly to interested parties.

Dental hygienists who participate in social action step out of their comfort zone and are challenged in extraordinary ways.[10] Members of the organization who have experience working on change initiatives are responsible for mentoring others in this process and using their leadership abilities to model the way.[16] Other important leadership practices are inspiring a shared vision, enabling others to act and celebrating accomplishments, even small ones.[16] Rallying the troops to celebrate and have fun helps everyone feel a sense of accomplishment and sustains the momentum of the initiative.

The last phase in the process is the evaluation phase. The evaluation consists of retrospectively reviewing the actions in the assessment, planning and implementation phases and reflecting on what worked, what did not and understanding the reasons for both. An evaluation of the outcomes can be judged as to whether or not they were accomplished or to what degree they were accomplished. Learning from this experience can forge the way for future endeavors and being more savvy and successful.

Synergy in Social Action Theory

The improvement of social problems, including access to oral health care, involves a long term commitment. This commitment requires social action that is sustainable throughout decades. *Synergy in Social Action* is a theory constructed from data collected from dental hygienists who were engaged in social action. Synergy is the perpetual momentum needed to sustain social action to improve access to oral health care. The key elements of the theory interact with each other to sustain the gears in motion (for reference, see Diagram 12.3 Synergy in Social Action Theory below).[10]

Diagram 12.3. Synergy in Social Action Theory

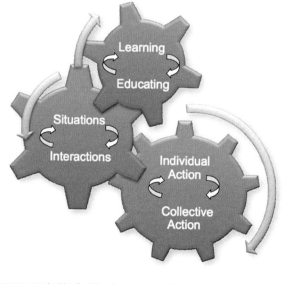

Diagram created by Dr. Ellen Rogo; information from Rogo EJ. Dental Hygienists as
Adult Learners and Educators in Social Action: A Grounded Theory. 2009.
Unpublished doctoral dissertation, University of Idaho.

In social action, dental hygienists are engaged in lifelong *learning* and *educating* to promote the social action movement, which represents the first element of the theory. Secondly, practitioners continue to learn in the context of their professional lives in each *situation* and *social interaction* they experience. Situations and social interaction are vital to the education of others within the profession and those outside of the profession to sustain the momentum. The last key element of the theory is the relationship between *individual action* and *collective action*. Individual action based on personal values and a commitment to oral health helps build a collective consciousness that fosters collective action. The Synergy in Social Action Theory is a means to understand the interaction of numerous elements that creates the perpetual momentum needed to sustain social action to improve access to care.

References

1. U.S. Department of Health and Human Services. About healthy people 2020 web page. Available at: http://www.healthypeople.gov/2020/about/default.aspx. Accessed May 5, 2011.

2. U.S. Department of Health and Human Services. Healthy people 2020 framework. Available at: http://www.healthypeople.gov/2020/Consortium/HP2020Framework.pdf. Accessed May 5, 2011.

3. U.S. Department of Health and Human Services. Oral health web page. Available at: http://www.healthypeople.gov/2020/topicsobjectives2020/objectiveslist.aspx?topicid=32. Accessed May 5, 2011.

4. U.S. Department of Health and Human Services. Oral Health in America: A report of the surgeon general. Rockville, MD: U.S. Department of Health and Human Services, National Institutes of Health, National Institute of Dental and Craniofacial Research. 2000.

5. Committee on Assuring the Health of the Public in the 21st Century. *The Future of the Public's Health in the 21st Century*. Washington, D.C.: National Academies; 2003.

6. McKinlay JB, Marceau LD. To boldly go . . . *American Journal of Public Health*. 2000;90:(1):25-33.

7. American Dental Hygienists' Association. Direct access states. Available at: http://www.adha.org/governmental_affairs/downloads/direct_access.pdf.

8. Prepared March 2011. Accessed May 5, 2011.

9. Gaston MA. Dental hygienists and access to oral health care. *J Dent Hyg*. 2004;78:323-324.

10. American Dental Hygienists' Association. Dental hygiene: Focus on advancing the profession. Available at: http://www.adha.org/downloads/ADHA_Focus_Report.pdf.

11. Updated June 2005. Accessed May 5, 2011.

12. Rogo EJ. *Dental Hygienists as Adult Learners and Educators in Social Action: A Grounded Theory*. 2009. Unpublished doctoral dissertation, University of Idaho.

13. American Dental Hygienists' Association. Bylaws. Code of ethics. Available at: http://www.adha.org/downloads/ADHA-Bylaws-Code-of-Ethics.pdf.

14. Updated June 2010. Accessed May 5, 2011.

15. Bensley, RJ, Brookins-Fisher J. *Community Health Education Methods: a Practical Guide*. Sudbury, MA: Jones and Bartlett; 2009.

16. Goleman D, Rosier RH, ed. Consortium for Research on Emotional Intelligence in Organizations. Emotional Competence Framework, 1998. Available at: http://eiconsortium.org/reports/emotional_competence_framework.html. Accessed May 11, 2011.

17. Hampton C, Nagy J, Wadud E, Whittman A. Fawcett SB, Berkowitz B, Nagy K, eds. The Community Toolbox. How to Respond to Opposition Tactics. Available at: http://ctb.ku.edu/en/tablecontents/sub_section_ main_1278.aspx. Accessed May 11, 2011.

18. Nagy J, Fawcett SB. Berkowitz B, Schultz J, eds. The Community Toolbox. An Overview of Strategic Planning or "VMOSA" (Vision, Mission, Objectives, Strategies, and Action Plans). Available at: http://ctb. ku.edu/en/tablecontents/sub_section_main_1085.aspx. Accessed May 11, 2011.

19. Kouzes JM, Posner BZ. *Leadership Challenge*. 4th ed. San Francisco, CA: Jossey-Bass; 2007.

Critical Thinking Exercises

1. Use a real or fictitious legislative initiative to change laws to increase access to dental hygiene care. Complete the steps in the assessment and planning phases in groups.

2. Role play with participants being a dental hygienist and a legislator or other decision maker about an oral health problem or professional issue. The role play can be used to practice focused communication strategies.

3. Conduct a debate on a professional issue such as preceptorship or mid-level providers (Advanced Dental Hygiene Practitioner vs. Community Dental Health Coordinator vs. Dental Therapist).

4. Do a search using an Internet search engine to locate the website for your state legislature. Search for the number of your district and identify your state legislators. Once you know your district or the name of your legislators, go to the Project Smart Vote website (http://www.votesmart.org/official_five_categories. php?dist=voting_ category.php), enter your zip code; this will result in a listing of legislators. Click on a name; this will take you to a screen with information about this person. Read his or her biography, voting record and issue positions. Make a judgment as to whether this person would be a strong supporter, lukewarm supporter or not support an oral health initiative.

5. Go to the Consortium for Research on Emotional Intelligence in Organization's website (http://www. eiconsortium.org) and read the emotional intelligence competencies. Have people rate their six best emotional intelligence competencies and their six worst. Have them write a journal for the two weeks to track how they worked to improve these competencies.

Key Concepts

1. The healthcare paradigm has shifted from a focus on individual health to population health.

2. Health interventions at all levels, including the micro, mesio and macro level, are the most effective approach to population health.

3. As oral healthcare professionals, dental hygienists have an ethical responsibility to the community and society to improve access to care.

4. Social action results from an awareness of a problem (e.g. access to care) and challenging the status quo by taking action to solve the problem.

5. The professional roles of educator and advocate are expanded for dental hygienists engaged in social action.

6. Using focused communication and emotional intelligence are two strategies to build relationships and support for social action initiatives.

7. The process of improving oral health at the community and policy level is assessment, planning, implementation and evaluation.

8. The Synergy in Social Action Theory is the interaction within and among the key elements of (1) learning and educating, (2) situations and social interactions and (3) individual action and collective action that sustain social action through perpetual momentum.[10]

Chapter 13: Business Etiquette in Dental Hygiene Practice

By Janice Hurley-Trailor, BS

Learning Objectives

The student dental hygienist and dental hygiene professional will learn the following key objectives from this chapter:

1. Explain the importance of first impressions in grooming, appearance and conversational etiquette to the health of the patient and the health of the practice.
2. Describe how to prepare for each patient in your daily appointment schedule and stay on time with each patient.
3. Describe how to protect patients' privacy.
4. Create statements about treatment plans that show respect for the patient and build a perception of value for the practice.
5. Evaluate one's professional attitudes and create a plan for ongoing professional development.

Overview

The dental hygienist's contribution to the health of the patient and the health of the practice cannot be overemphasized, and while clinical skills are critical, they are not enough. Patient acceptance of treatment, compliance and continuing care often depends on the dental hygienist's personal skills and emotional intelligence in observing proper business etiquette.

First Impressions

First impressions are lasting and highly influential. Patients often decide within minutes whether they have chosen the right dental practice and how comfortable they will be with the dental hygienist. On a typical day the clinician will welcome at least one new patient. That patient's willingness to return for future appointments and to refer others to the practice is often determined by his or her experience during the first appointment.

We have learned that 70% of the patient's final perception of his or her dental hygienist is formed on the first visit and is determined by the visual, verbal and personal energy they experienced. All three of these aspects can be modulated and refined.[1]

Personal Grooming

Hair for women should be worn up and off the neck and shoulders. Bangs should be restrained so they don't hang in the dental hygienist's face while he or she is working with a patient. All hairclips or ties should be a neutral color that closely matches hair color. It is important to be clean and well coifed at all times (for reference, see Figure 13.1 below for appropriate women's hair style for appropriate women's hair style).

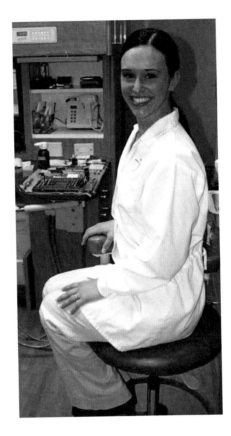

Figure 13.1. In regard to professional attire in dental hygiene, and in health care in general, it is recommended that clinicians wear their hair pulled up and off the shoulders. *Figure provided by and printed with permission from Janice Hurley-Trailor.*

Hair for men should always be well groomed. This includes facial hair and hair on the back of the neck as well as ear and nose hair. Contact with patients will be very close and intimate, and fastidious attention to daily grooming is key in presenting a professional image clients will find reassuring. Facial hair on men is fine as long as it is trimmed and maintained regularly.

Nails for women should be no longer than ¼-inch and have a clear or neutral nail color. Well manicured and naturally buffed nails are an excellent choice. If worn, acrylic nails should be kept shorter, clean and professional.

Nails for men should be trimmed regularly and trimmed very short. Perceived cleanliness by patients depends on the dental hygienist's ability to keep his hands visually appealing. Although clinicians will wear gloves when working inside a patient's mouth, there is almost equal time spent without gloves when patients will see the dental hygienist's hands.

Makeup is appropriate for the polished female dental hygienist. Eye shadow should be neutral, with blush and lipstick chosen for individual preferences. The goal of "well applied" makeup is to look both natural and prepared for the day.

Jewelry should consist of only small conservative earrings and a watch can be worn (if desired). As per the Centers for Disease Control guidelines, rings should not be worn due to their impingement with latex or non-latex gloves.

Scents, intended and unintended, are more of a consideration than ever. Clinicians need to remember the clinging power of the tobacco scent and any other unwanted odors and take measures to eliminate them. Likewise, refrain from using perfumes, colognes, aftershave lotions, etc., in the daily routine.

Chest exposure should be avoided at work by men as well as women. This can sometimes be a very real issue when men are assigned scrubs as the office uniform. An excellent solution for this would be for men to wear T-shirts underneath the scrub top.

Body art and piercings are fine for a day at the beach, but in the professional environment, these items can detract from what the clinician is trying to communicate and accomplish. The work environment has relaxed considerably in the last 10 years, however, the healthcare work place is fairly conservative. Dental hygienists should carefully consider a dental practice's employee manual before getting any visible tattoos or piercings. However, if religious or cultural traditions dictate one's appearance in any way, the clinician should be prepared to offer an explanation and seek out the most conservative way in which to express this.

Professional Attire

Identical uniforms should be worn by all clinical team members, no matter how long they have been employed. Any uniform assigned should be crisply pressed and clean. Solid colored lab jackets, properly hemmed and tailored, are always more professional looking than scrubs. The proper fit of a pant often has very individual criteria and should be selected on fit above all. Pants should all be from the same general material and exact color, but many times they need to come from different sources. Uniforms for the clinical team are determined by office policy and personnel guidelines. This important aspect of the practice should be reviewed annually for its effectiveness in portraying the desired practice image. Written guidelines in the office policy manual should be taken seriously and adhered to by each clinical team member. A consistent visual portrayal of cleanliness and orderliness should be an office goal (for reference, see Figure 13.2 on page 244 for proper office attire and name tag placement).

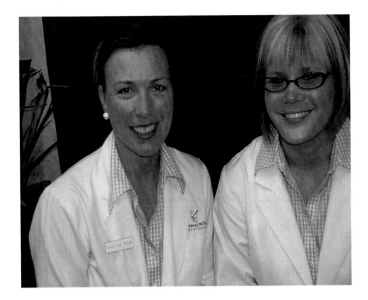

Figure 13.2. It is important that dental team members wear a name tag, as seen on the right side of the lab jacket of the dental hygienist pictured here. *Figure provided by and printed with permission from Janice Hurley-Trailor.*

Shoes should be selected by each individual for comfort and should adhere to the written office policies for color, material and safety.

Pace and Voice Tone

When the dental hygienist sounds sincere and caring, she or he wisely contributes to patient comfort and the success of treatment. The dental hygienist should make certain that he or she is not speaking too quickly. This common mistake often occurs because clinicians say certain routine things eight to ten times a day. It frequently happens that the dental hygienist can speak much faster than the patient listener can process in the information, so when the clinician wants to convey sincerity or instruction, he or she needs to remember to slow the pace of his or her speech enough for patient recognition and retention.

Voice tone is another important element. It has the greatest impact on how the message is received. As professionals, we work very hard on what to say, when how we say it can be more important. When the professional's voice tone is appropriate, patients will be forthcoming in sharing personal medical and dental health issues and perceptions of recommended dental treatment. When the tone is not appropriate, the clinician may find patients less willing to share. Phrases to avoid are "You need to" or "You should" so patients do not feel as though they are being directed by the dental professional. Dental hygienists are typically very passionate about communicating the value of recommended oral health services, but these phrases tend to have a parent-to-child connotation, even when said with the best of intentions.

The author noted that when recording the likes and dislikes related to oral healthcare delivery, one aspect patients frequently mention is that they highly appreciate it when their dental hygienist does not ask them questions while they have something in their mouth.

Professional Greetings

A key component to establishing professional image and relationship with each patient is the initial meeting. This most often takes place in the reception area of the dental practice. The best impression to give is one of warmth and professionalism, and it is more easily achieved by making the following preparation:

Before greeting the patient, review the patient's chart to become aware of his or her past dental experiences (identify if the patient is phobic or nervous coming to the dental office) as well as the patient's gender and age. This helps the dental hygienist to properly identify the patient in the reception area that will be under his or her care.

Then leave the patient's chart in the room (if the office still uses a paper chart) while going to get the patient. Dental hygienists need to remove all protective masks and eyewear, thereby removing all physical barriers that separate them from the patient during their communication process.

The dental hygienist should greet the patient by name and introduce his or herself, extending the right hand for a professional handshake (for reference, see Figure 13.3 below). Proper business etiquette requires that the process of the professional handshake include the following:

1. Make eye contact first.
2. Extend the right hand before getting too close to the patient, letting them know what to expect.
3. Keep an open palm until the web of the hand meets the web of the other's hand.
4. Apply gentle pressure, just enough to match the pressure of the recipient.
5. Let go of their hand after a second or two.
6. If there are cultural competence issues, they can be addressed as well.

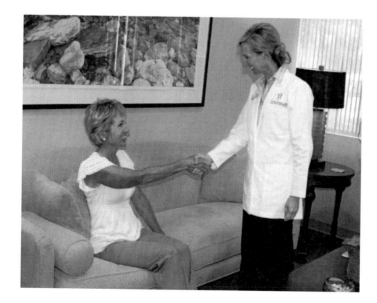

Figure 13.3. Dental hygienists should begin appointments with a professional greeting for new patients. Use a handshake and a warm smile to set the tone. *Figure provided by and printed with permission from Janice Hurley-Trailor.*

Components of a proper introduction include:

- A welcome: "Thank you for coming to our dental practice."
- The clinician's first name: "I am Susan."
- State his or her position in the office: "I am the registered dental hygienist who works with Dr. Jones."
- An invitation to join him or her: "Please come with me and we will start your appointment."

Connection Time

Effectively and appropriately connecting with patients will play a major role in professional success. Remember, it's the visual, the verbal and the physical energy patients perceive about the dental hygiene professional that influences how they feel about their visit and the dental or specialty practice. Here are several components of a successful patient visit:

The Physical Setup of the Room

Although the dental hygienist may be working in their own treatment room, this is not the place to display personal items such as family pictures or drawings. Appropriate material for the office may include certificates of graduation, continuing education documentation, the vision of the practice and awards and honors received in the profession. These should be displayed with the permission of the practice owner as long as they are uniformly displayed with the rest of the office décor. The dental hygienist's license should be displayed in a frame on the wall.

Keep counters clutter free, with the proverbial "place for everything and everything in its place." Have a place for patients to hang coats and place personal items, and offer to do this for them as they enter the operatory.

Proper room setup prepares the patient's chair height to be at eye level with the dental hygienist when he or she first begins.

Dental hygienists should not bib patients until after a "get acquainted" time has been conducted for the first three or four minutes after entering the operatory. The clinician should sit down in front of the patient with his or her outside knee close to the patient's chair, and his or her shoulders squared up to the patient's as much as possible. Start the conversation with information already gathered from the New Patient Phone Slip, if the office uses this, at the front reception area, or from information on the patient's clinical chart if he or she is an existing patient.

Patients will feel more relaxed and establish rapport if the first couple of minutes are focused on them; communicating that the dental hygienist is informed and interested in their dental wants and needs. Review the medical history and note which medications the patient is taking while they are sitting in the operatory chair. Patients will respond well when they can first listen to what the clinician knows about them and learns what to expect in today's appointment.

Safe Subjects to Discuss with Patients

Proper patient/provider conversations focus on the patient and his or her past dental experiences, present dental needs and future desires. The rule of thumb is to start the conversation with what the patient starts talking about, but remain conscious of the time constraints in the restricted schedule. It is not professional for the dental hygienist to use the patient's time to talk about his or herself or family. Many team members make the mistake of thinking that patients appreciate hearing about what is going on in their own lives, and they misuse time the patient is paying for to receive dental care, not to socialize. It is also inappropriate to start discussions or voice opinions on such subjects as religion, politics or the economy – nothing controversial and nothing depressing, please.

The patient's perception of value for his or her appointment, willingness to pay for treatment and readiness to make their next appointment is strongly affected by the dental hygienist's ability to communicate professionalism and value of their visit to the practice. Here are three verbal skills the professional can use to increase a patient's perception of value received for services rendered:

- Avoid using the word "just" when describing treatment needed. One wouldn't want to say that a patient needs "just two fillings." This is disrespectful to the patient who might feel very strongly about the negative physical or financial ramifications of having to get any dental treatment completed.
- Avoid using the word "only" when talking to the patient about treatment or finances. Patients can be easily (and rightly) offended when we use the word "only" before telling the patient the dollar amount of treatment.
- Do communicate practice loyalty. It is proper etiquette for the dental hygienist to consistently communicate his or her loyalty and respect for the dentist(s) and coworkers within the practice. Anything less than complimentary conversation pertaining to others is unprofessional and detracts from the patient's overall experience. An excellent response upon hearing a negative comment about a coworker from a patient would be to say, "My goodness! I am so surprised to hear that. That doesn't sound like Mary at all, but I will certainly look into that for you if you would like."

It is always important to respect the patient's finances. Each dental practice will have its own set of policies and procedures surrounding patient finances, but a consistent rule of thumb should be that the dental hygienist does not perform dental treatment before the patient has been informed of the charges. Informing patients of their recommended treatment and corresponding charges usually falls to the administrative team members, but the clinician will sometimes need or want to initiate treatment for a patient who has not yet been informed of the financial ramifications.

Synergism and Success

The Dental Hygienist's Mindset

Professional success will be determined largely by the dental hygienist's ability to work well with others. Being able to function together as a team with coworkers and the employer so that all parties have their needs met will allow the dental hygienist to be selective about his or her place of employment. Every office will have its own culture as well as office policies and procedures, but it is often the unwritten rules with which the clinician will need to consistently align his or her actions. The professional's likeability with both patients and coworkers is often as important as clinical skills.

Dental teams depend on one another for their individual and practice success. Dental hygienists do not function separately from others, but work in their own operatories to provide the necessary dental hygiene care for patients. In fact, in most situations, others will fill the dental hygienist's schedule and process all necessary paperwork. True respect and appreciation for other team members' work will serve the team well. Everyone should assist other team members if they have time to clean rooms or instruments, set up trays, and help out when possible to create a cooperative and enjoyable work environment.

Specific Career Builders

Commit to running on time with appointments. It is rude to patients and other team members to run behind. If time is not well managed this will be the most stressful thing the dental hygienist will face every day. The key to running on time is for the dental hygienist to understand that he or she is not there to talk to the patient about his or herself, and to ask few "open-ended" questions of the patient. Instead of an open-ended greeting, such as "How are you?" the dental hygienist might use a close-ended statement such as "It's good to see you."

Another key to staying within the allotted appointment time is to manage the transition time between patients. Allow ten minutes at the beginning of the appointment to receive the patient, even allowing for them to be a couple of minutes late. The dental hygienist should complete treatment time with the patient ten minutes before the end of his or her hour so the clinician can answer any needed questions, document the patient record, clean up the room and set up for the next patient. If dental hygienists find themselves running consistently behind, they should video tape appointments to see how much unnecessary talking or disruption may occur. The best time for the doctor to come into the room for the preventive exam is the middle 30 minutes of the appointment; the worst time is the last ten minutes of the appointment.

Participating in local dental hygiene associations (component or state level) is an excellent opportunity for career building and networking. Communicating excitement for the profession and what it has to offer should be the general tone of what dental hygienists have to say. Clinicians' involvement in professional association activities and health programs in the community optimize the importance of oral health.

Pitfalls to Avoid

When interviewing for a position, focus on the needs and wants of the employer. A long list of personal requests can be perceived as demands by the interviewer. Let the initial conversation flow to what the doctor is looking for first. Then the dental hygienist will be in a better position to ask his or her own questions. Sometimes dental hygienists may have fewer employment options than would otherwise be available because of perceived "demands" for which they were instructed to seek. While dental hygienists should know what a good practice fit would be for their situation, clinicians should first look at things from the employer's point of view.

While employed, complaints about an employer or other team members should never be public discussion. Dental hygienists will not want to participate in such discussions even if they were not the initiators of the conversation because that will never serve the practice well.

Speak well of patients and observe confidentiality and be in accordance with the Health Insurance Portability and Accountability Act (HIPPA), which was instituted in 1996 and protects the privacy of an individual's health information. This is the law and it cannot be breached. Sometimes team members feel inclined to share negative perceptions of patients when it is not information necessary to deliver treatment. Confidentiality is also at risk if the dental hygienist talks to patients about treatment scheduled for today or in the future in front of others. This most commonly takes place in the front desk area of the office. That is the place to say simply, "It was so nice to see you today. Sara will give you a print out of today's services," or "Sara will give you a receipt for today's services." Any communication from the clinical team to the front reception team should not be discussed verbally in front of the patient, but through computer documentation or a physical route slip that has already been generated to document the treatment plan and next appointment.

Work hard to stay active in the newest technology and training available. Interacting with other dental hygienists will help the clinician avoid stagnation in information or viewpoint. Burnout can occur if the professional feels isolated or uninspired by repetition, so clinicians must keep active by attending continuing education courses and participating in professional organizations.

As the dental hygienist serves patients and team members with both technical skill and professional etiquette, the dental hygiene profession will be enjoyable and rewarding.

References

1. Reiman T. *The Power of Body Language: How to Succeed in Every Business and Social Encounter.* New York: Pocket; 2007.

Recommended Resources

1. Please visit janicehurleytrailor.com for video examples of professional greetings, conversational skills and grooming.
2. Beckwith, Harry. *Selling The Invisible,* Warner Business Books, 1997.
3. Bixler, Susan, and Lisa Scherrer Dugan. *5 Steps to Professional Presence: How to Project Confidence, Competence, and Credibility at Work* (2e), Adams Media, 2000.
4. Hurley, Janice. "Seven Essentials for Office Grooming." Dental Practice Report, Sept 2007.
5. Pease, Allen and Barbara. *The Definitive Book of Body Language: The Hidden Message Behind People's Gestures and Expressions.* Bantam Books, 2007.

Critical Thinking Exercises

1. Define what you think it takes to be well groomed in the treatment room. Explain how you will allocate enough time in your day to come to work consistently well groomed.

2. Describe the patient's point of view throughout his or her time in the dental office. How will you focus on the patient's emotional needs as well as his or her clinical challenges?

3. Take turns role-playing the use of good listening skills with your dental team members. This will help in communication with the patients.

4. Give examples of "open ended" questions and "close ended" statements that could be utilized with your patients during their appointments.

5. Use the chart at the end of this chapter to evaluate your business etiquette skills (for reference, see Table 13.1 Evaluate Business Etiquette Skills below).

Table 13.1. Evaluate Business Etiquette Skills

	Rarely	Frequently	Usually	Always
My appearance is professional.				
I speak respectfully of others.				
I refrain from gossip and criticism.				
I protect the privacy of others.				
I prepare my operatory effectively.				
I greet patients professionally.				
My voice is warm and reassuring.				
I adhere to professional conversation.				
I give dental advice respectfully.				
I handle treatment costs politely.				
I manage my time effectively.				
I cooperate with all team members.				
I participate in professional organizations.				
I continue to participate in lifelong learning, self evaluation and goal setting for my career in dental hygiene.				

Table created by Janice Hurley-Trailor.

Key Concepts

1. The dental hygienist's business etiquette skills contribute to the health of the patient and the health of the practice.

2. First impressions are based on appearance, greeting and professional conversation.

3. Tone of voice and the pace of speech create a welcoming, supportive atmosphere.

4. Staying on time with each appointment is a matter of careful preparation and professionally focused conversations. Avoid asking open-ended questions or speaking about one's personal life.

5. Speak about treatment plans in a way that shows respect for the patient and builds a perception of value for the practice.

6. Working as a team member and treating colleagues with support and respect creates an enjoyable and successful work environment.

7. Speaking well of patients and protecting their privacy is essential.

8. Continuing education and professional associations help dental hygienists grow in their profession and keep work enjoyable.

Chapter 14: Leadership in Dental Hygiene

By Carol A. Jahn, RDH, MS

Learning Objectives

The student dental hygienist and dental hygiene professional will learn the following key objectives from this chapter:

1. List the four top traits of effective leaders.
2. Discuss the five exemplary practices of leaders.
3. Describe how the exemplary practices could be implemented into clinical practice.
4. Explain the power and influence of good communication.
5. Identify resources to increase self-awareness and leadership skills.

Overview

This chapter will focus on the key practices used by effective leaders. The content will highlight practical application for dental hygienists in the dental office setting. Skill sets and resources for implementation will be identified.

Leadership, for many, is something to look for externally. Many equate leadership with the person in charge, the one who is perceived to know the most, or even the "rugged individualist." Leaders are sometimes viewed as those with special inborn talents or charisma. What most people do not realize is that while some people may be born with natural leadership talent, for most, it is an acquired skill that almost anyone with the desire can develop.

Dental hygienists have enormous capacity and great opportunity for being leaders. Why? Because at the core of leadership is influence. The potential sphere of influence for a dental hygienist is 360 degrees (for reference, see Diagram 14.1 Dental Hygienist Sphere of Influence on page 253). Dental hygienists, within their practice, have the ability to influence patients, caregivers, co-workers, employers and sales representatives. Outside of the office setting, the reach can expand even farther in communities, states and the nation.

Leadership can enhance personal potential and individual effectiveness. It can help make the clinician more competent and more confident. The purpose of this chapter is to help dental hygienists increase their leadership skills for greater effectiveness and satisfaction in the workplace.

Diagram 14.1. Dental Hygiene Sphere of Influence

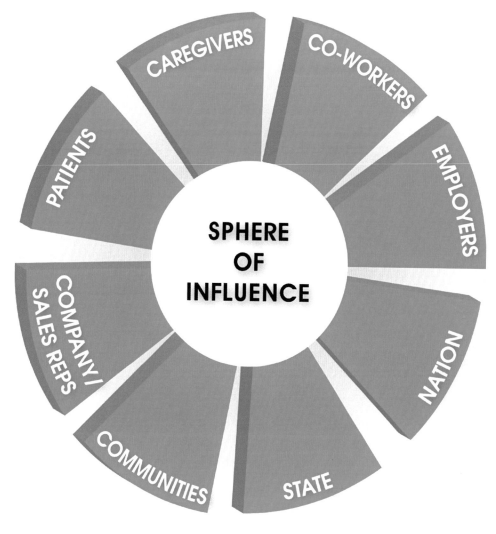

Diagram created by Carol Jahn.

The Traits of Effective Leaders

Leadership research has shown that over time, the four most consistent qualities that people look for in leaders are: honesty, forward-looking, competent and inspiring.[1] To sum it up, people want their leaders to follow through on promises, possess the skills and knowledge to get the job done, be passionate and be able to focus on the long-view. Leaders who are able to do this the most consistently develop the highest level of trust and credibility with people. Credible leaders enhance team spirit and drive commitment and ownership to the organization and/ or cause.[1]

Dental hygienists use many of these qualities in their daily interactions with patients. Let's take a look at a day in the life of "Molly," a registered dental hygienist with 12 years of experience who has spent the last eight years working for "Dr. Brown."

The first patient on Molly' schedule today is Henry Wilson age 62. Henry is a new patient to the practice and is scheduled for a one-hour appointment with Molly followed by a one-hour visit with Dr. Brown.

When Mr. Wilson comes for his appointment, Molly brings him to the treatment room and begins reviewing his medical history. His last dental visit was two years ago, and she discusses the need for a full set of radiographs. He agrees.

The radiographs are on the computer screen, and Molly begins her dental and periodontal assessments. During the probing, Mr. Wilson's mouth exhibits areas in the molar region in which several five – and six – millimeters pockets appear. He also has two isolated areas in which seven – millimeter pockets are revealed. There is extensive plaque, calculus and bleeding.

As Molly raises Mr. Wilson to a sitting position in the chair to discuss the findings, he tells her that no one has ever 'poked around' in his mouth in that manner before. He follows up by saying, "by the way, I think I tasted blood – did you make me bleed? I thought you were just going to clean my teeth?"

First, Molly acknowledges all of Mr. Wilson's issues before responding. Molly begins, "It sounds like you have some concerns about what we are doing today. What questions do you have?" She proceeds, "At our office, we are committed to providing our patients with the highest level of care. Dr. Brown and I regularly attend continuing education courses; we enjoy staying on top of everything in the dental field. One thing that is very important to us is patient education. We feel one of the best ways we can help you understand your dental needs is to conduct very thorough oral health assessments. We call all this 'poking around your mouth' probing. I was assessing the gum tissue and bone, or what is called the periodontal tissue. We measure the health of the bone, assess the gum tissue and the depth of the bone. What I found in the probing and in reviewing the radiographs is that around many teeth, you have lost bone. That can compromise the health of the tooth. The bleeding you noticed is a sign of gum disease; it tells us that you have infection and inflammation in those areas. The good news is that it is treatable; however a traditional cleaning will not be beneficial. To clear up the infection, reduce the inflammation and promote healing, you need a more thorough procedure called scaling and root planning, where we thoroughly clean each section of your mouth with dental hygiene instruments in two to four visits. Having these procedures will clear up your infection, help restore your periodontal health and give you the opportunity to keep your teeth for a lifetime."

Molly provides a great example of the leadership traits dental hygienists use every day with patients. Her direct communication about his condition and outcome displays both honesty and forward-thinking. By talking about the philosophies of the office she demonstrates competency and inspiration. What is also important to consider is that it isn't just Molly's choice of words but also her approach and how she presents the situation. Rather than promoting her plan for the patient, she begins by gently asking questions as well as carefully choosing the words for her reply. Molly also thinks about her body language by trying to engage with warm eye contact and keeping her arms at her side – to signify openness – rather than crossed.

Inquiry or asking questions versus advocacy or giving advice can be a powerful tool of influence with patients.[2] Inquiry conveys interest and a willingness to listen. Beginning with inquiry instead of advocacy, frames the provider-patient relationship as a partnership. Molly also exhibits leadership traits through the words she chooses. The influence of words is very powerful.[2] Molly uses the power of language in a compelling way to describe the benefits of the treatment she is proposing and thus influences her patient.

The Practice of Leadership

The behavior and skill set of leaders is most evident when consistently applied to everyday practice. Leadership researchers Posner and Kouzes discovered common patterns of action when reviewing personal best leadership experiences. They have found that in the process of leadership, the most successful leaders engage in what they refer to as the *Five Practices of Exemplary Leadership.* They are:[1]

- Model the Way
- Inspire a Shared Vision
- Challenge the Process
- Enable Others to Act
- Encourage the Heart

Model the Way

Model the Way focuses on setting an example through both actions and words. It epitomizes 'doing what you say you are going to do.' Effective leaders communicate with clarity their beliefs and values, and they demonstrate this by aligning their actions with values.

Let's see how Molly displays **Model the Way.**

Mr. Wilson looks at Molly, "so you aren't going to clean my teeth today?"

Molly replies, "No, that would not be one of the treatment options. What I will do . . ."

Before she can finish, Mr. Wilson, interrupts "I have options?"

"Yes, Mr. Wilson, when possible, all of our patients have treatment options. At our office, we are committed to providing you the best care possible. Would you like to hear your options?" Mr. Wilson nods and Molly continues. "Option 1 is a procedure called scaling and root planning. Because of the infection and inflammation, people are more comfortable if it is done with local anesthesia and conducted in two to four visits. It also allows us to get to the base of the infection and clean the area without causing you discomfort. This procedure has been shown to be very effective; the research supports it and so does my experience as a dental hygienist. Option 2 is the same as I

just discussed, plus the delivery of local antibiotics into the infected areas. Some studies have shown that people who have the addition of this therapy may get better results.

"Just having a simple cleaning – that isn't an option?" Mr. Wilson asks. "I don't understand."

"No, it isn't. A simple cleaning would not be enough to completely clear up the infection in your gum tissue. So even though your teeth might look better, deep down, where you can't see or even feel it, the infection could progress. Doing a cleaning instead of scaling and root planing would be like putting a bandage over an infection. For example, if you had an infection on your hand that was swollen, bleeding and emitting pus, wouldn't you want to do everything you can, including antibiotics to resolve that infection?

Molly begins her dialogue with Mr. Wilson by talking about the values of the office – providing the best care possible and offering treatment options. She aligns her values with her actions by explaining why a cleaning is not a potential alternative. She holds firm to her beliefs even though the patient presses about having a cleaning. Molly sticks to her principles because she is clear about both her personal values and the values of the office.

Inspire a Shared Vision

At the heart of Inspire a Shared Vision is one's ability to have excitement about the future and a willingness to share that passion with other people. Leaders with vision are compelling to be around as their ability to 'speak from the heart' is a powerful influence.

Now let's look at how Molly **Inspires a Shared Vision.**

Molly excuses herself from Mr. Wilson to brief Dr. Brown on the patient. As she returns to her operatory, she is paged by Sheila, the new office manager.

"Molly, did I just hear you say that you did not do a cleaning on Mr. Wilson?"

"That is correct." Molly replies.

"Well, that is going to affect today's production. And if Mr. Wilson is upset about this, you know, I'm the one who will hear about it," Sheila states.

"I understand your concern, and I know the way we do things here is different from your last office. Our goal with new patients is to build a relationship so that we have the opportunity to treat the patient for a lifetime. By taking our time with patients and educating them about the best treatment for them, including dental hygiene care, they have better clarity on their needs, treatment is accepted at a higher rate and we get more referrals."

When Molly responds to Sheila's concerns, she focuses on the long-term gain of the office rather than short term profit. Molly uses words like 'we' and 'our' rather than 'I' or 'me' to emphasize the collective or shared aspirations of the office. She paints a picture of what the future looks like when the team adheres to these goals. Molly shows Sheila she understands her concerns about profitability by finding common ground on that subject when she talks about treatment acceptance and patient references.

Challenge the Process

When effective leaders *Challenge the Process* it's not about complaining or whining; its purpose with an intention towards improvement of themselves and the organization. They look for ways to test the status quo and break-up routines and mindsets.

Molly shows how she **Challenges the Process.**

As Molly prepares for her next patient, Dr. Brown comes in. "Molly, can you talk to my patient, Mrs. Miller, about flossing? I just prepped a crown, and it was very difficult to take an impression due to the bleeding." Molly agrees and finds Mrs. Miller. "Hello Mrs. Miller, Dr. Brown tells me there were some challenges today getting the crown prep completed because of bleeding. Can you tell me about your homecare routine?"

"Well, Molly, I really do try to floss, but my teeth are so tight, the string seems to always break. If it breaks between the teeth, it feels like I have a boulder stuck in there."

Molly responds, "So it seems like I'm hearing you say that dental floss is not the best product for you. Have you tried anything else?"

"No, I haven't. I've looked at my local pharmacy, but they have so much, I wasn't sure what to get." Mrs. Miller states.

"I've got some ideas for you." Molly tells her as she picks up a small, interdental brush. "See this? In some places in your mouth, you have wide spaces – like here." She hands Mrs. Miller a mirror. "You put it through the teeth just like this to remove plaque biofilm between the teeth as well as food debris. Molly gives the interdental brush to Mrs. Miller to allow her to practice using this interdental cleaning device and see if she is comfortable in using it and provide her with instruction for use. Another consideration is a dental water jet." Molly shows her a unit and hands her a brochure. "It has been shown to work as well as dental floss and you can use it around all of your teeth. I'll call you in a couple weeks to see how your oral care cleaning methods are working for you. We can discuss how you feel and if we need to make other oral care changes, we will."

When Molly talks to Mrs. Miller about flossing, she challenges the process by breaking up the mindset that dental floss is the 'only way.' She partners with her patient in the process by giving her choices and allowing her to experiment with different product options. Further, Molly encourages her patient to take some initiative in the process if she finds that the recommended products are not for her.

Enable Others to Act

Effective leaders *Enable Others to Act* because they know that organizational success is a team effort. This is especially true in dental practices where strong teams know the value of collaboration in achieving peak performance.

Let's take a look at how Molly **Enables Others to Act.**

It's lunch time and Molly joins April, a newly graduated dental hygienist. As she is sitting down, April says, "Molly, can I ask why you are still using fluoride gel and trays? In school, we used fluoride varnish. I've been here a few months now, and I've tried the gel/tray thing, but don't like it. It's so messy."

"Gosh, April," Molly replies, "I am embarrassed to say, it's probably habit more than anything. I've seen several ads, but I just haven't taken the time to learn about it. As much as we focus on trying to practice evidence-based dentistry, I think I've just taken the way we do fluoride for granted. Why don't you tell me why you like varnish?"

"Well, for one it's really easy and there aren't as many restrictions with it as with gel." April answers.

"Is it as effective?" Molly asks.

"Yes, it is as effective as gel. Molly, would you talk to Dr. Brown about it for me?" April says.

Molly smiles, looks at April, and replies, "Actually April, I think you should talk to Dr. Brown. Why don't you get some product samples and information along with a couple of research studies and present it to her. Tell her why you like using it and how it will benefit our patients and the practice. You can even do a practice run on me first. And I promise you, if she asks me for my opinion on it, I'll back you."

"It's a deal." April replies.

Molly enables April to act by first asking questions and listening to April. She demonstrates trust and support for April by giving her the opportunity to present the idea to Dr. Brown. By offering to collaborate with April on the presentation, she helps her gain competence in her presentation skills as well as overall confidence.

Encourage the Heart

Good leaders know the importance of showing appreciation for and recognizing the contribution of others. They understand that it helps contribute to a shared sense of value and overall team spirit.

The day is almost over for Molly. Let's observe how she honors **Encourage the Heart**.

Molly's afternoon was a family affair: Mom and her four boys, ages 10, 8 and 6-year – old twins were all having professional cleaning appointments today and the 6-year-old twins were also having sealants applied to their first molars. Needless to say, it was a little wild and crazy, and Molly needed some additional help from Jo Ann, one of Dr. Brown's dental assistants. At the day's end the assistants are finishing up in the lab, and Molly comes in and sees Jo Ann.

"Thank you so much for the help, Jo Ann. I couldn't have done it without you. And Dr. Brown, thank you for allowing her to work with me today. It made a difference, and I appreciate it. We have a great team here! I feel so lucky to work with all of you!" Molly can see that there is a lot more work to be done. With Jo Ann helping her, instrument cleaning has backed up. Molly gloves up and helps the dental assistants.

Molly encourages her fellow team mates by not only thanking Jo Ann, but showing appreciation for Dr. Brown, who played a contributing role. Molly goes the extra mile, setting an example by showing pride and recognition for the dental team. She supports her colleagues by pitching in and helping them out as a way of returning the favor.

Developing Leadership Skills

Leadership is a process, and the skills that help people become effective leaders can be developed by anyone with time and effort. One of the most important pieces of leadership development is self awareness. Each person has distinct strengths and talents. Scientists from the Gallup Consulting Organization have shown that people who have the opportunity to focus on their strengths every day are six times as likely to be engaged in their jobs and three times more likely to report an excellent quality of life.[3] Developing awareness of personal strengths is the first step in maximizing potential. Another way to develop self-awareness is via personality testing. Assessments such as the Myers-Briggs Type Indicator, the DISC Profile or the Forte Communication Style Profile can help individuals learn more about themselves (for reference, see Table 14.1 Tools for Self Awareness on page 260).

Table 14.1. Tools for Self Awareness

ASSESSMENT TOOL	INFORMATION
Myers-Briggs Type Indicator® www.myersbriggs.com	• Developed in 1940's by Katherine Cook Briggs and Isabel Briggs Myers • Most widely used personality assessment in the world; more than 2 million people take the assessment annually • Promoted as a tool to help improve performance, reduce workplace conflict and improve communication • Demonstrated validity and reliability
DiSC® Personality Profile Test www.onlinediscprofile.com	• Developed through the work of William Moulton Marston circa 1928 • Taken by over 5 million people • Promoted as a tool to help people focus on their strengths and learn to use them in work/life situations • Demonstrated validity
Strength Finder www.strengthfinder.com	• Developed by Gallup scientists led by Donald Clifton based on 40 year study of human strengths • Number who have taken the assessment: unknown • Promoted as a way to discover one's top five talents and implement them on a daily basis • Validation – Unknown
The Forte System www.theforteinstitute.com	• Developed in 1978 by CD Morgan III • Number who have taken the assessment: unknown • Promoted as a tool to bring together lifetime communication strengths and understanding of personal and interpersonal preferences • Validation – Unknown

Table created by Carol Jahn.

Leaders are learners. Studying the art and science of leadership is another way to develop leadership potential. One area that can benefit nearly everyone, even established leaders, is to enhance communication skills. Whether it is the art of knowing how to craft a clear and influential message or the nuts and bolts of conflict management, effective leaders respect the power of words. The right words can be the difference between the dental hygienist showing empathy for patients and understanding how they feel. Words are the foundation of what people desire to create. The choice of words can sow the seeds of a victory garden, or they can generate fear, destroying all in its path. Effective leaders know that good communication is a key skill that builds relationships and expands the capacity for influence. Business literature is replete with resources designed to help people develop better communication skills (for reference, see Table 14.2 Communication and Leadership Tools on page 261).

Table 14.2. Communication and Leadership Tools

RESOURCE	WEBSITE
The Leadership Challenge, (4th Ed), 2007 Posner, B, Kouzes J. ISBN: 978-0-7879-8491-5	www.leadershipchallenge.com
Crucial Conversations: Tools for Talking When Stakes are High, Patterson K, 2002, Grenny J, McMillan R, Switzler A. ISBN: 0-07-140194-6	www.vitalsmarts.com
Difficult Conversations: How to Discuss What Matters Most, 1999, Stone D, Patton B, Heen S. ISBN: 0-14-028852-x	www.diffcon.com
Strength Finder 2.0, 2007, Rath T. ISBN: 978-1-59562-015-6	www.strengthfinder.com
Absolute Honesty, 2003. Johnson L, Phillips B. ISBN: 0-8144-0781-1	www.absolutehonesty.com
The EQ Edge: Emotional Intelligence and Your Success, 2006. Stein S, Book H. ISBN: 0470838361	www.eqedge.com
What Got You Here Won't Get You There. 2007. Goldsmith M. ISBN: 1-4013-0130-4	www.marshallgoldsmithlibrary.com

Table created by Carol Jahn.

The mastery of any skill involves practice. In addition to the dental office setting, dental hygienists can find leadership opportunities within their professional association, academic institution or other civic/private organization. Taking on a volunteer leadership role is a great way to develop one's self-awareness, discover passions and personal strengths, enhance skills and quite simply, practice the art of the profession. Volunteering provides the ideal situation to find a mentor; someone outside of the individual's work setting who can help enhance leadership and grow one's sphere of influence. Another way to gain insight and practice is through coaching. Personal and career coaches can help individuals set goals and achieve the skills for influential leadership (for reference, see Table 14.3 Resources for Mastery of Leadership Skills on page 262).

Table 14.3. Resources for Mastery of Leadership Skills

ORGANIZATION	INFORMATION
American Dental Hygienists' Association www.adha.org	Membership open to licensed dental hygienists
American Dental Education Association www.adea.org	Membership open to dental hygiene faculty or any supporter of dental/dental hygiene education
International Federation of Dental Hygiene www.ifdh.org	Membership open to dental hygienists of member countries such the US, Canada or Mexico and organizations such as ADHA
International Coach Federation www.coachfederation.org	Professional organization for accredited coaches Helps individuals find an accredited coach
The Leadership Challenge www.leadershipchallenge.com	Offers workshops and programs (fee-based) based on the book *The Leadership Challenge*
Vital Smarts www.vitalsmarts.com	Provides free web seminars and training programs (fee-based) based on the book *Crucial Conversations*

Table created by Carol Jahn.

Summary

Leadership is a learned skill that can be developed by anyone with the desire and motivation to lead. Dental hygienists have leadership opportunities with patients, co-workers, employers and countless other stakeholders who come into the dental practice. Developing leadership potential helps dental hygienists create a sphere of influence.

References

1. Kouzes JM, Posner BZ. *The Leadership Challenge*. 3rd ed. San Francisco: Jossey-Bass; 2002.
2. Whitney DK, Trosten-Bloom A. *The Power of Appreciative Inquiry: A Practical Guide to Positive Change.* San Francisco, CA: Berrett-Koehler; 2010.
3. Rath T. *Strengths Finder 2.0.* New York: Gallup; 2007.

Critical Thinking Exercises

1. You have started a new position in an established dental practice. The dental hygienist who preceded you was there for many years. Most of the instruments are old and dull including the ultrasonic inserts. Develop a plan using some of the Five Models of Exemplary Leadership to construct a plan for influencing your employer to purchase new instruments.

2. Reflect on the daily discussions that you have with patients. What percentage of your conversation is about giving advice and what percent is about inquiry or asking questions? Develop a script reframing your advocacy into inquiry statements to use with patients.

3. Your employer has just implemented a procedure where each staff member will take turns leading a staff meeting. You were the first one to be selected to lead the first meeting. Develop a meeting objective and agenda highlighting the areas that will be discussed with the entire team and any additional steps you need to take prior to initiating the meeting in order to make it successful.

Key Concepts

1. Leadership is about influence, and dental hygienists influence patients on a daily basis. The ones who do so most effectively follow through on promises, possess the skills and knowledge to get the job done, are passionate and are able to focus on the long-view.

2. An effective leader will Model the Way by communicating with clarity his or her beliefs and values and demonstrating this by aligning his or her actions with values.

3. Leaders with who Inspire a Shared Vision create excitement about the future and are willing to share that passion with those around them.

4. An effective leader will Challenge the Process with an intention towards improvement of his or herself and the organization.

5. An effective leader will Enable Others to Act because he or she values collaboration and knows that organizational success is a team effort.

6. Good leaders know that showing appreciation for and recognizing the contribution of others contributes to a shared sense of value and overall team spirit.

7. Leadership skills can be developed by anyone with time and effort. Each person has distinct strengths and talents that contribute to overall effectiveness.

Chapter 15: Dental Hygiene is a Business of Dentistry

By Christine A. Hovliaras, RDH, BS, MBA, CDE, and Colleen Rutledge, RDH

Learning Objectives

The student dental hygienist and dental hygiene professional will learn the following key objectives from this chapter:

1. Determine how the economy has affected the practice of dentistry.
2. Understand the value of the dental hygiene department and that it is a business within dentistry.
3. Evaluate new technological advances that can be applied to the practice of dentistry.
4. Learn the rationale and technique for three commonly placed local delivery agents.
5. Understand the role of risk assessment in periodontal therapy.
6. Discover the financial impact of non-surgical periodontal therapy.
7. Assess dental hygiene productivity and the sales of products and services to enhance the profitability of the practice.

Overview

This chapter will discuss the importance of the dental hygiene department and its effect on the practice of dentistry. Dental hygienists play an enhanced productive role in the practice of dentistry by providing lucrative professional services. These services assist patients in improving their oral health through recare and periodontal therapy appointments. Oral wellness is an essential part of overall wellness, and inflammation in the mouth must be reduced to prevent the link to other systemic diseases such as cardiovascular disease, diabetes, respiratory illnesses and issues with pregnancy.

As stated in the Surgeon General's 2000 report, Oral Health Care in America a "silent epidemic" of dental and oral disease has affected large numbers of people in the United States.[1] Furthermore, the Secretary of Health and Human Services summarized the findings by portraying the mouth as a "mirror for general health and well-being and the association between oral health problems and other health problems." Articles like the February 2004 cover of Time magazine: "The Secret Killer: The Surprising Link between Inflammation and Heart Attacks, Cancer, Alzheimer and Other Diseases" began to emerge, and the article entitled, "Health: The Fires Within," brought the issue to mainstream media. Dental journals published articles citing research suggesting that oral bacteria may contribute to a host of systemic diseases including cardiovascular disease, diabetes, pre-term/low birth weight babies, atherosclerosis, osteoporosis, stroke, stomach ulcers, and pneumonia.[2] Dental hygienists are the front line providers and dental health educators. They perform a multitude of procedures and therapy, depending on their state practice regulations (e.g., local anesthesia, administration of nitrous oxide, laser, local delivery placement, fluoride and sealant application, oral cancer screening), recommend *products and systems for oral disease prevention and provide thorough patient education through effective communication and leadership in the practice.*

Today's Economy

Current unemployment is higher now than at any other time in the U.S. since 1983.[3] Current unemployment as of February 2012 is 8.3% and the economic recession, which began in December 2007, has continued to affect the job security of many people both in the U.S. and globally (for reference, see Figure 15.1 for a graph of unemployment rates from January 2007 until January 2012 on page x). The economic crisis appears to be lasting longer than expected, and this steady cycle of uncertainty continues to unfold.[4]

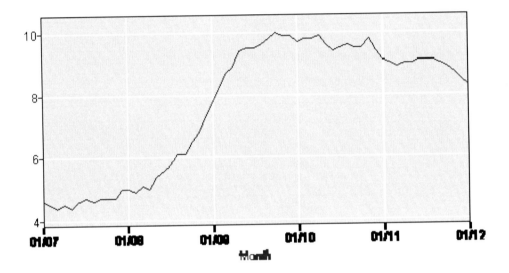

Figure 15.1. Bureau of Labor Statistics Unemployment Rates from January 2007 through January 2012. *Figure available from Bureau of Labor Statistics website at http://data.bls.gov/pdq/SurveyOutputServlet.*

Current unemployment is due to a major downfall in the housing market with current homes selling for less than their market value; foreclosures and short sales increasing; the difficulty of obtaining mortgages in the presence of credit card debt; the lack of an adequate down payment on mortgages; the complication of obtaining a line of credit, which has been stopped due to the downturn in the economy; and the increase in costs for everything from energy and food, to clothing and other daily and monthly expenses. People are experiencing decreased work hours and complete job loss, which results in the loss of medical and dental benefits and the unemployed are trying to pay their bills on a limited income.

In this difficult and challenging economic time, how are dental practices being affected and what is happening to the dental hygienists working in the dental hygiene departments across the U.S. and globally? One of this chapter's authors experienced the crisis when she lost a three-day-a-week dental hygiene position because her experience commanded more money than a new dental hygienist who was working one day a week at that same practice. Despite the author's expertise and valuable skill in the profession, the dentist terminated her and hired the new clinician in her place. Other dental hygienists have shared with one of the chapter's authors that their hours were reduced, and there were no raises or bonuses for 2011; others were also terminated.

Is there a better way to handle this tough economy? Can professionals work as a cooperative dental team by putting business strategies into place that do not reduce work hours? As dental hygienists, can we offer an enhanced business approach to the dental hygiene department and the value that this department brings to the practice?

The answer is yes! So what has to be done next?

The Value of the Dental Hygiene Department

In the midst of an economic recession, the weekly team meeting takes on an even more important role. It is the communication tool that educates the entire team about the impact of the economy on the practice. It is of vital importance that the dentist and the dental team, including the dental hygiene department, review the weekly schedule. The team must determine which patients will be coming to their appointments and what type of previous dental/restorative/cosmetic treatment was diagnosed to be scheduled to be completed but was not carried out. The team also can review what type of services may now be considered during each patient's dental hygiene professional cleaning appointment.

In a 2009 survey conducted by Dental Economics and Dr. Roger Levin, Dr. Levin stated that the dental hygiene department is the second largest production center of the practice. It is the gateway of opportunity for the practice, and having a strong dental hygiene team is needed to carry out the goals of this department.[5] With the current economic crisis, would the dental hygiene department be the No. 1 production center of the practice? It is something to think about especially if patients who have lost their insurance are putting off restorative treatment due to financial instability.

Goals of the Dental Practice and the Dental Hygiene Department

The goals of the practice need to be defined by the dentist and shared with the dental team. Professional Savvy, LLC, has developed a Career Tools CD for dentists that assists them in defining the key vision and goals for the practice and what the dental hygiene team, the dental assistant team and front office team should accomplish that year for the dental practice and subsequent years (1 to 3 years, 4 to 6 years and 7 to 9 years). See Chapter 6: Career and Professional Development for more information on these new tools. The Career Tools CD for the dentist, dental specialist, dental hygienist and dental assistant can be purchased at www.professionalsavvychd.com. The dental goals need to be discussed with the dental hygiene team so they understand exactly what type of restorative, cosmetic and implant dentistry the dentist(s) would like to conduct with their patients. The dental hygiene team understands the goals and then identifies the goals for the dental hygiene department, which would be reviewed in detail with the dentist. Once agreement of the dental hygiene goals are reached, then the dental hygiene team would carry out next steps with the patients in the practice.

Medical Overview, Screening Assessments and Dental and Periodontal Charting

A thorough review of the patient's medical history must be conducted to identify previous and existing medications, systemic diseases and medical issues the patient is currently experiencing. As well, the dental team should review any medical interactions with dental treatment the patient might experience and the necessity of premedication prior to dental and dental hygiene services. Several adjunctive salivary diagnostics are available to test for periodontal pathogens, caries and HPV (e.g., BANA Test, MyPerioPath®, MyPerioID® PST®, OraRisk®, etc.). Conducting a blood pressure assessment on the patient may also be considered due to hypertension being a risk factor to cardiovascular disease and stroke.[6]

The sequence of the appointment is an important consideration. A routine dental recare appointment can be broken down into three parts:

1. Diagnostics

First, the dental hygienist must gather all the diagnostics. Without doing this first, it's like driving a car blindfolded to an unknown location without a map. This critical step includes updating the medical history, doing a periodontal risk assessment, salivary diagnostic testing, oral cancer screening (dentist will follow up during exam) and taking blood pressure. Taking appropriate radiographs (full mouth series (FMX), horizontal/vertical bite wings (BW's)) should be done at the beginning of the appointment as well, as the images are used not only to detect dental decay and pathology, but also to evaluate bone levels and supporting tooth structures. Lastly, a full (6 point) periodontal charting (manual or technologies like Florida Probe®, periopal® or Dental R.A.T.™) should be recorded and used in conjunction with all other diagnostic and clinical observations in order to determine a treatment plan. The information gathered during this portion of the dental hygiene visit determines the difference between a professional prophylaxis and periodontal therapy – it is important that dental hygienists 'probe first' before they pick up a scaler or ultrasonic device!

2. Clinical Treatment

Once a treatment plan is developed, then it's time for the actual treatment to begin. It would be suggested to have the patient conduct a 30 second pre-procedural rinse (essential oils or chlorhexidine) and then use ultrasonic therapy throughout the entire mouth followed by hand scaling. (See Figure 15.2 of author conducting a professional prophylaxis on patient on page 269).

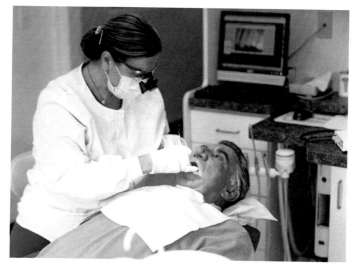

Figure 15.2. Christine Hovliaras conducting a professional prophylaxis on a patient. *Figure provided by and reprinted with permission from Christine Hovliaras.*

Next polishing is conducted and therapeutic polishing may be necessary for desensitization. If this is the case, conduct polishing first. Patients may be more comfortable when polishing first with a desensitizing prophy paste (ProClude®, Enamel Pro®, Nova Min®, Colgate® Sensitive Pro-Relief™ Desensitizing Paste, etc). The latter part of the clinical portion of the appointment includes flossing, irrigation, application of local delivery agents if necessary, oral hygiene instruction and if conducting periodontal therapy and local delivery agents, it may be necessary to provide post-operative instructions.

3. The Dentist Examination

Utilizing a caries detection technology (DIAGNOdent, SOPROLIFE), dental patient education (Casey) and the intraoral camera will help to easily communicate restorative needs to the patient and increase patient compliance. Complete the appointment by establishing a recare frequency and enter treatment into the computer or write it in the patient's chart. When clinicians conduct oral cancer screening (remember a chemiluminescent light source is most effective during first ten minutes), they should notify the dentist when they are ready for an exam to be conducted. While waiting for the dentist, the clinician should schedule the patient's next appointment and prepare a take-home bag of oral hygiene supplies for the patient (for reference, see Form 15.1 Perio-Therapeutics' Dental Hygiene Department Sequencing Protocol on page 270).

Form 15.1. Dental Hygiene Appointment Sequence Protocol

PERIO-THERAPEUTICS & BEYOND
Dental Hygiene Appointment Sequence Protocol

I. Gather all Diagnostics*:

1. Review and update medical history and take blood pressure and pulse.
2. Conduct a risk assessment (PreViser™ software or written form).
3. Take appropriate radiographs (full mouth series (FMX), horizontal or vertical bitewings (BW's)).
4. Conduct full (6 point) periodontal charting (manual, Florida Probe®, periopal®, Dental R.A.T.™ 2.0).
5. Treatment plan using all the above information.

*The information gathered during this portion of the dental hygiene visit determines the difference between conducting a prophylaxis or periodontal therapy.

II. Routine Clinical Treatment:

1. Conduct a 30 second pre-procedural rinse.
2. Provide ultrasonic therapy throughout the entire mouth including tongue disinfection.
3. Hand scale the mouth with instruments.
4. Polish (note: if polishing is necessary for desensitization, the therapeutic polishing would be conducted FIRST – Nova Min®, ProClude®, Enamel Pro®, Colgate® Sensitive Pro-Relief™ Desensitizing Paste).
5. Flossing and irrigation utilizing medicament if necessary.
6. Place any necessary isolated local delivery agents. IMPORTANT! If the clinician is placing several local delivery agents during a "prophy" then he or she may have missed the early periodontal diagnosis.

III. Prepare for the Dentist Exam:

1. Utilize caries detection technology any suspected areas of decay (DIAGNOdent, SOPROLIFE).
2. Utilize dental patient education software (Casey).
3. Identify any incomplete restorative treatment.
4. Use intraoral camera to communicate restorative needs.
5. Enter today's treatment and any treatment plan under the appropriate provider.
6. Establish recare frequency or need for periodontal therapy.
7. Conduct oral cancer screening (e.g. ViziLite® Plus with TBlue®, VELscope Vx, etc) examinations.
8. Notify the dentist when the exam needs to be completed.
9. Schedule next appointment.
10. Provide oral hygiene instruction/give patient appropriate oral care supplies or literature to take home.

Radiographs should be assessed to determine previously diagnosed treatment, and new radiographs taken to determine if new dental diseases are diagnosed. When a dental restoration or dental issue is diagnosed, the use of an intraoral camera is recommended to identify the dental issue, show the picture of the dental issue to the patient describing what is currently going on and then determine next steps for treatment. A picture is worth a thousand words when utilizing intraoral images, and when the patient sees it and experiences it – there should not be the challenge of having to literally "sell" the treatment to the patient. At this point, patients should understand the importance of what the dental hygienist is recommending.

With today's advances in computerized software technology, the use of Dentrix's G5, Carestream Dental's SoftDent and Practiceworks practice management software programs make the entire team's job easier in scheduling and managing patient appointments, conducting digital radiographs, assessment of dental and periodontal concerns to help determine a treatment plan and next steps. Conducting a periodontal probing of patients is vital to assess their periodontal health and determine any suspicious areas that are four millimeters or more in depth. This information should be captured in a computer chart or written in the patient's chart if the dental office is not paperless. Use of various technologies featuring the Florida Probe®, periopal® and the Dental R.A.T.™ system can be introduced to make periodontal probing easier in practice.

Technologies in Periodontal Charting

There are several products available to simplify periodontal evaluation and charting. The Florida Probe® offers "constant-force" accuracy with an educational component and data analysis. Dental R.A.T.™ is a foot-operated mouse that provides hands free-periodontal charting and periopal® offers voice-activated periodontal charting. All systems run on in-operatory dental software computers. The Ultrasonic Periodontal Probe, not yet available in the U.S., is a non-invasive periodontal probe that uses ultrasound imaging technology with an intra-oral ultrasound beam probe.

Risk Assessment

Comprehensive periodontal risk assessment reveals important medical factors that are essential to determining a patient's true periodontal status. Without the knowledge of risk factors, clinicians tend to default to a "prophy" and miss the diagnosis of periodontal therapy. It is critical to employ this step as there is little to go on to differentiate between gingivitis and early periodontal disease. Common risk assessment factors are: smoking, genetics, diabetes, cardiovascular disease, stress, diet and nutrition, hormone imbalance and high blood pressure to name a few (for reference, see Form 15.2 Risk Assessment Form on pages 272-273).

Form 15.2. Periodontal Risk Assessment Questionnaire

Periodontal Risk Assessment Questionnaire

Name _____   Date _____

Do you now or have you ever used the following:

	Amounts per day	Used for how many years	If you quit, list what year
☐ Cigarette	_____	_____	_____
☐ Cigar	_____	_____	_____
☐ Pipe	_____	_____	_____
☐ Chewing	_____	_____	_____

IF YOU ARE A PATIENT WHO HAS DIABETES:

Is your diabetes under control?　☐ Yes　☐ No

Are you prone to diabetic complications?　☐ Yes　☐ No

How do you monitor your blood sugar? _____

Who is your physician for diabetes? _____

IF YOU ARE NOT A PATIENT WHO HAS DIABETES:

Any family history of diabetes?　☐ Yes　☐ No

Have you had any of these warning signs of diabetes?

☐ frequent urination　　　☐ excessive thirst

☐ excessive hunger　　　☐ weakness and fatigue

☐ slow healing of cuts　　☐ unexplained weight loss

Tobacco Use

Tobacco use is the most significant risk factor for gum disease.

Blood Sugar

Diabetes

Gum disease is a common complication of diabetes. Untreated gum disease makes it harder for patients with diabetes to control their blood sugar.

Do you have any risk factors for heart disease or stroke?

☐ Family history of heart disease   ☐ Tobacco use   ☐ Obesity

☐ High cholesterol   ☐ High blood pressure

If you have any of these other risk factors it is especially important for you to always keep your gums as healthy as possible.

Are you taking or have you ever taken any of the following medication:

☐ Antiseizure medications. (such as Dilantin®, Tegretol®, Phenobarbital, etc.)

     ☐ Yes   ☐ No

   If you answered yes, are you still taking the anti-seizure medication?

     ☐ Yes   ☐ No

   Other Medication: _____

☐ Calcium Channel Blocker blood pressure medication. (such as Procardia®, Cardizem®, Norvasc®, Verapamil®, etc.)

   Other: _____

☐ Immunosuppressant therapy (such as Prednisone, Azathioprine, Cyclosporins, Corticosteriods (Asthma-Inhalers), etc.)

   Other: _____

Is there an immediate family member(s) who currently has or had gum problems in the past? (e.g. your mother, father, or siblings):

☐ Yes   ☐ No

Heart Attack/Stroke
Untreated gum disease may increase your risk for heart attack or stroke.

Medications
A side effect of some medications can cause changes in your gums.

Family History/ Genetics
The tendency for gum disease to develop can be inherited.

Perio-Therapeutics & Beyond

267-241-5833   www.PerioAndBeyond.com

Risk assessment software is available for periodontal disease, oral cancer and caries through PreViser. This is an ideal tool for offices that are paperless and are serious about risk assessment. Educational videos are available at PreViser University: http://previser.net/university/default.htm.

If a patient has periodontal pocketing of four millimeters or greater, an assessment should be made to the patient's periodontal status and if current recare visits should continue to take place at six months or occur more frequently at three or four months. A determination if the patient should undergo periodontal therapy such as debridement, scaling and root planning and placement of local delivery agents in practice must be considered. The dentist should be working collaboratively with a periodontist for patients with moderate-severe periodontitis in order to optimize periodontal health. It is always best to refer to a periodontist when a patient presents with severe chronic periodontitis, furcation involvement, vertical/angular defects, aggressive periodontitis, acute periodontal conditions, progressive recession and peri-implant disease.[7]

New, Recare and Periodontal Therapy Appointments in Practice

The number of new patients on the dental hygienists' schedule can vary. Some practices appoint a new patient on the dentist's schedule and new patients aren't recorded under the dental hygienists' production. As noted by one of the chapter author's during numerous consultation sessions, in practices in which new patients are scheduled with the dental hygienist first, a comprehensive examination may not count toward the hygiene production. Insurance driven practices tend to have higher monthly new patient numbers, whereas fee-for-service practices may be a bit lower

The ratio of services within the dental hygiene department is important. As a general rule of thumb, 30 to 33% of services should be in periodontal therapy procedures (for reference, see Box 15.1 with periodontal codes in the 4000s below) with the remaining 67 to 70% in recare, exams, radiographs, etc. Often times dental offices are only providing 1 to 15% in periodontal services. From this information one can see how much untapped potential lies within every dental practice! Here's an example of how one of the chapter author's dental practice clients actually surpassed the goal of 33% periodontal/67% recare ratio.

Box 15.1. Periodontal Codes in the 4000's

PERIODONTAL CODES IN THE 4000'S

D4341 – Scaling and Root Planing of 4 or more teeth

D4342 – Scaling and Root Planing of 1 to 3 teeth

D4355 – Full Mouth Debridement

D4381 – Locally Applied Antimicrobial Agent

D4910 – Periodontal Maintenance

This client actually started out better than most dental practices, with 24% periodontal therapy services/76% recare, exams, radiographs, etc. After implementing a strong non-surgical periodontal therapy program, the practice surpassed the author's consultation expectations by increasing the ratio of services to 37% periodontal and 63% recare, exams, radiographs, etc., which surpasses the anticipated standard in the profession.[8]

As stated above, one-third of dental hygiene production should be in periodontal therapy services. To determine how a dental practice ranks in this parameter, one should add the total monthly production of all periodontal procedures (refer back to Box 15.1) and divide it into the total dental hygiene production.

Dental Hygienists as Production Leaders

Generally speaking, dental hygienists are expected to produce three times their salary or 33% of dental hygiene production. Many clinicians are experiencing cutbacks of their hours or are being terminated and don't realize why. In order to increase job security and understand the business side of dental hygiene, dental hygienists should track their production, especially in the current economic climate.

First, ascertain what the actual production is per hour and compare that to the hourly salary. To determine the production per hour, take the clinician's daily total production (not including the doctor's exam) and divide it by the number of hours worked.

An example would be: $1200 daily production divided by 8 hours =$150 /hour production. If clinicians are making $35, they are certainly producing three times their hourly production rate.

However, if the production is below 33%, then the day is probably full of "prophylactic appointments." To rectify this situation, the dental hygienist should start doing the things that are addressed in this chapter. Begin immediately by doing full-mouth, six-point periodontal charting on each patient and then treatment plan by quadrant. When clinicians consider doing more periodontal therapy in conjunction with locally applied antimicrobials, they will find that production will easily increase. Strategies like the ones mentioned in the chapter will not only ensure clinicians' job security, but might even earn them a raise at the next review!

One the authors of this chapter was trying to determine what a fair hourly rate would be once she started doing more periodontal therapy cases and incorporating locally applied antimicrobials routinely. The formula above was used. Here is an example of how the hourly rate was determined (note: a six-month daily production average was used): $1570 daily production divided by 8 hours = $195/hr. An hourly rate of $65/hour was determined to be fair when using the formula because it was three times the production. (See Figure 15.3 one of the author's conducting periodontal treatment on a patient on page 276).

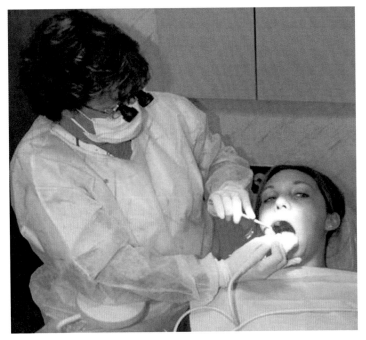

Figure 15.3. Colleen Rutledge conducting periodontal therapy on a patient. *Figure provided by and reprinted with permission from Colleen Rutledge.*

Take it a step further. Consider adding one day a month providing ONLY periodontal therapy services. What would a fair hourly rate be to do periodontal therapy cases ONLY all day long? Let's use the formula: $3835 daily production for periodontal therapy ONLY divided by 8 hours = $479/hr. An hourly rate of $159/hour is fair. Motivated yet? For reference, see Figure 15.4 Periodontal Therapy Program on next page).

Options for Production Success

There are several ways to increase dental hygienists' salaries besides hourly once they are producing at periodontal therapy levels. Here are some options to consider:

Quarterly Periodontal Therapy Bonuses
1. If working on periodontal therapy model all day, (refer, again, to Figure 15.4 Periodontal Therapy Program) calculate each dental hygienist's production (do not include exams and radiographs 2. Subtract the overhead (gross salary, the cost of all local delivery agents, etc.).
2. The remaining production is split accordingly: 1/3 goes back into the practice, 1/3 for the doctor and 1/3 for the dental hygienist.

Bonus for Surpassing Daily Production Quota
The dental hygienist is compensated 33% of the amount remaining after the daily production goal is met. Run a six-month report to determine average daily production.

Figure 15.4. Periodontal Therapy Program

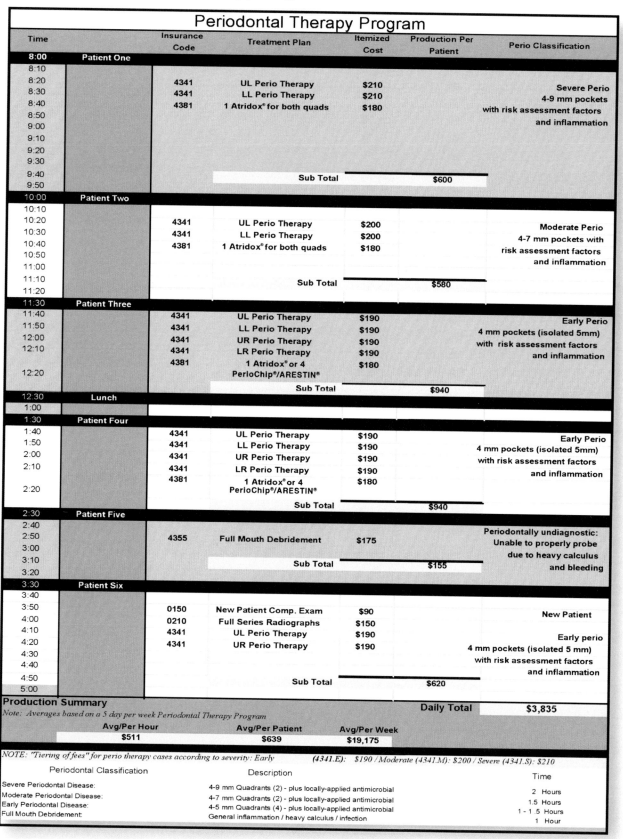

Time		Insurance Code	Treatment Plan	Itemized Cost	Production Per Patient	Perio Classification
8:00	Patient One					
8:10						
8:20		4341	UL Perio Therapy	$210		Severe Perio
8:30		4341	LL Perio Therapy	$210		4-9 mm pockets
8:40		4381	1 Atridox® for both quads	$180		with risk assessment factors
8:50						and inflammation
9:00						
9:10						
9:20						
9:30						
9:40			Sub Total		$600	
9:50						
10:00	Patient Two					
10:10						
10:20		4341	UL Perio Therapy	$200		Moderate Perio
10:30		4341	LL Perio Therapy	$200		4-7 mm pockets with
10:40		4381	1 Atridox® for both quads	$180		risk assessment factors
10:50						and inflammation
11:00						
11:10			Sub Total		$580	
11:20						
11:30	Patient Three					
11:40		4341	UL Perio Therapy	$190		Early Perio
11:50		4341	LL Perio Therapy	$190		4 mm pockets (isolated 5mm)
12:00		4341	UR Perio Therapy	$190		with risk assessment factors
12:10		4341	LR Perio Therapy	$190		and inflammation
		4381	1 Atridox® or 4	$180		
12:20			PerioChip®/ARESTIN®			
			Sub Total		$940	
12:30	Lunch					
1:00						
1:30	Patient Four					
1:40		4341	UL Perio Therapy	$190		Early Perio
1:50		4341	LL Perio Therapy	$190		4 mm pockets (isolated 5mm)
2:00		4341	UR Perio Therapy	$190		with risk assessment factors
2:10		4341	LR Perio Therapy	$190		and inflammation
		4381	1 Atridox® or 4	$180		
2:20			PerioChip®/ARESTIN®			
			Sub Total		$940	
2:30	Patient Five					
2:40						Periodontally undiagnostic:
2:50		4355	Full Mouth Debridement	$175		Unable to properly probe
3:00						due to heavy calculus
3:10			Sub Total		$155	and bleeding
3:20						
3:30	Patient Six					
3:40						
3:50		0150	New Patient Comp. Exam	$90		New Patient
4:00		0210	Full Series Radiographs	$150		
4:10		4341	UL Perio Therapy	$190		Early perio
4:20		4341	UR Perio Therapy	$190		4 mm pockets (isolated 5 mm)
4:30						with risk assessment factors
4:40						and inflammation
4:50			Sub Total		$620	
5:00						

Production Summary				Daily Total	$3,835

Note: Averages based on a 5 day per week Periodontal Therapy Program

Avg/Per Hour	Avg/Per Patient	Avg/Per Week
$511	$639	$19,175

NOTE: "Tiering of fees" for perio therapy cases according to severity: Early   (4341.E): $190 / Moderate (4341.M): $200 / Severe (4341.S): $210

Periodontal Classification	Description	Time
Severe Periodontal Disease:	4-9 mm Quadrants (2) - plus locally-applied antimicrobial	2 Hours
Moderate Periodontal Disease:	4-7 mm Quadrants (2) - plus locally-applied antimicrobial	1.5 Hours
Early Periodontal Disease:	4-5 mm Quadrants (4) - plus locally-applied antimicrobial	1 - 1.5 Hours
Full Mouth Debridement:	General inflammation / heavy calculus / infection	1 Hour

Straight Percentage

1. Twenty-five percent of anything conducted in the dental hygiene operatory (this would include exam, radiographs, whitening, night guards, sealants, etc.).
2. Thirty-three percent of all procedures limited to preventive and periodontal procedures (recare, periodontal maintenance, periodontal therapy, full mouth debridement, local delivery agents

Hourly Rate Plus Commission for Periodontal Procedures

1. Hourly rate PLUS
2. Ten percent of all procedures in the 4000 category for periodontal procedures (for reference, see Box 15.1 on page x). This rewards the progressive, skilled and more competent dental hygienist to diagnose, treatment plan, schedule and treat "more challenging" patients.

Locally Applied Antimicrobials

1. Ten percent of all local delivery agents placed (ARESTIN®, PerioChip®, Atridox®) in the form of a bonus at the end of each month

Assisted Hygiene

1. One dental hygienist working two rooms with a dental hygiene assistant: Pay the hygienist 30% of the combined room production (minus the assistant's salary).
2. Two hygienists with one dental hygiene assistant shared between them: Pay $10 for each additional patient seen. Example: If the RDH usually sees 12 patients when practicing solo and with an assistant they are able to see 15, the RDH would be compensated an extra $30 that day.[8]

See Chapter 16: Assisted Dental Hygiene for more information about utilizing an assisted dental hygiene model in practice.

Dispel the "Loss Leader Myth"

Dental hygiene departments can easily transform from "loss leaders," producing $600 to $800 daily, to "production leaders" achieving $2,500+ when employing a comprehensive periodontal therapy program.

Many practices maintain a *mechanical* model, which focuses on removing calculus, plaque biofilm, stain and performing root planing one quarter of the mouth at a time. Treatment plans will commonly segregate each quadrant of therapy by two weeks. In reality, many cases never come to fruition until months later, at which time the initial quadrants have become re-infected by bacteria from the latter quadrants.

Research now directs dental professionals to a *medical* model, decreasing the bacterial load in the entire mouth, with treatment completed within 24 to 48 hours.[9] Although longer appointments are necessary, proper use of ultrasonics increases efficiency, rendering one or two one-and-a-half hour appointments rather than four one hour appointments. The incorporation of local delivery agents during initial therapy as well as maintenance enhances clinical outcomes and substantially augments the services and profitability of the dental hygiene department.

Practices offering services based on current research and trends in periodontal therapy see an increase in their hourly production rate ranges of $90 – $120 when integrating periodontal therapy into a traditional hygiene program (see Figure 15.5, Integrating Periodontal Therapy into the Traditional Dental Hygiene Program on page 280). For a different approach, one may take the dental hygiene department to the next level by implementing a Periodontal Therapy Day once a month seeing hourly production soar from $150 to $400 (see Figure 15.4. Periodontal Therapy Program on page 277). Embracing this model, dental hygiene departments can flourish into indispensable channels of both quality and profitability.

Figure 15.5. Sample Dental Hygiene Schedule Integrating Periodontal Therapy into Traditional Dental Hygiene Program

Integrating Periodontal Therapy with a Traditional Hygiene Program

Time	Patient Number	Insurance Code	Treatment Plan	Itemized Cost	Production Per Patient	Perio Classification
8:00	Patient One					
8:10						
8:20		4341	UR Perio Therapy	$200		
8:30		4341	LR Perio Therapy	$200		Moderate perio
8:40		4381	1 Atridox® Treatment	$180		4-5 mm pockets
8:50						
9:00			Sub Total		$580	
9:10						
9:20						
9:30	Patient Two					
9:40		0120	Periodic exam	$50		
9:50		1110	Adult Prophy	$90		
10:00		0274	4 BW's	$70		Recare
10:10		4381	2 ARESTIN® or PerioChip®	$90		
10:20			Sub Total		$300	
10:30	Patient Three					
10:40		0120	Periodic exam	$50		
10:50		1110	Adult Prophy	$90		
11:00						Recare
11:10			Sub Total		$140	
11:20						
11:30	Patient Four					
11:40		0120	Periodic exam	$50		
11:50		1110	Adult Prophy	$90		Recare
12:00		4381	1 ARESTIN® or PerioChip®	$45		
12:10			Sub Total		$185	
12:20						
12:30	Lunch					
1:00			Lunch 12:30 - 1:30			
1:30	Patient Five					
1:40		0120	Periodic exam	$50		
1:50		1110	Adult Prophy	$90		Recare
2:00		4381	1 ARESTIN® or PerioChip®	$45		
2:10			Sub Total		$185	
2:20	Patient Six					
2:30		0120	Periodic exam	$50		Overdue pt with gingivits
2:40		4355	Full Mouth Debridement	$175		heavy calculus and
2:50		210	Full Series Radiographs	$150		bleeding
3:00			Sub Total		$375	
3:10	Patient Seven					
3:20		0120	Periodic exam	$50		
3:30		1110	Adult Prophy	$90		Recare
3:40		9999	Power Toothbrush	$100		
3:50			Sub Total		$240	
4:00	Patient Eight					
4:10		0120	Periodic exam	$50		
4:20		1110	Adult Prophy	$90		Recare
4:30		4381	2 ARESTIN® or PerioChip®	$90		
4:40			Sub Total		$230	
4:50						
5:00						

Production Summary | | | | | Daily Total | $2,235 |

Note: Averages based on a 5 day work schedule

Avg/Per Hour	Avg/Per Patient	Avg/Per Week
$298	$279	$11,175

NOTE: "Tiering of fees" for perio therapy cases according to severity: Early (4341.E): $190 / Moderate (4341.M): $200 / Severe (4341.S): $210

Periodontal Classification	Description	Time
Severe Periodontal Disease:	4-9 mm Quadrants (2) - plus locally-applied antimicrobial	2 Hours
Moderate Periodontal Disease:	4-7 mm Quadrants (2) - plus locally-applied antimicrobial	1.5 Hours
Early Periodontal Disease:	4-5 mm Quadrants (4) - plus locally-applied antimicrobial	1 - 1.5 Hours
Full Mouth Debridement:	General inflammation / calculus; infection in all quadrants	1 Hour

Local delivery agents that dental hygiene departments recommend and utilize will help to show numbers in terms of profitability. Dental hygienists should keep track of their profitability in the practice to determine the production they are bringing in especially in this bad economic time.

Local Delivery Agents

It is important to address systemic considerations and optimize clinical outcomes in periodontal therapy cases as the goal when incorporating any adjunctive therapies. The local delivery agents discussed in this chapter are all approved by the U.S. Food and Drug Administration (FDA) as biodegradable, bioadhesive and require no refrigeration. They are indicated in periodontal pockets of 5 mm or greater and can be placed at the time of initial non-surgical therapy or as a secondary treatment for non-responsive sites.

PerioChip®

PerioChip® is 2.5 mg chlorhexidine gluconate and is distributed by Adrian Pharmaceuticals. It was the first non-antibiotic, local delivery agent. The orange-brown, rectangular chip measures 4 mm by 5 mm and is inserted directly into a single site (e.g. #12 ML) infected pocket. PerioChip® may be reinserted after three months with no interdental cleaning for ten days after placement and can be easily placed with cotton pliers or a pressure-sensitive instrument called 'Laschal' (for reference, see Figure 15.6 of placement of PerioChip® below).

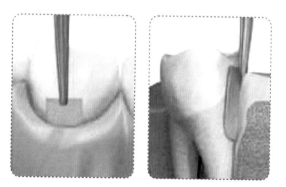

Figure 15.6. PerioChip® 2.5 mg Chlorhexidine Gluconate. *Figure provided by Colleen Rutledge and reprinted with permission from Adrian Pharmaceuticals. Figure available from the British Dental Journal at* http://www.nature. com/bdj/journal/v195/n4/full/4810497a.html.

ARESTIN®

ARESTIN® is an antibiotic comprised of 1 mg. minocycline powder manufactured by OraPharma, Inc. The handle/ cartridge system makes placing minocycline powder easy, with the best result obtained when the end of the plastic cartridge is flattened. The tip of the cartridge is placed at the base of the pocket, where the red-complex bacteria are the most virulent, in order to be most effective. A handle is used to express the minocycline into single site periodontal pockets (e.g., #12 ML) and may be reinserted three months after placement. Patients are advised not to floss in the treated area for ten days (for reference, see Figure 15.7 of placement of ARESTIN® on page 282).

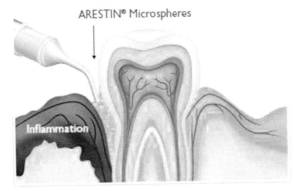

ARESTIN® Microspheres

Inflammation

Figure 15.7. ARESTIN® 1 mg Minocycline. *Figure provided by Colleen Rutledge and reprinted with permission from Orapharma, Inc. Figure is available at* http://www.arestin.com/effectiveness/.

Atridox®

ZILA, a division of Tolmar distributes Atridox®, which is 10% doxycycline hyclate antibiotic gel that flows into periodontal pockets then quickly hardens to a wax-like substance, slowly releasing the antibiotic to the infected area. It is an antibiotic and treats multiple sites making it an excellent choice when copious pockets are present, as in the case with initial non-surgical periodontal therapy cases. With proficient use, 15 to 30 pockets can be treated making it a prudent and effective choice for both patients and dental practices (for reference, see Figure 15.8 of placement of Atridox® below).

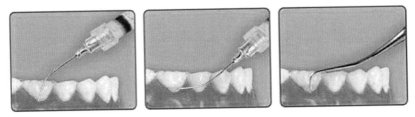

Figure 15.8. Atridox, 10% doxycycline hyclate. *Figure provided by Colleen Rutledge and reprinted with permission from Zila, a Tolmar Company. Figure available at http://www.zila.com/93/HOW%20TO%20USE/.*

Ordering and Pricing Information for Local Delivery Agents

As a rule, the higher the quantity purchased, the greater the profit to the practice. PerioChip® can be ordered at 1-866-PerioChip and distributed by: Adrian Pharmaceuticals. There are 20 chips per box. This product can be used just like ARESTIN® (for single sites) and is great to use when a patient is allergic to tetracycline, prefers no antibiotics or is pregnant (consent from the obstetrician/gynecologist is recommended). The box is small enough to be kept in the top drawer of the most frequently used dental hygiene operatories or in the central supply closet.

ARESTIN® is distributed by the Henry Schein Company and comes with 24 cartridges in a box and can be ordered at 1-866-273-7846. Ordering ten boxes reduces the dental practice's cost to $17.08 per cartridge as of 2012 pricing.

Atridox® is distributed by Zila, a division of Tolmar and comes with six syringes per box. Atridox® can be purchased at 1-877-865-6271. Dental offices would benefit from ordering at least six boxes; especially at the onset of integrating local delivery agents within the dental hygiene department. The cost to the dental practice per treatment (or per patient) would be reduced to approximately $59 as of 2012 pricing.

Many clinical factors should be considered when choosing which local delivery agent to use. Having said that, let's look at two scenarios, all things being equal clinically (for reference, see Figure 15.9 on single and multiple application of a local delivery agent).

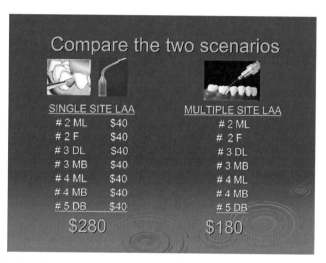

Figure 15.9. This figure illustrates the cost comparisons of a single versus a multiple site local delivery agent. *Figure provided by and reprinted with permission from Colleen Rutledge.*

The national average fee for Atridox® is $180 (using pricing available in 2012). The cost to the practice is about $68 per syringe, so the practice makes approximately $112 on each Atridox® application. As one can see by the chart above, using a multiple site antimicrobial is the best economic choice for both the patient and the practice. The above scenario saves the patient $100, thus increasing patient compliance and more importantly enhances periodontal therapy clinical results (for reference, see Figure 15.10 on the rationale for recommending Atridox® to patients).

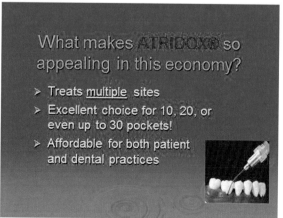

Figure 15.10. This figure illustrates the benefits of utilizing Atridox® with patients who require a local delivery agent. *Figure provided by and reprinted with permission from Colleen Rutledge.*

Impact of Incorporating Non-Surgical Therapies: A Case Study

Dental accountants and consultants understand the economic impact of periodontal services within the dental hygiene department. When analyzing a production analysis report, one can quickly see how frequently "codes in the "4000s" are being used. Dental hygiene departments flourish and production increases when the 4000s codes are cited routinely.

In the September 2008, *Dental Economics* featured an article by practice management consultant Linda Miles: "Trust, Delegate and Celebrate," which profiled a dental office in Cary, NC. This dental office had two dentists and three dental hygienists within the dental hygiene department producing $44,000 per month. After a year of implementing effective communication, scheduling and practice management consulting, the hygiene department increased by $10,000 up to $54,000 per month. After implementing a periodontal therapy program, independent hygiene consulting: *Perio-Therapeutics & Beyond www.PerioAndBeyond.com*, this practice now has four full-time dental hygienists (16 days per month each) who now average over $84,000 per month.[8]

Additional Case Studies: Four Dental Practices

Many dental offices across the country are still operating with a 1980's treatment protocol, leaving patients uninformed and untreated. It's more than just about "saving teeth" – it's about the patients total body health. For reference, see Figures 15.11a through 15.11d below, which illustrate the chapter author's consulting work that was completed with four dental practices – three practices that employ three hygienists and one that employs one full-time and one part-time hygienist), (two that are one-dentist practices and two that are two–dentist practices). These figures show the revenue generated by employing a periodontal therapy model.

Client #1: 2 DDS / 3 RDH

Client # 1	Pre-consult 6 mo total	Post consult 6 mo total	Revenue increase 6 mths post consult
arestin	27	99	$ 4,464
atridox	0	12	$ 2,916
SRP 4341	3	16	$ 5,161
SRP 4342	6	21	$ 3,300
			$ 15,841

* this client incorporated Oral Cancer Screening technology as well and increased production by an <u>ADDITIONAL</u> $17,159

Client # 2: 2 DDS / 3 RDH
Texas

Client # 2	Pre-consult 6 mo total	Post consult 6 mo total	Revenue increase 6 mths post consult
arestin	42	134	$ 4,464
atridox	0	27	$ 2,916
SRP 4341	39	100	$ 5,161
SRP 4342	13	63	$ 3,300
*PCht 0180	69	268	$ 3,980
			$ 24,720

* this client incorporated Oral Cancer Screening technology as well and increased production by an <u>ADDITIONAL</u> $8,710

Client # 3: 1 DDS / 1.5 RDH
Virginia

Client # 3	Pre-consult 6 mo total	Post consult 6 mo total	Revenue increase 6 mths post consult
arestin	0	55	$ 1,925
atridox	0	19	$ 3,420
SRP 4341	11	57	$ 13,048
SRP 4342	3	52	$ 9,702
periochip	0	35	$ 1,400
P Mt 4910	41	64	$ 2,484
			$ 31,979

Client # 4: 2 DDS / 3 RDH
Pennsylvania

Client # 4	Pre-consult 6 mo total	Post consult 6 mo total	Revenue increase 6 mths post consult
debr 4355	12	19	$ 1,015
periochip	0	32	$ 1,280
arestin	0	130	$ 5,200
atridox	0	52	$ 9,360
SRP 4341	12	44	$ 6,240
SRP 4342	16	147	$ 16,375
P Mt 4910	1	11	$ 1,210
Pchrt 0180	0	17	$ 1,275
			$41,955

Figures 15.11 a-d. These additional case figures illustrate the revenue that three, two-dentist and one-dentist practices achieved with the dental hygienists implementing a non-surgical periodontal therapy program in conjunction with local delivery agents in practice. *Figure provided by and reprinted with permission from Colleen Rutledge.*

Ensuring Patient Compliance with Thorough Education and Oral Hygiene Instruction

Once the professional prophylaxis or periodontal care provided during the appointment is over, it is very important to review the steps the patient's role in conducting proper oral hygiene procedures at home. The office should have a list of products that are recommended for flossing, interdental cleaning devices, manual toothbrushes or power toothbrushes (for reference, see Figure 15.12 of Christine Hovliaras conducting flossing instruction on a child patient).

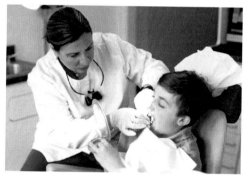

Figures 15.12. Christine Hovliaras teaching flossing technique to a child patient. *Figure provided by and reprinted with permission from Christine Hovliaras.*

Toothbrushes

The Chairside Guide developed with dental hygienists assists in understanding the patient's oral care needs and recommending the type of toothbrush that can be used to provide the best oral health outcomes and promote strong patient compliance. The Toothbrush Assessment Guide can be first be completed by patients about what their oral care habits are. Next the dental hygienist will conduct an oral health assessment on the patient, determine risk factors and recommend toothbrush products to improve the patient's oral health and offer instructions for proper flossing and toothbrushing. The Chairside Guide helps dental hygiene professionals to select toothbrushes from the Colgate toothbrush product line. It is a very efficient tool to consider utilizing in practice at the beginning of the appointment and doesn't take a lot of time to complete. It also helps to bring the dental hygienist and patient into a collaborative working relationship regarding the patient's oral care needs. See Figures 15.13 and 15.14 on pages 286-291 for a more detailed tool that can be used with patients to improve their oral hygiene care.

Figure 15.13 Colgate® Toothbrush Assessment Guide

How do you rate your oral care habits?

We can provide you with an oral care plan during today's visit. Simply fill out this form and present the information to your dental professional.

Name:_____ Date Completed:_____

My oral care habits

Please circle the best description for each category.

The toothbrush I am currently using is___	Manual	Electric rechargeable	Battery-powered
The toothbrush bristles are___	Soft	Medium	Hard
I brush___ per day	Once	Twice	More than twice
I usually brush for___minutes	Less than one	One or two	More than two
I floss___	Never	Occasionally	Daily
I clean my tongue___	Never	Occasionally	Daily

I use the following (circle all that apply): floss picks, interdental brush, gum stimulators, other _____

My oral health self-assessment

Circle the description that best applies to you.

The amount of plaque on my teeth is ___	Heavy	Medium	Light
Bleeding and/ or swollen gums	Severe	Mild to moderate	None
Brushing my teeth is ___	Difficult	Slightly hard	Easy
I have the following (circle all that apply):	Braces	Fillings	Implants or partial or full dentures
	Dry mouth	Sensitive teeth	Receding gums
	Bad breath	Heartburn	Tooth decay
I regularly (circle all that apply):	Use smokeless tobacco	Smoke	Drink alcohol

This review will help you and your dental professional discuss how you can lower your risk.

Dear Professional, review risk factors and determine risk for the following oral diseases/conditions:

	At risk		Notable risk factor
Caries	☐ Yes	☐ No	_____
Periodontal diseases	☐ Yes	☐ No	_____
Dentin hypersensitivity	☐ Yes	☐ No	_____
Other	_____		_____

This will enable you to discuss ways to reduce risk factors with your patient, including at-home care.

This self-assessment does not replace an examination by a dental professional. Please give this self-assessment to your dental professional or dental hygienist and discuss the results.

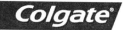 **YOUR PARTNER IN ORAL HEALTH**

Recommended products and instructions for improved oral health

Take this section with you after reviewing your oral care history with your dental professional.

If you have...	These are the right products.
Questions about brushing technique	_____
Visible plaque	_____
High rate of cavities	_____
Lack of tongue cleaning	_____
Bad breath	_____
Trouble holding toothbrushes	_____
Bleeding or swollen gums	_____
Lack of regular flossing	_____
Plaque between teeth	_____
Recurring debris between teeth	_____
Receding gums	_____
Evidence of wear on tooth enamel	_____
Sensitive teeth	_____
Dry mouth	_____
Children under the age of 6	_____
Braces	_____
Postoperative dental procedures	_____

Additional home care instructions

_____

_____

Proper oral health

In addition to regular dental checkups, you can improve your oral health with proper brushing and flossing.

Steps to brush more effectively

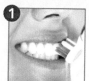 **1** Place the toothbrush at a 45° angle towards the gumline.

 2 Use gentle, short strokes, moving the brush back and forth against the teeth and gums. Continue inside every surface of each tooth in a similar way.

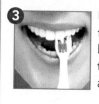 **3** Use the tip of the brush to reach behind each front tooth, on the top and bottom.

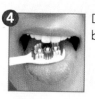 **4** Don't forget to brush your tongue.

Remember to clean between your teeth

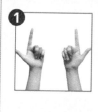 **1** Hold a short amount of floss between your thumb and fingers, and insert it between your teeth. Be careful not to apply too much force to the gums.

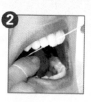 **2** Curve the floss around each tooth in a 'C' shape and gently move it up and down, including under the gumline.

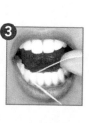 **3** Use a new section of floss for each tooth.

 4 Use an interdental brush to clean hard-to-reach places between teeth.

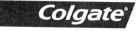 *Colgate®* YOUR PARTNER IN ORAL HEALTH

Figure 15.13. The Colgate® Toothbrush Assessment Guide developed by Colgate-Palmolive Company to assist dental hygienists in assessing the oral care habits, determine risk factors, reinforce flossing and toothbrushing instruction and recommendation of toothbrush products to their patients. *Figure provided by and reprinted with permission from the Colgate-Palmolive Company.*

Figure 15.14 Colgate® Chairside Guide

Reference guide for risk assessment of brushing efficacy

After your professional dental examination and procedures, discuss your patient's oral care habits. Together, you can enact a plan for effective oral hygiene.

Help your patients choose the right tool for their oral care needs

If your patient has...	Recommend a brush that offers...	Available Colgate® products
Improper brushing technique	Improved plaque removal, regardless of brushing technique	Colgate® 360°® Surround
Lack of tongue cleaning	Reduction in breath volatile sulfur compound levels	Colgate® 360°® Series of Toothbrushes
Halitosis	Removal of odor-causing bacteria on the tongue	
Manual dexterity problems	Ergonomic handles, kinetic cleaning power	Colgate® 360°® Sonic Power
Interproximal plaque	Significantly greater interproximal access	Colgate Total® Floss
Constant debris between teeth		
Gingival recession	Softer bristles than an ordinary flat-trimmed toothbrush	Colgate 360°® Sensitive Pro-Relief®
Evidence of abrasion or wear	Less wear on exposed root surfaces vs soft toothbrush	
Dentin hypersensitivity	Gentle care for already irritated gums	
Children under the age of 6	Special features for child compliance	Colgate® Smiles™ Toothbrushes for Kids

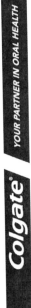

Colgate® / *YOUR PARTNER IN ORAL HEALTH*

Colgate® has the right tool for your patient's unique oral care needs

	Daily Oral Care		Pediatrics	Sensitivity	Interproximal
	Colgate® 360°® Surround	Colgate® 360°® Sonic Power	Colgate® Smiles™	Colgate 360°® Sensitive Pro-Relief®	Colgate Total® Floss
Indication	Designed to remove plaque, regardless of brushing technique	Designed for patients who cannot brush effectively with a manual brush	Designed for your pediatric patients	Designed for patients with tooth sensitivity	For healthy gums and better oral health
Special Features	Multi-height, Surround-Clean™ bristle design cleans both sides of teeth to the gumline, significantly reducing interproximal plaque[1]	AAA battery-powered Produces 20,000 strokes per minute Ergonomic handle	Protects gums and teeth Special child-sized handles Extra-soft bristles Bristles indicating toothpaste dosage	Ultra-soft bristles 48% softer than ordinary flat-trimmed toothbrushes[3] Produces significantly less wear on sensitive tooth surfaces[3]	Micro-crystalline coating slides easily between teeth Single-strand Teflon fiber for nonshredding
Evidence	Removes up to 89% more plaque than ordinary flat-trimmed toothbrushes[1]	Bristles remove over 96% more bacteria than an ordinary flat-trimmed toothbrush[2]	81% of parents surveyed believe their child is more interested in brushing[2]	Produces significantly less wear on teeth vs soft toothbrush[4] Significantly reduced tooth sensitivity after 8 weeks[5]	Regular flossing with brushing reduces gingival bleeding by 67%[6]

References: 1. Mankodi S. Data on file. July 2010. Colgate-Palmolive Company. **2.** Data on file. Colgate-Palmolive Company. **3.** Standard laboratory testing of bristle stiffness versus Oral-B® Indicator® Soft. Data on file. Colgate-Palmolive Company.
4. Li N, Ersen E, Hefferren JJ. Data on file. 2006. Colgate-Palmolive Company. **5.** Schiff T, Wachs G, Petrone M, et al. Compendium. 2009;30(4):234-240. **6.** Graves RC, Disney JA, Stamm JW. J Periodontol. 1989;60:243-247.

Colgate® / *YOUR PARTNER IN ORAL HEALTH*

Figure 15.14. The Colgate® Chairside Guide developed by Colgate-Palmolive Company to assist dental hygienists in understanding their patients' oral care needs and recommending the right toothbrush for their patients' needs. *Figure provided by and reprinted with permission from the Colgate-Palmolive Company.*

Patient compliance in conducting oral care techniques are crucial to the outcome of their periodontal health depending on whether the patient returns to the practice at three, four or six months.

Toothpastes

As toothbrush selection is important to assist patients in their toothbrushing needs, so is choosing the right toothpaste for patients a dental hygienist is treating. Identify what the patient's oral health issue is and then determine what is the best toothpaste to recommend to help patients with their oral care need. For example, for a patient who has tooth sensitivity the dental hygienist should recommend a toothpaste that provides an ingredient to reduce tooth sensitivity such as Sensodyne®, Crest Sensitive® or Colgate® Sensitive. If a patient is cavity prone, then a toothpaste with fluoride should be recommended, and the dental professional can determine whether a prescription fluoride toothpaste should be considered. A patient suffering from plaque accumulation as well as the development of gingivitis should be recommended a toothpaste that has been approved by the American Dental Association (ADA) for reducing plaque and gingivitis (Colgate Total®). Patients who require more vigilant care in helping to decrease cavities should consider prescription fluoride toothpastes. It is important to read the clinical research to know that a toothpaste product has been clinically tested with patients to support the product claims.

Mouthrinses

The dental hygienist should assess if an adjunctive therapy such as fluoride mouthrinse (Fluorigard®), a fluoride and xylitol mouthrinse (Restore, CariFree®) or an antimicrobial mouthrinse (LISTERINE®) should be recommended in addition to brushing and flossing if the patient needs improved oral health beyond those two mechanical cleaning tools.

Selling Products in the Dental Hygiene Department

There are many practices will sell products that are of great need to their patients and then determine if the dental hygiene department can sell this product in practice and obtain a commission on the sale of it. Practices sell power toothbrushes and/or battery operated flossing devices, oral irrigation systems and at-home bleaching systems. Some dental practices are offering whole body wellness services knowing that the oral cavity is part of a whole system. These products include vitamin and mineral tablets and supplements, superfruit antioxidant juices for enhanced nutritional wellness as well as massage therapy, acupuncture, reflexology, meditation/stress reduction and cosmetic enhancements.

Conclusion

Dentistry is a specialty, however it has become integrated with the medical side of health and wellness. Dental hygienists play a critical and important role in the first line of defense for the health of the whole body. The responsibilities that dental hygienists offer to patients to assess, understand oral care concerns, diagnose new oral care needs, treatment plan and offer the right plan for improving patients' oral and systemic health cannot go unnoticed. The dental hygienists' presence must be valued and appreciated in each and every dental and specialty practice they work in across the U.S. and globally.

References

1. U.S. Department of Health and Human Services. Oral Health in America: A report of the surgeon general. Rockville, MD: U.S. Department of Health and Human Services, National Institutes of Health, National Institute of Dental and Craniofacial Research. 2000.

2. Gorman C, Park A, Dell K. Health: the fires within. *Time Magazine*. February 23, 2004. Available at http://www.time.com/time/covers/0,16641,20040223,00.html and http://www.time.com/time/magazine/article/0,9171,993419,00.html. Accessed March 29, 2012.

3. U.S. Bureau of Labor Statistics Unemployment Rates from January 2007 through January 2012. Available at: http://data.bls.gov/pdq/SurveyOutputServlet. Accessed March 29, 2012.

4. Carson E. Jobs Recession Now 49 Months: Longest Since WWII [online article]. *Investors.com*. Available at: http://news.investors.com/article/603791/201203090838/ jobs-recession-is-longest-since-depression.htm. Accessed March 29, 2012.

5. Levin R. Part 2 – 2009 Salary Survey with Dentists [online article]. *Dental Economics*. Available at: http://www.dentaleconomics.com/index/display/article-display/371137/articles/dental-economics/volume-99/issue-11/features/part-2-2009-dental-economics-levin-group-practice-survey.html. Accessed March 29, 2012.

6. McCauley S. Screenings During Dental Hygiene Appointments [online article]. *Dentistry iQ*. September 15, 2011. Available at: http://www.dentistryiq.com/index/display/article-display/8009132297/articles/dentisryiq/rdh-products/evillage-focus/2011/09/screenings.html. Accessed March 29, 2012.

7. Krebs K, Clem D. Guidelines for the management of patients with periodontal diseases. *J Periodontol*. 2006 Sep;77(9):1607-1611.

8. Miles L. Trust, Delegate, Celebrate [online article]. *Dental Economics*. Sept 2008. Available at: http://www.dentaleconomics.com/index/display/article-display/341052/articles/dental-economics/volume-98/issue-9/features/trust-delegate-and-celebrate.html.

9. Miles L. *Dynamic Dentistry: Practice, Management, Tools and Strategy for Breakthrough Success*. Virginia Beach, VA : Link Publishing; 2003:107-108.

10. Quirynen M, De Soete M, Boschmans G, et al. Benefit of "one-stage full-mouth disinfection" is explained by disinfection and root planing within 24 hours: a randomized controlled trial. *J Clin Periodontol*. 2006 Sep; 33(9):639-647. Epub 2006 Jul 20.

Recommended Reading

Perio-Therapeutics & Beyond (www.PerioAndBeyond.com) offers the following DVD and CD's to assist dentists and dental hygienists in enhancing production and keeping abreast of new information in periodontal therapy:

1. *Dispel the Loss Leader Myth: Blueprints to Double Your Hygiene Production*
2. *Treatment Planning Non-Surgical Periodontal Therapy Cases*
3. *Incorporating Locally-Applied Antimicrobials: Rationale and Technique Tips for ARESTIN®, PerioChip®, Atridox®*
4. *What's New in Ultrasonics? Exploring Piezoelectric Technology*
5. *Implementing Periodontal Therapy into Daily Practice*
6. *New Trends in Periodontal Therapy*
7. *"Do-It-Yourself" Dental Hygiene Department Consulting Package*

Critical Thinking Exercises

1. Determine what the dental and dental hygiene goals are for the practice for this year and put your plan of action into place.

2. Identify what your patients' oral care needs are, how you are currently satisfying their needs and what needs improvement.

3. Track your daily dental hygiene production to determine the goals for recare and periodontal therapy cases in the practice that the dental hygiene department can communicate with the dentist. Determine if the dental hygiene department is meeting daily and weekly production needs.

4. Run a monthly 'procedure by provider' report to determine what percentage of the dental hygiene services provided are in the periodontal therapy code range.

5. Continue to take continuing education courses to stay abreast of the trends in dentistry, periodontal therapy and new products being offered to dental hygienists in improving patients' oral hygiene.

Key Concepts

1. The economic recession is affecting dental practices across the country by patients losing their jobs and their dental insurance and because patients frequently do not identifying the importance of oral care as a part of their total systemic health.

2. The dental practice should define goals for the practice, the dental hygiene department and the administrative team in order to achieve annual, weekly and quarterly goals for the year.

3. The dental hygienist should conduct an accurate oral health assessment of each patient that includes: an oral health examination, periodontal probing and radiographic interpretation of what type of dental and dental hygiene treatment patients will need to improve their oral health.

4. The importance of conducting a six-point periodontal charting will help to assess periodontal therapy cases in the practice.

5. Three technologies that assist dental hygienists with periodontal charting are the Florida Probe®, periopal® and Dental R.A.T.™

6. The three most commonly placed local delivery agents are ARESTIN®, Atridox® and PerioChip®, which are site specific antimicrobial therapy for patients with inflamed periodontal pockets (5mm or greater in depth).

7. Risk assessment is a critical component in treatment planning early periodontal therapy cases.

8. A financial impact in the dental hygiene department is realized by providing non-surgical periodontal therapy.

9. The goal for periodontal services in the dental hygiene department is 25 to 33% of the total hygiene production. The dental hygienist should consider tracking daily, weekly, monthly and quarterly production on dental hygiene services to provide the dentist with the value of the dental hygiene department.

Chapter 16: Assisted Dental Hygiene

By Richard A. Huot, DDS

Learning Objectives

The student dental hygienist and dental hygiene professional will learn the following key objectives from this chapter:

1. Increase the potential for better patient care.
2. Involve all members of the dental team to enhance the dental hygiene experience for the patient.
3. Provide more services for the patient during the scheduled appointment time.
4. Increase the productivity of the dental hygienist, indirectly improving the financial well being of the hygienist and the well being and health of the patient.
5. Decrease the stress of the dental hygienist by providing team support before, during and after the scheduled appointment time.

Overview

Over the past several decades, the practice of dental hygiene has undergone numerous changes in the complexity and scope of responsibility. With the advent of electronic health records, modern equipment and instruments facilitating patient treatment and the evolution of digital dental radiology, today's dental hygienist is managing more aspects of dental care. This requires a better coordination of the entire dental hygiene delivery of care with the dental team.

Although assisted dental hygiene is not a new concept, the emphasis on a designated staff member whose primary duties include assisting and augmenting the various dental hygiene duties is. It is a concept that is needed now more than ever.

This chapter will outline the steps needed to maintain and run a successful assisted dental hygiene department in any healthcare setting.

What Is Assisted Dental Hygiene?

Defined broadly, assisted dental hygiene is or involves a clinical setting in any type of dental health care system that incorporates the use of a designated dental assistant. This assistant's primary role is to augment and assist the dental hygienist before, during and after the patient dental hygiene appointment.

The hygiene assistant can be "shared" with another dentist or dental hygienist, can work out of one or several treatment rooms, or possibly during some treatment days, be solely designated to one dental hygienist in the course of the entire treatment time segment.

Some of the duties assigned to the dental assistant would encompass all that is legally allowed under general, direct or indirect supervision, as outlined in the statutes of that particular state, territory or other public health setting.

The most common duties delegated to the assistant on behalf of the dental hygienist/dental team would include:
1. Reviewing the medical and dental health history and recording a baseline blood pressure.
2. Taking and processing radiographs by either analog or by digital radiography.
3. Providing chairside "four handed" assisting to facilitate the appointment.
4. Preparing and conducting infection control procedures in cleaning the dental hygiene treatment room prior to and after the patient appointment.
5. Application of preventive treatment modalities such as topical fluoride treatments, fluoride varnishes, pit and fissure sealants and provision of oral hygiene instructions.
6. Recording treatment and clinical observations in the analog or digital records.
7. Scheduling future maintenance visits for patients and/or their family members, or future restorative/ treatment planning visits with the dentist.

Why an Office Would Consider Assisted Dental Hygiene

Implementing assisted dental hygiene may or may not be intuitive for every practice. The dental practices that would be the most successful in transitioning to that practice modality would most likely be offices that already incorporate expanded dental functions in all other aspects within the dental delivery (and optimally utilize dental assistants in a variety of other capacities).

Since each state Board of Dentistry has different rules regarding the use of dental auxiliaries, a good initial step would be to thoroughly review the list of allowable duties for each position description in the dental practice. All states have a website for their respective Boards of Dentistry, and the laws pertaining to delegable duties, along with a list of those duties, are readily available on the website.

The first step for progressive dental practices wishing to include assisted dental hygiene as part of their protocol is to decide what specific duties the dental hygiene assistant will perform and what educational qualifications are necessary to provide these duties.

The reasons why a practice would consider assisted dental hygiene include:
1. Increased emphasis on periodontal health and preventive periodontal maintenance by the dental practice. Today's consumers are increasingly aware of their overall health because of the amount of information available on the Internet and through social networking. The message consumers receive is that they can participate in decision-making regarding their health and have a say in leading healthy lives. Today, most patients are better educated about dental treatment procedures and alternative treatments. This particularly applies to the area of preventive health.

Dental practices that want an increase in appointment demand will emphasize:

- Frequent professional cleaning appointments;
- Thorough periodontal health assessments that include yearly six-point periodontal probing of each tooth; and
- Maintain a successful preventive maintenance program.
  Supporting this demand will require an efficient and productive treatment schedule.

2. The competitive nature of the dental market for common procedures, such as prophylaxis, exams and radiographs, increasingly puts pressure on keeping fees for these procedures relatively low, making it ever more difficult to compensate dental hygienists fairly for the services provided. Rising employee costs such as healthcare benefits, pension plans and other offered benefits make it challenging to ensure a completely full daily schedule in order to run a profitable dental hygiene department.

3. A successful preventive maintenance program will require more appointments, increasing the workload and demand for additional dental hygiene production hours. This may or may not be possible in a particular geographic location due to workforce demographics.

4. Since dental hygienists earn a competitive salary and the employment of dental hygienists is expected to grow 36% through 2018, dental hygiene is a profession that is in demand for the future.[1] Instituting a salary and bonus system is necessary to compensate a dental hygienist who has the use of a full-time assistant. More on this type of compensation will be forthcoming later in this chapter.

5. With a flexible schedule in the dental practice, and multiple interchangeable treatment operatories, more than one treatment room can be used by a dental hygienist. This allows for greater productivity and higher utilization of treatment time, as opposed to a single room setup with breakdown times that interfere with patient treatment time. Assisted dental hygiene can greatly expand the production of any dental practice schedule, regardless of time.

6. Assisted dental hygiene may also serve as a career recruitment strategy. Last, but certainly not the least is the ability of a dental assistant who is interested in pursuing a dental hygiene career. By assisting the dental hygienist, the assistant can observe firsthand the clinical skills necessary to become a registered dental hygienist. The author has had firsthand experience in this area, as four former dental assistants eventually pursued dental hygiene careers after being utilized as dental hygiene assistants.

In turn, dental hygiene graduates who have had experience as dental hygiene assistants are more apt to utilize an assistant themselves once they are practicing. This approach enhances the quality of the dental hygienist's work and provides optimum patient benefit. Some of the most productive and well managed dental practices have a well run team of professionals who are being utilized to the fullest of their licensed or regulated capacities. This scenario creates an environment of learning and cooperation among team members that projects extreme professionalism to the dental patients and offers an excellent standard of care.

Essential Elements of Assisted Dental Hygiene

There are five essential elements to a successful Assisted Dental Hygiene Program:
1. The Dentist
2. The Dental Hygienist and Assistant
3. The Dental Team
4. The Office Design
5. The Compensation

Each of these requirements is essential to create and sustain a successful department, which can be consistently applied to every clinical setting, and can be repeated with any staff member of the dental team regardless of staff turnover, due to geographical moves, family needs, etc.

The Dentist. Not all dentists are alike! The nature of dental education has changed dramatically over the past two decades. The various clinical and life experiences that dental students are exposed to will have great bearing on their use of auxiliaries in a dental practice.

In the early 80s, dental assisting and dental hygiene programs were increasingly not affiliated with dental schools, for a variety of demographic and philosophical reasons. Many programs were developed for the rapidly increasing student population that attended community college and junior colleges, to appeal to a career-type educational track. The majority of dental schools today have dental students performing clinical requirements without the use of a chairside assistant within the clinical educational model for the dental training done at the main dental school facility. Until the students work in an externship clinical outreach environment, they are not exposed to the concept of having a full-time assistant for the dental procedures they perform. If a dental student is fortunate enough to experience high utilization of dental auxiliaries and support staff in dental school, it is more likely that an assisted dental hygiene program will be implemented in the dental practice in which the graduate student eventually works.

Likewise, dentists experience a higher success rate with assisted dental hygiene programs if they reside in a state that has comprehensive expanded function responsibilities.

The management philosophy of the dentist and dental practice manager is extremely important in the successful implementation of the assisted dental hygiene program. The dentist has to have a proper outlook and mindset when increasing the delegation of additional responsibilities among the dental team that will increase productivity and efficiency of the dental practice, and not necessarily drive costs up. The ability to implement change and guide it through the process is essential in the initial stages, and leadership and encouragement from the dentist at these points is crucial to the success of the program.

It is critical for dentists to be able to delegate some of the implementation of the problem and not try to "micromanage" the entire process. There is a tendency by team members to resist change if they feel they were not properly consulted on the original concept. The dentist will ensure success when he or she convinces the staff that they will benefit from the changes.

It is also important for general dentists to institute a soft tissue periodontal therapy program, and the benefits it will provide for their patients. It is estimated that 80% of the adult population has some form of periodontal disease.[2] If this is the case, then most dental hygienists would be doing two to four quadrants of periodontal debridement per day just to meet the demand. If patient treatment is accepted, patients like to keep appointment times to a minimum, so treating two quadrants per visit makes good business sense, increases compliance, improves oral health and enhances a productive dental hygiene schedule.

The concept of an "interruptive" dental hygiene exam also must be introduced by the dentist, and this has been successfully used in the author's practice for over 20 years. By coming into the dental hygiene treatment room at any point in the appointment, the dentist aids the dental hygienist in keeping the schedule, and can discuss treatment options and dental needs. This process also reinforces the patient's treatment plan throughout the remainder of the appointment, solidifying and validating the acceptance process.

The Dental Hygienist and Dental Assistant. One of the most critical requirements for the assisted dental hygiene department is the right "chemistry" and work environment for the hygienist-assistant team. Much like a dentist-assistant team, the hygienist-assistant team must work well together, and have a positive professional relationship to be productive and for patients to observe and perceive they are receiving the best care. As stated previously, an assistant with a keen interest in pursuing a future dental hygiene career is a logical and very often key choice. Another good selection would be an assistant who can update the medical history and patient's medications, enjoys taking radiographs, and helping the dental hygienist in these tasks. Dental hygienists who see the value of having someone helping them to be more productive, and, at the same time, reducing the stress level of always having to see patients on time, will ensure the team's success. The dental hygienist and the dental hygiene assistant focus on improving productivity and the importance of improving patients' health outcomes in the practice.

Most dental hygienists who utilize two treatment rooms know that this provides a major benefit in improving time management and also examination of the patient by the dentist and then beginning the next patient.

Dental assistants should be fully comfortable knowing that their primary duty will be to one or two dental hygienists, and that they may be called upon to split the workload between the dentist and the dental hygienist(s), depending on the work week and the demands of the schedule.

The Support Staff. One of the critical preliminary steps before implementing assisted dental hygiene in any dental practice is the "buy-in" by all team members prior to seeing any patients under this system. A special staff meeting several months prior to implementation is highly recommended, and during this meeting the goals and objectives should be outlined precisely. Distribution of a simple outline at the meeting and allowing ample time for questions and overcoming objections is a must for a successful placement of this program into existing dental office procedures. It is important that this process also be evaluated on an ongoing basis to determine things that can be improved to make it successful as well as team building exercises.

A clear outline of what is expected from each member of the staff under the new format will alleviate most fears of change, and a gradual schedule change on certain days might prove to be the easiest way to implement the program.

Most important of all, patients must feel that the focus of the dental practice is still centered on them, despite the obvious acceleration of time use and delegation. The patient must also perceive that the quality of the treatment has remained the same or improved in order to be satisfied with the new approach. All team members should be able to answer questions that patients may have concerning their treatment plan so that patients are comfortable with the next steps to improve their oral or dental health.

A well-known industry standard is that 33% of the dental office production should be coming from the dental hygiene department.[3] Dental hygiene production consists of all preventive therapy including dental sealants, periodontal debridement, scaling and root planning, placement of local delivery agents, and if offered, cosmetic bleaching. This production figure does not include the exam done by the dentist.

Since teeth whitening has become a popular elective procedure in the dental practice, the author feels that the dental hygienist/assistant team is the best source of knowledge to discuss this treatment modality with patients. Many team members are female, and women are the chief healthcare decision makers (58%) in the majority of United States families, according to the Kaiser Family Foundation.[2] As a dental professional, dental hygienists have to understand the patient's needs and incorporate that learning in what will be presented to patients as part of case acceptance for their dental and dental hygiene needs. This collaborative communication and rapport created between patient and staff will create a higher acceptance rate. It will also increase the practice's referrals and profitability based upon restorative, cosmetic and dental hygiene treatment rendered.

Finally, the team must be fully committed in keeping the dental hygiene schedule full at all times in terms of recare and periodontal therapy appointments. This means that all members of the staff need to strive to successfully schedule patients who are overdue on their preventive maintenance appointments, to include direct contact in the form of follow-up phone calls and reminder letters. If the dental hygiene schedule is full, the dentist will be assured of keeping the restorative schedule full, since roughly 50% of the entire dental work done by the dentist is derived from the existing hygiene population.[4] Additionally, the dental team can also generate non-restorative procedures (bleaching, oral care product sales) too.

The Office Design. An area that can be easily overlooked, but is vital to a successful assisted dental hygiene program, is the actual office design and layout of the treatment rooms. Many advances have been made in the area of dental facility design, especially in the delivery style surrounding the dental unit, i.e., the supporting equipment such as computer screens, ultrasonic cleaners, tray setups, etc.

Each operatory should be designed to allow for four-handed dentistry rather than single operator delivery. Most offices can now be constructed so that all rooms are interchangeable to provide dental and dental hygiene treatment. This is to take advantage of times or days in the schedule where dental hygiene could be the only type of dental treatment performed. Roughly ten minutes of each appointment block is used to first prepare each room and then break down the used space per patient. The use of multiple rooms allows the hygienist to move smoothly from room to room, and see at least two more patients per day depending on the planned treatment. This allows the practice to increase the availability and flexibility of their preventive maintenance schedule, which patients perceive as great customer service, and adds to the quality of their dental treatment experience.

Keeping in mind that an excellent office design produces good patient flow, the dentist must inventory existing operatory set ups prior to initiating assisted dental hygiene. This will allow the dentist to determine if any additional equipment or tray setups will be required to meet the demands of increased patient flow. As mentioned previously, supplies and equipment should be located in the same location in all treatment rooms for time efficiency and patient usage.

To minimize time in the treatment rooms, many functions previously taken care of in dental hygiene rooms can now be done by staff members in the consultation room. It is helpful if the consultation room is located next to the main reception area. This is also an excellent place to conduct new patient interviews in a professional, private and quiet setting.

The Compensation. In order to remain competitive in the dental hygiene employment market, it is crucial that dental hygienists be adequately compensated for the treatment they provide in the dental practice. Since the industry standard for percentage compensation as a proportion of production is in the 29-33% of production range,[4] the author has compensated his dental hygienists on a percentage of production only for one specific case, in which an employee requested a base salary due to family financial constraints.

Every state has its own employments laws, and since dental hygienists may have different benefit package requirements, it is best for dentists to utilize professional accounting/human relations advice prior to offering this concept to their dental hygiene employees.

A fair dental fee schedule is extremely important, including a specific list of procedures to be compensated and how that is accomplished.

Summary

Many successful dental practices have incorporated an assisted dental hygiene modality into their practice schedule in order to provide their dental hygienists with a more effective means of implementing dental and dental hygiene services. The modality increases production and helps patients to improve their overall health and well being. Assisted dental hygiene provides a rewarding effort to the entire practice, and outstanding oral health care to their patients.

References

1. Bureau of Labor Statistics website. Occupational Outlook Handbook, 2010-2011 ed. "Dental Hygienists." Available at http://www.bls.gov/oco/ocos097.htm. Viewed Feb. 1, 2012.
2. US Dept of Health and Human Services. *Periodontal (Gum) Disease: Causes, Symptoms, and Treatments.* NIH Publication No. 06-1142. January 2006.
3. McKenzie S. In lean times, remember Rule of 33. *e-Management Newsletter.* December 4, 2009. Issue 404.
4. McKenzie S. Dental teams: Make the most of your doctor's 'Great ideas.' *e-Management Newsletter.* December 18, 2009. Issue 406.

Critical Thinking Exercises

1. Calculate the total amount of dental hygiene production generated by each dental hygienist. This amount should represent (three times) as compared to the total salary and benefit package the dental hygienist currently makes in the practice.

2. List the current duties that a dental hygienist has prior to seeing a patient both in and out of the treatment operatory, and determine how many of those duties could easily and appropriately be delegated to an expanded function dental assistant.

3. Describe the process you would use to reactivate a current patient of a practice that is overdue in their preventive maintenance regimen. Identify all the steps that would be involved in that process.

4. Analyze your state practice act to determine the services which may be legally delegated to the dental hygiene assistant and those of which are in the purview of the registered dental hygienist.

Key Concepts:

1. With the changes anticipated in healthcare reform, all delivery systems for dental hygiene services will be looking for more efficient ways of delivering more care in a shorter time period.

2. The dental hygiene professional should embrace the concept of assisted dental hygiene as a way to more effectively deliver care to their patients, much like the dentist embraced the concept of four-handed dentistry decades ago. This practice has led to an expanded function role for the dental assistant and more efficient and cost effective delivery of oral health care for the patient.

3. The practice of assisted dental hygiene will more accurately reflect the level of education that dental hygienists have by making sure that the type of procedures specifically performed by the dental hygienist is to the broadest scope allowed by current dental hygiene licensing law.

4. Identify services to be performed by the dental hygienist and those which may be delegated to the dental hygiene assistant by law.

5. The dental hygiene provider will be able to apply the concept and develop a plan to convert traditional dental hygiene practice to the assisted dental hygiene practice model.

Glossary of Terms

Glossary of Terms

A

5 As: An evidence-based approach to tobacco cessation that establishes a framework whereby the provider asks patients about their habit, advises them to stop, assesses their readiness to stop, assists them in the stopping process and arranges follow-up during the course of the intervention.

AAR (Ask, Advise, Refer): A model for assisting patients with tobacco cessation, which modifies the 5 As and incorporates the use of quitlines as a referral mechanism. This model was developed by the American Dental Hygienists' Association (ADHA). It provides an alternative approach to tobacco cessation deemed compatible with the practice of dental hygiene.

Abandonment: The termination of treatment by a healthcare provider without just cause.

Abduction: To move away from the midline of the body.

Abrasion: The act of producing scratches or grooves on a surface resulting in the removal of material.

Abrasive: An agent or material abrading a surface such as pumice polishing paste with grit.

Absolute Risk Reduction (ARR): The ARR is the difference in the risk of an event occurring between two groups of patients in a study. For example, if 6% of patients die after receiving a new experimental drug, and 10% of patients die after having the old drug treatment, then the ARR is 10% – 6% = 4%.

Abstinence: Refraining from tobacco use.

Academy of Laser Dentistry (ALD): Is the international organization of clinicians, researchers and academicians for laser dentistry and its mission is to improve the health and well being of patients through the proper use of laser technology.

Accreditation: A process by which a professional association or nongovernmental agency grants recognition to a school/university or health care institution for demonstrating the ability to meet predetermined criteria for the establishment of standards.

Acidogenic: An organism that secretes acid.

Aciduric: An organism that tolerates living in acidic conditions.

Acoustic Streaming: Unidirectional fluid flow caused by ultrasound waves when using ultrasonic devices.

Acoustic Turbulence: Tip stroke causes water to accelerate, producing an intensified swirling effect, which disrupts biofilm. Higher power settings increase this action with ultrasonic devices.

ADA Seal of Acceptance: A strictly voluntary program of the American Dental Association to which dental product companies may submit products for review. These companies commit significant resources to meeting the requirements of the program including submission of product information, data from clinical trials designed according to specifications which support safety and effectiveness of the product as well as promotional claims.

Adherence: Encourages patients to take a more active role with becoming involved within their own oral care.

Administrator/Manager: An individual who has responsibilities in administration and works as a manager in an oral health care environment.

Advanced Dental Hygiene Practitioner (ADHP): The ADHP is a licensed dental hygienist educated at the master's degree level. In addition to the full range of dental hygiene clinical services, ADHPs will administer minimally invasive restorative services and will also have limited prescriptive authority. ADHPs will be educated in health promotion and disease prevention, provision of primary care, case and practice management, quality assurance and ethics, which will provide a comprehensive approach to the delivery of oral healthcare services.

Adverse Drug Effects: Undesirable or unwanted negative side effects associated with medication use; dose-related.

Adverse Drug Events: Undesirable or unwanted negative events associated with medication use, including allergic reaction, drug interactions or idiosyncratic reactions.

Advocacy: The ability to give advice.

Advocate: An individual who publicly supports or recommends a particular cause, policy or law.

Aerosol: Atomized particles suspended in air.

Agency for Health Research and Quality (AHRQ): The AHRQ mission is to improve the quality, safety, efficiency and effectiveness of health care for all Americans. As one of twelve agencies within the Department of Health and Human Services, AHRQ supports research that helps people make more informed decisions and improves the quality of health care services. AHRQ was formerly known as the Agency for Health Care Policy and Research.

All-Ceramic Restorations: A restoration designed to cover the entire outer surface of the tooth composed entirely of a ceramic material.

American Academy of Pediatric Dentistry (AAPD): Governing body that advocates policies, guidelines and programs that promote the oral health and oral health care of children.

American Dental Association (ADA): The ADA is the professional association of dentists dedicated to serving both the public and the profession of dentistry. The ADA promotes the public's health through commitment of member dentists to provide quality oral health care, accessible to everyone.

American Society of Anesthesiology (ASA): The American Society of Anesthesiologists is an educational, research and scientific association of physicians organized to raise and maintain the standards of the medical practice of anesthesiology and improve the care of the patient.

Amplitude: Distance of tip movement per stroke; the power knob adjusts the amplitude in ultrasonic devices.

Analog Data: Analog data is characterized by a continuous grayscale from black to white.

Angular Cheilitis: Fissuring or cracks in commissures of the lips usually caused by Candida albicans although nutritional deficiencies especially vitamin B can contribute. A side effect of antibiotics can also cause candidiasis.

Anticipatory Guidance: An understanding that genetics may have a significant role in a child's predisposition to obtaining dental caries.

Antimicrobial: A substance that kills or inhibits the growth of microorganisms such as bacteria or fungi.

Antiplaque or Antigingivitis Agents: Chemotherapeutic agents added to dentifrices and mouthrinses to prevent or reduce the pathogenic effect of plaque and/or inflammation of the gingiva.

Aphthous Ulcer: Painful oral ulcer that frequently recurs in episodes. An aphthous ulcer is also known as a canker sore.

Assessment: A systemic collection, analysis and documentation of the oral and general health status and patient needs. The dental hygienist conducts a thorough, individualized assessment of patients with or at risk for oral disease or complications.

Assisted Dental Hygiene: Assisted dental hygiene defined broadly would be a clinical setting in any type of dental health care system that incorporates the use of a designated dental assistant whose primary role is to augment and assist the dental hygienist before, during and after the patient dental hygiene appointment.

ATP: (Adenosine TriPhosphate) an energy molecule present in high concentrations within organisms that require great stores of energy (like Mutans Streptococci).

Author: An individual who writes a book or other text materials that will be published.

Autism: Autism is a severe and lifetime disorder characterized by major impairment in mutual social interactions, communication skills and repetitive patterns of interests or behaviors.

Auto Tune: Machines that automatically adjust the frequency of the insert.

Autoimmune Diseases: A condition in which the immune system attacks healthy cells.

Autonomy: The person's right to make their own decisions and act independently.

Avulsed Tooth: A tooth that has been knocked out of the mouth due to an injury.

B

Bacterial Culture: Growing bacteria in an incubator on specially designed nutrient rich compounds.

Balanced Life Elements: The basic principles that add up to a balanced, satisfying lifestyle. These include Personal, Professional, Professional Community, Health, Wellness and Community elements.

Bass Toothbrushing Method: A sulcular-cleaning method to clean the teeth and gingival tissue.

Behavior Management: Pharmalogical and nonpharmalogical techniques used by dental health care professionals to alleviate the patient's fear associated with dental procedures.

Behavioral Interviews: A job interview focused on discovering how an individual behaves or acts in specific employer-related situations.

Bell's Palsy: Paralysis of the facial nerve.

Beneficence: The core value that promises beneficial treatment will be rendered by the professional.

Benefits: A service provided by employers for employees that is in addition to wages or salary.

Biofilm: Formation of bacteria into an organized matrix that attaches itself to a site in the oral cavity.

Biomarkers: Substances used as an indicator of a biologic state.

Black Hairy Tongue: Papillae on the dorsal tongue become elongated and are brown to black in color. Chromogenic bacteria and changes in the microbial flora are the cause of black hairy tongue coupled with other predisposing factors.

Bloodborne Pathogens Standard: The Occupational Safety and Health Administration (OSHA) standard requiring employers to protect employees who have occupational contact with blood and body fluids.

Board of Dentistry: A board that licenses and regulates dentistry and its related professions in a particular state.

The board licenses dentists, registered dental assistants, limited registered dental assistants, dental hygienists, teachers, interns and residents studying dentistry. The board also issues the following permits: parenteral conscious sedation, general anesthesia and specialty (advertisements).

Bradycardia: Slow heart rate.

Bradypnea: Slow respiration rate.

Buccal Mucosa: A mucous membrane of tissue inside the mouth that covers the cheek.

C

CAM: Complementary and Alternative Medicine is diverse medical and healthcare systems, practices and products including such resources perceived by their users as associated with positive health outcomes.

Candidiasis: Is an infection caused by a species of yeast called Candida, usually Candida albicans. People who have low immune function can develop candidiasis of the mouth.

Capability: The ability to undertake a given action.

Carcinogenesis: The process by which normal cells undergo changes that lead to the development of a malignant tumor.

Care Planning: Establishment of realistic goals and treatment strategies to facilitate optimal health.

Career Success: A measurement of daily, weekly and yearly achievements that are aligned with personal and professional goals that have been purposefully chosen.

Caries Indicator: A marker, sign, or symptom specific to the disease or condition, dental caries.

Caries Management by Risk Assessment (CAMBRA): Strategies for prevention of dental caries based on an assessment of risk factors related to the patient's oral and medical condition and history followed by specific treatment recommendations including behavioral, chemical and minimally invasive procedures.

Cariogenic: The term given to anything that is thought to cause dental caries.

Carpal Tunnel Syndrome: Chronic pain, numbness or tingling in the hand, caused by compression of the median nerve at the wrist. Can be caused by occupational risk factors or medical conditions.

Case Presentation: Discussion of the entire care plan with other members of the dental team and presentation to the patient provides a complete understanding of the patient's oral health status and needs by all those involved.

Casein Phosphopeptide-Amorphous Calcium Phosphate (CPP-ACP): A compound containing protein, calcium and phosphate that is able to remineralize early caries lesions.

Causative Risk Factor: A factor effective, as a cause or agent for the onset of disease; producing an effect.

Cavitation: Bubble formation in liquids caused by rapid movement as in ultrasonic technology.

Cerebral Palsy: Cerebral Palsy (CP) is a permanent, non progressive neuromuscular disorder caused by damage to the immature brain.

Cetylpyridium Chloride: An antiseptic agent, cationic quaternary ammonium compound, used in mouthrinses as an antimicrobial agent.

Chain of Infection: Conditions that must exist before any disease can be transmitted. Breaking the chain at any point stops the transmission of disease.

Chair-side Mentoring: A dental hygiene professional who would provide oral health education and counseling to a patient.

Charge-coupled Device (CCD): Solid-state, silicon chip detector that converts light or x-ray photons to electrons.

Chemical Dependency: Generic term relating to psychological or physical dependency, or both, on an exogenous substance.

Chemotaxis: The phenomenon in which cells, bacteria and single or multicellular organisms direct their movement according to certain chemicals in their environment.

Chemotherapeutic Agents: An agent which includes a chemical of natural or synthetic origin and used for its specific action against disease, usually against infection.

Chemotherapeutic Mouthrinse: Mouthrinse formulations that contain a chemical ingredient or drug that targets the treatment of disease or condition that is selectively toxic to the causative agent of the disease, such as a virus, bacterium, fungi or other microorganism.

Chlorhexidine Gluconate: A chemical antiseptic that kills microbes associated with gingivitis by altering bacterial membranes, most commonly delivered in prescription mouthrinses at a concentration of 0.12% in the U.S.

Cleanser: A non-abrasive means to polish enamel and/or materials. An alternative minimally invasion option.

Clinical Contact Surface: A surface in the healthcare practice that has the highest level of contamination. Defined as any surface that is touched by contaminated hands, aerosol, instruments, devices or other items in the course of providing dental care.

Clinical Diagnosis: When the oral health professional's diagnosis comes from the clinical appearance alone.

Clinical Simulation: An environment that serves as a resource to learners and instructors during the development, implementation and evaluation of simulation activities.

Colgate® Toothbrush Assessment and Chairside Guide: The Colgate® Toothbrush Assessment Guide developed by Colgate-Palmolive Company to assist dental hygienists in assessing the oral care habits, oral care issues and disease risk assessment in the recommendation of toothbrush products to their patients. The Chairside Guide assists dental hygienists in understanding their patients' oral care needs and recommending the type of toothbrush for their patients' best oral health outcomes and promote strong patient compliance.

Collaboration: A process of interaction or working together with one or more individuals or groups of people to achieve a common goal.

Collaborative Dental Hygiene Practice (CDHP): CDHP is also known as independent or unsupervised dental hygiene practice. Under a written agreement with a collaborative dentist, dental hygienists can provide oral health promotion and disease prevention education, oral health assessment and clinical, preventive and therapeutic services for patients without a dentist's direct supervision. CDHP is a new approach to promote oral health, lower cost of oral health care and improve access to oral health care for under-served populations.

Comfort Zone: The behavioral state where an individual carries on in an anxiety-free environment where a level of comfort is obtained.

Commitment: The act of commitment, pledging or engaging oneself in a promise to do something.

Communication: Speaking, listening, nonverbal face and body language, reading and writing skills that allow for the exchange of information.

Community Balanced-Life Element: One of the basic principles of a balanced, satisfying lifestyle. The Community element encompasses that portion of individuals' lives in which they spend time volunteering to support the community in which they live through activities not related to their profession.

Compensation: Something given or received as an equivalent for services, debt, loss to injury, etc.

Competence: The ability to do something successfully through the scope of one's knowledge and ability.

Complementary Metal Oxide Semiconductor (CMOS): Solid-state detector similar to the charge-coupled Device (CCD) with built-in control functions, smaller pixel size and lower power requirements.

Compliance: Willingness of the patient to follow oral care recommendations.

Confidence: The belief in oneself and one's abilities, self-confidence and power within themselves.

Confidentiality: Keeping information gleaned from a patient private. This is the responsibility of a healthcare professional as outlined by the code of ethics and the legal system.

Consent for Treatment Form: A written list given to parents that outlines the risks of treatment and non-treatment of their child so they can make an informed discussion to proceed or decline treatment.

Contacts: An acquaintance or colleague from whom an individual can gain information, networking, resources, etc.

Continued Care (CC) Appointment: Is a dental prophylaxis performed on transitional or permanent dentition that includes scaling and polishing procedures to remove coronal plaque, calculus and stains.

Continuing Education Units (CEU): Credits that are applied to each continuing course that is presented by a speaker.

Continuing Education: A program where courses or education is provided to enhance the knowledge base of a new or experienced learner in a specified area of study.

Contrast: The difference in densities between various areas on a radiographic image.

Contributing Risk Factor: A factor that may contribute or increase the chance of the onset of disease; tendency to have it occur.

Control Group: A control group is the group in a scientific experiment in which the factor being tested is not applied so that it may serve as a standard for comparison against an experimental group where the factor is applied. It is useful to make conclusions more accurate or precise, provided that both the control and the other experimental group(s) are exposed to same conditions apart from the factor being tested.

Coping Skills: Skills that individuals utilize to offset daily challenges and disruptions.

Cosmetic Recontouring: The alteration of the shape of a tooth to create a more harmonious appearance.

Counseling: Use of an interactive guidance process focusing on the needs, problems, or feelings of the patient and helping them to understand what their oral healthcare needs are in order to improve their oral health and wellness.

Cover Letter: A letter sent with the job seeker's resume that provides information about where the applicant saw the job posting listed and identifies key skills and expertise about the applicant to the employer or human resource department for the potential job.

C-Reactive Protein: A protein produced by cells in the liver as a response to inflammation.

Criteria: Guidelines that state what the dental health professional should or should not do.

Cultural Competence: The integration of knowledge about individuals and groups of people into specific standards, policies, practices and attitudes to increase the quality of services. Cultural may include customs, beliefs, values and institutions of racial, ethnic, religious or social groups.

Cultural Tailoring: The application of cultural competence to programmatic efforts by anticipating and planning for the needs, preferences or circumstances of particular cultural groups.

Culture: Human behaviors, perceptions and beliefs unique to a specific group and passed from generation to generation or from one to another within the group.

Curet: A periodontal instrument that is used to remove calculus deposits from the crown and root surfaces. The working end consists of a rounded toe and back and is semicircular in cross-section.

Curriculum Vitae (CV): A summary of the job seeker's educational and academic experiences, teaching and research, publications, presentations, organizational affiliations, professional positions, awards, honors and other work related information. The CV is a longer version of the resume that is utilized in academic, educational and research/scientific positions.

D

Dampening: Slowing ultrasonic vibrations by pressing too hard against the tooth.

Daily Hygiene Production: The total dollar amount excluding exams that is produced by a dental hygienist during the course of a workday.

Dental Biofilm: A cooperative, communicating mass of non-mineralized bacteria, highly organized as bacterial colonies within a self-produced matrix (biofilm) and found in the oral cavity; also called plaque biofilm.

Debridement Curets: Curets that are used in the removal of plaque and calculus deposits.

Debridement: The mechanical removal of bacterial plaque and clinically detected calculus in a patient's mouth in order to conduct an accurate periodontal assessment.

Declination Angle: In dental loupes, the steepness at which the scope is angled downward on the loupes.

Decubitus: A position as if lying in bed.

Density: Overall degree of blackness or image darkening of an exposed film; comparable to brightness in digital imaging.

Dental Assistant: An auxiliary to the dentist. The dental assistant assists dentists' and dental hygienists' in preparing the patient for treatment, sterilizing instruments, passing instruments to the dental professional, holding and utilizing a suction device, etc. Dental assistants can obtain a certification and take the Dental Assisting National Board after completing the Dental Assisting Program or after two years of full-time employment.

Dental Biofilm: A cooperative, communicating mass of non-mineralized bacteria, highly organized as bacterial colonies within a self-produced matrix (biofilm) and found in the oral cavity; also called plaque biofilm.

Dental Director: A dentist who oversees the responsibilities and management of the dental practice.

Dental History: A form or questionnaire used to gain knowledge concerning the patient's immediate problem or concern, his or her previous dental care, attitude toward oral health and the type of personal oral hygiene he or she practices on a daily basis.

Dental Hygiene Care Plan: The development of a dental hygiene care plan is critical to the oral health care of the patient. This process requires systematic and critical attention to detail as well as open communication between the patient and dental hygienist.

Dental Hygiene Department Analysis: Specific information gathered from a dental practice in order to access the proficiency of the dental hygiene department with emphasis on the ratio of periodontal therapy services compared to other preventive procedures.

Dental Hygiene Diagnosis: The dental hygiene diagnosis is an integral part of the dental hygiene process of care and allows the dental hygienist to use critical decision making skills to reach conclusions about the patients needs related to oral health and disease that fall within the dental hygiene scope of practice as defined by the American Dental Hygienists' Association.

Dental Hygiene Process of Care: The dental hygiene process of care provides a framework through which individualized needs of the patient can be met. The five components of the dental hygiene process of care are assessment, dental hygiene diagnosis, planning, implementation and evaluation.

Dental Hygiene Production: The total amount of procedures produced by the dental hygienist to determine the dollar amount that represents. This is calculated by using the ADA CDT © procedure listing commonly listed on the particular facility's fee schedule.

Dental Hygiene Prognosis: The dental hygiene prognosis is a prediction of the possible outcomes that can be anticipated from the chosen dental hygiene intervention. It is usually determined after the dental hygiene diagnosis and before the development of the dental hygiene care plan.

Dental Hygienist: The dental hygienist is a preventive professional who has graduated from an accredited dental hygiene program in an institution of higher education. This professional provides educational, clinical, research, administrative and therapeutic services supporting the total health of a person through the promotion of optimal oral health as defined by the American Dental Hygienists' Association (ADHA).

Dental Lasers: Dental lasers are a family of instruments. Some lasers are used for surgery, some to cure restorative materials and enhance tooth bleaching, and others to remove tooth structure for elimination of disease and restoration – different lasers for different procedures. All lasers require eye protection. Safety glasses with special lenses will be provided.

Dental Practice-Based Research Network (DPBRN): A consortia of dental practices conducting trials to compare various clinical methods and committed to improving clinical dental practice.

Dental Sealants: A composite material placed in the deep grooves of teeth to help prevent dental decay.

Dental Specialist: A particular specialist (pediatric dentist, periodontist, prosthodontist, orthodontist, etc.) in the treatment of dentistry.

Dentifrice: A dentifrice is a paste, liquid or powder used for oral hygiene. When used on a toothbrush, a dentifrice is called toothpaste.

Dentist: A licensed and registered dental professional who goes to graduate school to learn the practice of dentistry and who evaluates, diagnoses, and treats diseases, conditions and injuries of the oral cavity (teeth, jaw and mouth).

deQuervain's Syndrome: Inflammation of the sheath or tunnel that surrounds the two tendons that control movement of the thumb. Stabbing pain is felt on the thumb side of the wrist.

Desensitizing Agents: Chemicals added to dentifrices, varnishes or resin adhesives to reduce dentinal hypersensitivity by occlusion of the dentinal tubules or altering tubule structure and forming microprecipitates.

Diabetes: A group of diseases allowing for abnormally elevated serum glucose levels.

Diabetic Retinopathy: A serious medical condition of a diabetic patient that causes progressive damage to the retina of the eye.

Diagnosis: A statement identifying the cause and nature of a condition, situation or problem through evaluation and examination.

Diet: Eating habits, or the pattern of food intake.

Dietary Supplements: Vitamins, minerals and herbal preparations used as a part of medication therapy.

Differential Diagnosis: A systematic method of identifying oral health issues by ruling out one or more suspected lesions using tests or procedures to make a final diagnosis.

Digital Cameras: Single lens reflex cameras, often called extraoral cameras, used to take photos of patients.

Digital Data: Characterized by discrete segments of information called pixels (picture elements).

Digital Radiography: Digital x-rays systems, encompassing primarily sensor-based systems and phosphor plate systems.

Digital Sucking: Finger or thumb sucking.

Diode Laser: A soft-tissue dental laser that can perform procedures that electrosurge, as scalpels and dental instruments did in the past. The diode laser operates at a range from 810nm to 1064nm.

Direct Access to Care: The dental hygienist can initiate treatment based on his or her assessment of the patient's needs without the specific authorization by a dentist, treat the patient without the presence of a dentist, and can maintain a provider-patient relationship.

Direct Composite Restorations: The placement and shaping of a composite dental material in a malleable form on a prepared tooth and then allowing it to harden.

Director of Hygiene: A dental hygienist who oversees the responsibilities and management of the dental hygiene department.

Disability: A specific physical, functional, mental or emotional disorder that results in significant limitations in performing daily self maintenance activities, or a disorder that requires the use of special equipment or devices.

Disaccharides: Simple double sugars such as sucrose, lactose and maltose that can be used as a food source by cariogenic bacteria.

Disinfection: Killing of most microorganisms; more resistant organisms such as bacteria spores not inactivated.

D-MORT (Disaster Mortuary Response Team): A team of experts in the field of victim identification and mortuary services. This team can be utilized for large scale disasters to assist in the identification of deceased individuals that need to be claimed by loved ones.

DOS-Based: Older software that was designed to run on MS-DOS, a computer operating system that predated Microsoft Windows.

Down Syndrome: A genetic disorder that can range in severity from moderate to serious cases that causes lifelong intellectual disability, developmental delays and other medical issues.

Drug Abuse: Any use of a drug that results in negative physical, psychological, economic, legal and/or social consequences to the user or to other persons affected by the user's behavior.

Drug Addiction: A chronic disorder leading to negative physical, psychological or social consequences from compulsive use of substance; characterized by continued use despite negative effects encountered by use.

Drug Allergy: Hypersensitivity reaction to a medication; unpredictable and not dose-related.

Drug Interaction: A negative result in the efficacy of a medication when one or more drugs are taken at the same time.

E

Eating Disorders: A constellation of disorders most commonly found in young women, which can seriously impact general and oral health and require a multi-disciplinary approach to management.

Economic Recession: An economic recession is a business cycle contraction, a general slowdown in economic activity over a period of time.

Editorial Director: An individual who reviews and edits manuscripts for a professional journal, writes articles and identifies topics of discussion for future issues of a professional journal.

Educator: An individual who is involved in the development of curriculum and presents this information to students through an educational process of learning.

Element: A basic principle or entity of an object or subject.

Embrasure Space: Space created between two adjacent teeth by the curvature of the contact area.

End-Rounded Bristles: Rounded toothbrush filaments to prevent injury to the oral tissues.

Environmental Tobacco Smoke (ETS) or Passive Smoke: Tobacco smoke present in room air resulting from ignited tobacco products burning in an ashtray or exhaled by a smoker.

EPA-Registered Surface Disinfectant: All liquid chemical disinfectants used on noncritical surfaces as well as gaseous sterilants are regulated by the Environmental Protection Agency (EPA), and federal law requires that any product used is registered with the EPA.

Epigenetic Alteration: Modifications to genes other than with DNA.

Epilepsy: Epilepsy is not a disease; it is a symptom of a brain dysfunction characterized by an abnormal, excessive neuronal discharge.

E-portfolio: A collection of work that students would post on the Internet regarding their academic work and achievements in their respective field of study.

Ergonomics: The application of human physiology to the design of objects, systems and environment to maximize worker productivity and reduce injuries.

Erosion: Chemical attack to the enamel surface from biofilm: bacterial plaque, cariogenic beverages, tooth whitening, procedures and acid reflux/regurgitation (GERD).

Erythema Multiforme: Ulcerated crusted lips and tongue that accompany a skin rash that shows characteristic iris or target lesions.

Erythroplakia: A clinical term that is used to describe an oral mucosal lesion that appears as a smooth red patch or a granular red and velvety patch.

Essential Oils: Volatile oils from plants, such as thymol, menthol and eucalyptol, used in mouthrinses as antibacterial agents to prevent or reduce plaque formation or kill bacteria associated with gingivitis.

Esthetic Dentistry: Esthetic dentistry is the branch of dentistry that deals with dental treatments whose goal is to improve the appearance of the teeth.

Ethics: The philosophy of morals and values and their impact on what is considered right and wrong.

Etiquette: The customs of polite behavior among members of a group or profession.

Evidence-Based Decision Making: A decision-making process based on sound scientific evidence.

Evidence-Based Practice: Evidence-based practice utilizes research based on the scientific method of inquiry with the goal of applying valid and reliable research for clinical practice.

Evidenced-Based: Oral care treatment and recommendations that are based on scientific support, patient circumstances/condition, the clinician's judgment and patient preferences.

Experimental Group: An experimental group is the group in a scientific experiment in which the factor being tested is applied so that it may serve as a standard for comparison against a control group where the factor is not applied.

Exposure Control Plan: A plan required by OSHA that includes a detailed written explanation of how the office plans to prevent exposure to bloodborne pathogens (and other diseases as well) and minimize exposure incidents to blood and other potentially infectious materials (OPIM) in the dental office.

F

Facial: Pertaining to the lip side of the mouth.

Family Support: The formal or informal processes that a family utilizes to support one another.

Feedback: Verbal and nonverbal responses during the communication process.

Fidelity: An ethical concept in healthcare that revolves around the duty to fulfill all commitments made to the patient.

Fiduciary Relationship: When individuals work in complete confidence with one another in regard to a particular transaction or each other's general business affairs.

Filaments: Bristles are bunched together to form tufts. Filament diameter, length and number relate to the firmness of the bristles per tuft. End rounded filaments produce less tissue irritation and abrasion.

Fissured Tongue: The grooves that appear on the dorsal surface of the tongue and can be derived from a hereditary condition.

Fixed Metal Substructure Prostheses: A restoration designed to cover the entire outer surface of the tooth composed of a metal substructure covered by an esthetic porcelain outer layer.

Floss Handles: Adjunct device that holds the floss. Come in many shapes and aid those who experience difficulty with flossing.

Floss Threaders: Nylon filament with a loop for threading a length of floss between adjacent teeth.

Fluoride: Fluoride is the negatively-charged ionic form of the element fluorine, an abundant element in the earth's crust. It is an anion which is able to lower the solubility of hydroxyapatite and is added to toothpastes, mouthrinses, varnishes, cavity liners and other professional and consumer dental products to prevent dental caries or slow its progression.

Focal Trough: Image layer or plane of focus that corresponds to the shape of the average jaw; located between the x-ray source and image receptor.

Follow-up Communications: After initial communication is made between the job seeker and a potential patient or colleague, additional communication is conducted by telephone, email or texting to determine if a task or project is completed.

Food Fiber: The non-digestible carbohydrates found in food; cannot be used as a food source by cariogenic bacteria.

Fordyce Granules: Small, elevated ectopic sebaceous glands that can develop on the oral mucosa or lip area.

Forensic Dentistry: The process of examination and evaluation of dental evidence that may be used in legal cases, crime scenes and identification of a perpetrator in an unexpected attack.

Frequency: Number of times per second the insert tip vibrates back and forth per second.

Front Desk Manager: An individual who oversees management of the front office team in a dental or specialty practice.

Fulcrum: A stabilizing position for the clinician during instrumentation.

Functional Shank: The part of the shank of the instrument that extends from the closest bend to the handle to the last bend before the working end.

Furcation Space: Anatomic area of multirooted teeth where the roots join together.

G

Gingival Abrasion: Damage to the gingival tissue as a result of aggressive toothbrushing.

Glare Technique: Used to test the sharpness of an instrument. A sharp instrument does not reflect light; whereas, a dull instrument reflects the light and produces a glare.

Glucans: A sticky substance produced by bacteria that allows the adherence to tooth surfaces.

Goals: The result or achievement toward which and effort is directed.

Golden Proportion: The golden proportion is a mathematical progression observed repeatedly in nature and is considered to be universally esthetically appealing.

Granular Cell Tumor: A rare benign tumor most commonly found on the tongue.

Greater Palatine Nerve Block: Interruption of the passage of impulses through the greater palatine nerve anesthetizing the posterior palatal tissues.

Grit: Particle size of an abrasive material.

H

Handle: The part of the instrument that is used for holding the instrument and houses the shank and working end.

Health Balanced-Life Element: One of the basic principles of a balanced, satisfying lifestyle. The Health element encompasses that portion of individuals' lives in which they spend time exercising and pursuing other health-related activities including, adequate nightly sleep, periodic doctor and dentist visits, dietary considerations, etc.

Health History: A form or questionnaire used to ascertain information that could reveal diseases, allergies and physiological state of the patient that may contraindicate certain kinds of dental and dental hygiene therapy.

Health Insurance Portability and Privacy Act (HIPPA): The "Health Insurance Portability and Privacy Act" was enacted by Congress in 1996 and is the federal law that allows people to take insurance with them after they leave a job and also establishes strict privacy standards for the handling of medical records for each individual.

Health Literacy: The ability to read, understand and act on health information. "The ability to obtain, process, and understand basic health information and services needed to make appropriate health decisions" (Institute of Medicine report).

Hemangioma: Well circumscribed, sessile based, blue lesion that occurs from birth or is associated with a trauma that involves the blood vessels and blood pooling in the area upon healing.

Hematoma: Red to purple area caused by some kind of trauma, typically found on the labial mucosa of upper lip.

Hemostasis: The change from a fluid to a solid state.

Hirshfeld Files: Periodontal files that are designed to crush and remove tenacious calculus deposits and are designed with long shanks that are easily adaptable. Great for furcations.

Historical Diagnosis: A systematic method of identifying oral health issues through the use of a patient's personal history (age, sex, race, occupation), family history, history of the presenting condition, drug history, medical/dental history and any combination of one or several of these features with the clinical aspect.

Horizontal Scrub Toothbrushing Method: Horizontal strokes with a toothbrush placed at 90-degree angle to the tooth surfaces.

Host Modulation: Agents or drugs used to limit the immune systems response to a pathogenic or foreign body.

Host Response: The reaction of the body's immune system to a pathogen or injury.

Human Papilloma Virus (HPV): A species of human viruses that are transmitted by sexual contact. High risk strains, particularly HPV-16, are major etiologic agents for the development of oropharyngeal cancer.

Hz: Abbreviation for hertz; one cycle per second.

I

Idiosyncratic Reaction: An adverse drug effect in which the reaction to a medication is qualitatively different from what is expected.

Immunoassay: A method of detecting cariogenic bacteria in a patient's mouth. A sample of saliva is treated with chemicals and then placed on a test strip containing antibodies which attach to the bacterial cells and produce colored lines if the bacteria are present.

Implants: A cylindrical shaped titanium device surgically placed into the jaw bone, which integrates with the jaw and is used to support a dental restoration.

Implied Consent: A form of consent inferred from the patient's actions and the particular situation to a course of treatment proposed.

Incipient Lesion: A white spot lesion on a tooth caused by the sustained presence of bacteria producing acid on that surface. The lesion is white due to a lack of calcium and phosphate in the tooth crystals.

Indirect Composite Restorations: The placement of a laboratory manufactured composite dental restoration in a cured form on a prepared tooth.

Inflammation: The body's response to injury, bacteria or foreign bodies.

Informed Consent: It is the legal and ethical responsibility of the dental professional to obtain an informed consent before implementing treatment. The process of informed consent is to explain to patients their treatment needs, the potential risks and consequences of related procedures. Informed consent can be verbal or written depending on the treatment involved.

Informed Refusal: A decision made by the patient to refuse proposed treatment based upon an understanding of the facts and possible implications of not following the professional recommendation.

Infraorbital Nerve Block: Interruption of the passage of impulses through the infraorbital nerve anesthetizing the soft tissue and maxillary anterior teeth.

Inquiry: To ask open-ended questions.

Insurance Coordinator: An individual who handles patients' insurance, submitting and documenting insurance claims and payment of claims in a dental or specialty practice.

Interdental Brushes: Variable size brushes designed to facilitate cleaning between adjacent teeth, bridges, implants or orthodontic appliances where space allows.

Interdisciplinary Collaboration: Involves researchers, students and teachers with the goals of connecting and integrating several academic schools of thought, professions or technologies; along with their specific perspectives – in the pursuit of a common task.

International Standards Organization (ISO): Founded in 1947, the organization promulgates worldwide industrial and commercial standards for machinery and products.

Interruptive Dental Hygiene Examination: The process of performing a dental exam by the dentist on each preventive maintenance visit to establish the patient of record and then allow the dental hygiene therapy to proceed on schedule.

Intervention: A clinical procedure, such as periodontal debridement or topical fluoride application.

Interview Thank You Letter: A letter sent to the person or people one interviewed with for a potential job to thank them for the time spent with them for the interview.

Interviews: A formal meeting in which one or more persons question, consult or evaluate an individual who is seeking a future job.

Intraoral Cameras: Wand-shaped video cameras used to record still images and videos taken inside the oral cavity.

Inventor: A person who develops or creates a new idea, device, process or machine that addresses the answer to a problem or concern.

Invisible Thermal Radiation: Is on one end of the electromagnetic spectrum. It contains the Near-Infrared, Mid-Infrared and Far-Infrared Spectrums with a range of 750nm+. These longer wavelengths do not enter the nuclei.

In-Vitro Research: Research in which a human is not used, and which can include a test tube or an inanimate object, whereas an in-vivo research involves a procedure within the human body.

Iron Deficiency Anemia: A blood disorder that can be caused by inadequate intake of iron, poor absorption, and gastrointestinal bleeding are but a few.

Irritation Fibroma: A slow growing fibrous nodule on the oral mucosa can be caused by cheek biting or other occurrences such as dentures.

J

Job Burnout: The result of experiencing stress characterized by physical and emotional exhaustion where an individual is not happy or satisfied in their career.

Job Satisfaction: The level of contentment that one feels toward their job being enjoyable and rewarding.

Jurisprudence: The philosophy of law. Rules of conduct as put forth by the state or federal statutes.

K

kHz: Abbreviation for kilohertz; one thousand hertz.

Kilovoltage: Potential difference between the anode and cathode in an x-ray tube; controls the quality or penetrating power of the x-ray beam.

L

Laboratory Diagnosis: A systematic method of identifying oral health issues through the use of patient samples of blood, urine analysis or laboratory cultures.

Lavage: To wash out.

Leadership: The ability to influence and develop a learned skill.

Leukoplakia: A clinical term used to identify a white plaque-like lesion of the oral mucosal that cannot be wiped off and cannot be diagnosed as any other disease on a clinical basis.

Life-long Learning: The continuous development of skills and knowledge of individuals throughout their lifetime.

Line Pair: A bar and its interspace of equal length; used to quantify the resolution of an image.

Lingual: Pertaining to the tongue side of the mouth.

Lipopolysacharides (LPS): A toxic substance on the outer cell wall of gram-negative bacteria.

Local Anesthesia: An amide or ester agent that blocks the passage of impulses through nerves.

Local Delivery of Antibiotics: Antibiotics injected or placed into the periodontal pocket to kill bacteria.

Locally Applied Antimicrobial: Site specific chemotherapeutic agents that kill microbes or affect the growth and multiplication of microorganisms.

Long Buccal Nerve Block: Interruption of the passage of impulses through the long buccal nerve anesthetizing the buccal soft tissue of the mandibular molars.

Loupes: Magnifying lenses that are used in conjunction with normal eyewear to allow for better observation of the teeth and gingiva.

M

Macro Level Health Interventions: Interventions that focus on broad systems and policies that influence health.

Macular Degeneration: Is a disease associated with aging that destroys sharp and central vision.

Magnetostrictive Ultrasonics: A machine that uses low voltage to expand and contract a metal stack producing a magnetic field and vibration.

Magnification Systems: Combination of a dental microscope and a computer and monitor, allowing the magnified image to be viewed on a computer screen.

Management Philosophy: The particular philosophy that each dental practice manages the clinical and business aspects of the dental practice. This varies by owner, clinician(s), and is dependent on several business and procedural policies.

Mandibular Nerve Block: Interruption of the passage of impulses through the inferior alveolar nerve anesthetizing the mandibular teeth.

Manual Tuning: A manually tuned ultrasonic machine that allows the clinician to adjust the frequency or number of strokes the insert makes each second.

Matrix Metalloproteinase: An enzyme found in different tissues that is responsible for remodeling or healing.

Maxillary Nerve Block: Interruption of the passage of impulses through branches of the maxillary nerve anesthetizing the maxillary teeth.

Mechanical Oral Hygiene Devices: Objects used to remove deposits and clean debris from oral structures.

Mechanical Plaque Control: Techniques for removal of dental biofilm through means of mechanical friction intended to prevent or dislodge colonies of pathogenic oral bacteria which combine and communicate within the biofilm to cause oral diseases such as dental caries and gingivitis.

Median Rhomboid Glossitis: Rectangular erythematous area, anterior to the circumvallate papillae ending at the junction of the anterior and middle thirds on the dorsal tongue. The surface is smooth because there are no filiform papillae. Recently defined as hyperplastic candidiasis.

Medication List: A complete list of all prescription, over-the-counter and dietary supplements that a patient discloses as a part of the comprehensive health history. The list includes name of the drug, dose, indication for use, and name of the prescriber.

Mentee: An individual who is being mentored.

Mentor: An individual who provides guidance, counseling and mentoring skills and experience to a mentee.

Mesio Level Health Interventions: Interventions that focus on the family, community, living and working conditions.

Meta-Analysis: A statistical method used to combine the results of several studies that address a set of related research hypotheses and their results are mathematically combined to compare the reliability of the results.

Meyer-Briggs Type Indicator: An assessment of the psychometric questionnaire designed to measure psychological preferences in how people see the world and make decisions.

MI Paste™ and MI Paste™ Plus: Is a series of products based upon Recaldent (CPP-ACP) technology. GC America parent company, GC Dental, first introduced MI paste in late 2002 in Australia. This Minimum Intervention Paste can treat a variety of oral health conditions but especially for reducing high oral acids levels from bacterial plague and excessive cariogenic beverages and prevent plaque accumulation and buffering acids.

Micro Level Health Interventions: Interventions that focus on the individual.

Micro Streaming or Acoustic Streaming: Unidirectional fluid flow caused by ultrasound waves.

Micro Ultrasonics: A prophylactic and/or therapeutic treatment procedure designed to remove biofilm and calculus from the tooth surface using thin precision ultrasonic tips.

Microtrauma: Physiological microscopic damage that occurs in the musculoskeletal system due to numerous ergonomic risk factors.

Milliamperage: Adjusts the number of electrons flowing in an electrical circuit; controls the number of x-rays generated.

Minimally Invasive Polishing (MIP): An evidence-based discipline that applies the philosophy of the preservation of hard and soft tissue in the oral cavity by polishing with the least abrasive agent and assessing if polishing needs to be incorporated into an oral prophylaxis procedure.

Mission Statement: A statement that captures the purpose of a person's day to day activities, goals and career objectives.

Monosaccharides: Simple single sugars such as glucose, fructose and galactose that can be used as a food source by cariogenic bacteria.

Morals: Standards of right or wrong usually based on inherent character, theological principles and ethical positions.

Mortuary Science: The study of dead bodies through mortuary work.

Motivational Interviewing (MI): A communication and counseling technique that can be employed with tobacco cessation. This approach requires the provider to be empathic and possess the abilities to assist the user in identifying reasons for or discontinuing the habit, rolling with patient resistance and helping the patient establish self-efficacy.

Multicenter Practices: A dental practice that has multiple centers in which to practice dentistry.

Multidisciplinary Management: The evaluation and management of patients by a team of clinicians, all of whom bring their particular expertise and focus to play in the care of the patient to provide the optimal outcome.

Multidisciplinary: Involving two or more academic or fields of study; professional disciplines working together.

Multimodality Treatment: The use of multiple different approaches to treat a single disease entity. In oral cancer this includes surgical resection, radiation and chemotherapy.

Muscle Imbalance: Response to unbalanced posture. Groups of muscles become long and weak, while the opposing muscle groups become short and strong, holding the body in non-neutral posture.

Musculoskeletal Disorder (MSD): Work-related pain or injury to the musculoskeletal system resulting from microtrauma that accumulates at a rate faster than the body can repair it.

Myalgia: Muscle pain.

N

Nanometer: Is a measurement that is 10 to the negative 9 . . . otherwise known as a billionth of a meter and is identified as "nm."

National Institute of Dental and Craniofacial Research (NIDCR): An agency within the National Institutes of Health with the mission to improve oral, dental and craniofacial health through research, research training and the dissemination of health information.

National Institutes of Health (NIH): An agency within the Department of Health and Human Services with the mission to seek fundamental knowledge about the nature and behavior of living systems and the application of that knowledge to enhance health, lengthen life and reduce the burdens of illness and disability.

ND YAG Laser: A soft tissue dental laser that can perform procedures that electrosurge, as scalpels and dental instruments did in the past. Originally used for most soft tissue procedures, and in recent years has been the second choice to diode lasers and usually operate at 1064nm.

Networking: A supportive system to share information and services among individuals and/or groups having a common interest or specific area of expertise.

Neurotransmitters: Chemical substances in the brain that are affected by tobacco use and transmit messages from one neuron to another's receptors.

Nicotine Addiction: Chronic, cyclic often compulsive use of tobacco products that are known to cause harm; may be characterized by difficulty with abstinence or controlling usage; users typically experience cravings, physical and psychological dependencies and withdrawal symptoms upon abstinence.

Nicotine Gum: An over-the-counter gum that releases nicotine and aids in smoking cessation.

Nicotine Lozenge: An over-the-counter lozenge that releases nicotine and aids in smoking cessation.

Nicotine Nasal Spray: A prescription nicotine containing liquid that is used nasally by the patient to aid in smoking cessation; most often used in nicotine dependence centers.

Nicotine Patch: A transdermal form of nicotine withdrawal therapy; available as an over-the-counter (OTC) product.

Nicotine: A poisonous, addictive stimulant that is the chief psychoactive ingredient to tobacco.

Noncompliance: Lack of willingness for following oral care recommendations.

Nonmaleficence: The promise of "do no harm" in the healthcare relationship.

Non-Surgical Periodontal Therapy: A conservative method of treating and managing periodontal disease with the use of ultrasonics, scaling, root planning, locally applied antimicrobials and other adjunctive modalities.

Nicotine Replacement Therapies (NRT): Pharmacologic adjunctive therapy (gum, lozenge, patch) containing nicotine that can be used for cessation. Some alternatives are over the counter (OTC).

Nursing Bottle Caries: Is a rampant form of dental decay caused by sleeping with a bottle containing a fermentable carbohydrate or sleeping on the mother's breast. Also known as Early Childhood Caries (ECC).

Nutrition: The systemic effects of food on the body.

O

Obesity: Medical condition of excess body fat >30 kg/mm body mass index.

Objective Assessment Data: Observations of the patient presented by the practitioner.

Objectives: Strategies or steps that are utilized to attain an identified goal.

Occupational Exposure: Exposure to blood/body fluids/OPIM while performing employee duties.

Odds Ratio: The odds ratio is a way of comparing whether the probability of a certain event is the same for two groups.

Online Courses: Continuing education courses that may be provided by colleges/universities, professional organizations and oral care manufacturers that are presented on the computer.

Open-Ended Questions: An unstructured group of questions that an individual would answer in his or her own words during a job interview. These questions usually begin with how, what, where, when and why.

OPIM: Other potentially infectious material.

Oral Health Needs: Conditions that require interventions to create an optimal state of the mouth without evidence of disease.

Oral Hygiene or Oral Physiotherapy (OPT): The use of a toothbrush, interdental stimulator, floss, irrigating device or other adjunctive aid to maintain oral health.

Oral Mucositis: Inflammation of the oral mucosa caused by head and neck radiation therapy and chemotherapy.

Orthognathic Surgery: Orthognathic surgery is an operative procedure used to correct skeletal disharmonies of the jaw and face by fracturing and repositioning bony segments.

Osteoradionecrosis: A disease state of bone destruction and lack of repair mechanisms that occurs in irradiated bone as a result of the post radiation triad of hypovascularity, hypocellularity and hypoxia.

Over-The-Counter (OTC) Products: Products that can be purchased by the consumer without a prescription and are available for oral care products.

P

Panel Interviews: A job interview where an individual is interviewed by a panel (group) of interviewers.

Papilloma: A small, slow growing benign lesion of squamous epithelium, caused by a human papillomavirus (HPV).

Passion: A powerful emotion or feeling an individual possesses.

Paternalism: The concept of "doctor knows best." Having the health professional make the final decision with regard to treatment instead of the patient.

Pathogenesis: The development of the disease process.

Patient Activation and Scheduling Systems: Software-based systems that automatically send electronic appointment reminders such as emails or texts.

Patient Education Systems: Software based systems that use high-end graphics to demonstrate dental procedures to patients.

Peer-Reviewed Journals: Published journals that review submitted manuscripts by a qualified individual or group of individuals within a relevant field of study.

Perception: The result or product of perceiving derived from sensory processes while a stimulus is present.

Perio-Aid: A brand of toothpick holder that positions the toothpick at a proper angle for cleaning in difficult to access places such as cervical and interproximal areas.

Periodontal Diagnosis: Is a diagnosis made of patients' periodontal conditions based upon their medical and dental history, assessment of periodontal probing measurements and completion of digital or standard radiographs.

Periodontal Pathogens: Bacteria responsible for periodontal disease.

Periodontal Surgery: Periodontal surgery is an operative procedure used use to correct abnormalities of the soft and hard tissues surrounding the teeth.

Periodontal Therapy (PT) Appointment: Is the incorporation of lasers into a periodontal procedure that used to be referred to as scaling and root planning.

Perlite: Perlite particles are expanded volcanic glass that readily become blunted or disintegrates during 15 seconds of polishing forming a superfine polishing paste that increases tooth luster.

Personal Balanced-Life Element: One of the basic principles of a balanced, satisfying lifestyle. The Personal element encompasses that portion of individuals' lives in which they spend time with family and friends.

Personal Community: The community boundaries that contain the people who live and work together. As a balanced-life element, the Community element encompasses that portion of individuals' lives in which they spend time serving others outside their family and their profession.

Personal Responsibility: The state of being responsible for a personal obligation.

Phagocytosis: The cellular process of engulfing solid particles by the cell membrane.

Pharmacologic History: A review of the patient's medication list, medication use behaviors, compliance and risks for adverse drug events, adverse drug effects and complications arising from medication use.

Photostimulable Phosphor Plate (PSP): Polyester base coated with a crystalline halide emulsion. The plate converts x-ray energy into stored energy that is released when scanned with a helium-neon laser beam.

Piezoelectric Ultrasonics: A machine that uses high voltage causing crystals to expand and contract producing vibration.

Pleomorphic Adenoma: A benign mixed tumor of salivary gland origin. It is the most common salivary gland tumor.

Polishing: The act of producing a smooth and lustrous surface on an object through a process of abrasion with an abrasive consisting of super fine grit particles.

Polypharmacy: Individuals taking multiple medications prescribed to treat one or more systemic conditions simultaneously.

Pooled Estimates: An estimate obtained by combining information from two or more independent samples taken from a population believed to have the same mean.

Population Health: A focus on the health outcomes of an entire population with similar personal or environmental characteristics.

Porcelain Laminate Veneers: Are a thin custom-made shell of tooth-colored porcelain that is chemically bonded to the buccal surface of the teeth to change the color, shape, size or length of a tooth.

Portfolio: A portable case that is used to carry a notepad/pen and important documents related to a business task or endeavor.

Power Toothbrushes: Toothbrushes with direct power or a battery source.

Practice Management Software: Software systems that handle all aspects of front and back office systems, such as billing, scheduling, reports, charting and treatment planning.

Practice Research Coordinators: Individuals who coordinate events within a practice-based network.

PracticeWorks: A practice management software program for dental offices developed in 1993 in Indianapolis, IN. It was one of the first Windows programs available in the dental industry, following shortly on the heels of Dentrix.

Preceptorship: In relation to dental hygiene education, it means to have a practicing dentist train a worker on the job to perform dental hygiene duties, instead of going through a two – to four-year formal, accredited education program and national and regional examinations to obtain a license as defined by the American Dental Hygienists' Association.

Preterm/Low Birth Weight Baby: A baby born before the 37th week of gestation. Low birth weight is less than 2,500 grams at birth.

Preventive Maintenance Program: The entire program of routine and ongoing periodontal care encompassing all providers in a dental practice, and the business and procedural processes involved with it.

Primary Herpetic Gingivostomatitis: Initial infection with the herpes simplex virus. It is characterized by painful erythematous and swollen gingiva and multiple tiny vesicles on the lips and oral mucosa.

Primary Tumor: Tumor that arises from the mucosa of the upper aerodigestive tract, usually of histology consistent with squamous cell carcinoma.

Privacy: The state of being free of being observed or disturbed by others; patients' legal and ethical right to protect their personal information, including their contact information and dental treatment plans.

Productivity: The rate of production measured by a common set of benchmark data typical for that industry's profession.

Professional Balanced-Life Element: One of the basic principles of a balanced, satisfying lifestyle. The Professional element encompasses that portion of individuals' lives in which they spend time at work or participating in work-related travel and events, professional development activities, continuing education, or their volunteer time with work-related organizations.

Professional Community: A community in which people from a professional expertise interact with one another. As a balanced-life element, the Professional Community element encompasses that portion of individuals' lives in which they spend time volunteering to support their profession.

Professional Involvement: Utilization of an individual or group's expertise or information to obtain professional influence in a specified area of expertise.

Professional Negligence (Malpractice): Failure to exercise a degree of care that an educated professional would have exercised under identical circumstances.

Professional Responsibility: The state of being responsible for a professional commitment or obligation.

Professional Savvy™ Career Assessment Test: A tool that is utilized to assess a dental professional's personal skills, career satisfaction, education, training and certification and selection of a mentor for career success. This test can be used for students, front office colleagues and practicing dental professionals.

Professional Savvy™ Career Goals Development Plan: A tool that is utilized to define a dental professional's vision, identify their current position, salary/benefits, lifelong learning, mentorship, networking and investments, yearly goals and objectives, job satisfaction and future goals and objectives of their career. This plan can be used for students, front office colleagues and practicing dental professionals.

Professional Savvy™ Career Tools CDs': Professional Savvy, LLC, has developed a line of CD's for dentists, dental specialists, dental hygienists and dental assistants to assist them in setting a vision for their career as well as goal attainment for one to three, four to six and seven to nine year time periods. Professional Savvy also offers separate tools for the front office management colleagues and dental, dental hygiene and dental assisting tools.

Professional Speaker: An individual who presents a speech, lecture or course pertaining to a specific topic.

Prognosis: An expected course and outcome of a disease; likelihood of recovery from a disease determined by the nature of the specific conditions.

Pro-Inflammatory Mediators: The production of proteins by inflammatory cells that enhance the body's response to injury or pathogens.

Protective Factor: Biologic or nonbiologic behaviors, agents or conditions that reduce the likelihood of a disease or condition and increase the likelihood of health.

Protégé: An individual who receives support and protection from an influential person or mentor who assists in furthering the protégé's career.

Provisional Patent: A type of utility patent that is filed with the United States Patent and Trademark Office (USPTO).

Public Health Role: An individual who promotes the prevention of oral diseases and promotes health wellness through organized community efforts.

Pulmonary Disease: Disease of the respiratory tract, including asthma and chronic obstructive pulmonary disease.

P-Value: A p-value is a measure of how much evidence occurs against the null hypothesis. Researchers will reject a hypothesis if the p-value is less than 0.05.

Pyogenic Granuloma: Not a true granuloma, this is a response to an irritant, often calculus, heavy plaque, a popcorn shell, foods with seeds or hormonal changes.

Q

Quality Assessment: The evaluation of a certain aspect of care in comparison to established criteria and the passage of judgment on quality based on that comparison.

Quality Assurance: Encompasses those activities designed to maintain or improve a standard of excellence in dental care. More specifically, quality assurance concentrates on the philosophy of each member of the dental team, the quality of care rendered to the patients and the marketing of the practice.

R

Radiographic Diagnosis: A method of identifying oral health issues through the use of radiographs to establish a diagnosis in bone or tooth structure.

RAM (Random Access Memory): Temporary memory of the computer in which programs and information are stored.

Randomized Controlled Trial (RCT): A study in which people are allocated at random (by chance alone) to receive one of several clinical interventions. One of these interventions is the standard of comparison or control. The control may be a standard practice, a placebo ("sugar pill"), or no intervention at all.

Ranula: A mucoseal like lesion that forms unilaterally on the floor of the mouth. It is associated with the sublingual and submandibular glands.

Real-Time Teleconsultation: Real-time teleconsultation uses videoconferencing equipment to provide instantaneous interaction between a dentist, dental hygienist or patient in a remote clinic and a dentist or specialist in a larger community who provides support or supervision in clinical examination, diagnosis and treatment planning.

Receptor: Any device or medium that transforms x-ray energy into a latent image that can be made visible by processing.

Recommendations and References: A letter from a former employer to a potential future employer describing an individual's qualities, dependability and work.

Recreational Drug Use: Substance abuse.

Refereed Journals: A journal that uses an editorial review board to review papers submitted for publication with the goal of identifying errors or inconsistencies within the manuscript.

Regional Metastasis: Focus of cancer that has spread to the lymph nodes draining the primary tumor.

Relapse: Situation where patient reverts to previous behavior (e.g., returns to tobacco use after a period of abstinence).

Relationships: A connection or association occurring between more than one person.

Relative Dentin Abrasivity (RDA): A method of measuring the erosive effect of abrasives in toothpaste on tooth dentin. The values obtained depend on the size, quantity and surface structure of abrasive used in toothpaste. International Standards Organization (ISO) stipulates that the RDA of toothpaste should not exceed 250, but most toothpastes in developing countries ≤ 100.

Relative Enamel Abrasivity (REA): A method of measuring the erosive effect of abrasives in toothpaste on tooth enamel. The lower REA, the less abrasive the toothpaste.

Relative Risk Ratio: Relative risk (RR) is the risk of an event (or of developing a disease) relative to exposure. Relative risk is a ratio of the probability of the event occurring in the exposed group versus a non-exposed group.

Repetitive Task: A task performed with the hands or fingers that involves the same fundamental movement for more than 50% of the work cycle allotted to perform the task.

Research: The systematic investigation of materials, products, initiative or information to establish facts and reach conclusions.

Researcher: An individual who uses scientific experimentation and methodology to interpret hypotheses or facts in dental hygiene or dentistry.

Resolution: Measures how well a radiographic image reveals small objects that are close together; measured in line pairs per millimeter.

Resources: The ability to provide an individual with materials, assets and information necessary for effective operation.

Respect (of Colleagues): The admiration of a person who has shared his or her achievements, expertise and/or values with others.

Respiratory Hygiene/Cough Etiquette: New component of Standard Precautions designed to reduce the spread of respiratory infections.

Resume: A one to two page summary of a job seeker's education, work experience and professional skills that an individual would provide to a potential employer with a cover letter.

Risk Assessment: A qualitative and quantitative evaluation gathered from the assessment process to identify the risks to the oral and general health. The data provides the clinican with information to develop and design strategies for preventing or limiting disease and promoting health.

Risk Factor: A variable which has been associated through research findings with an increased risk of disease or infection.

Risk Management: An integral element in quality dental care that includes accurate record keeping, proper communication skills implemented with patients, and reduce or minimize the risk of legal action or malpractice claims in the dental practice environment.

Rotator Cuff Impingement: Painful tendonitis of the supraspinatus tendon in the shoulder due to repetitive lifting, overhead reaching or abduction.

S

Salary: A fixed amount of money or compensation that is paid to an employee by an employer in return for work performed.

Screening Interviews: A type of job interview that is conducted to determine if an individual has the qualifications needed to do a position for which a company, practice or organization is hiring. This is usually the first interview in the hiring process.

Selective Polishing: A decision process through patient assessment to determine the need to remove plaque biofilm and stain from teeth and/or restorative material during an oral prophylaxis procedure.

Self-Efficacy: Capability of an individual to create positive change; i.e., have self-belief in the ability to abstain from tobacco use.

Self-Motivated: To undertake a task or activity without the supervision of another.

Self-Regulation: The ability to regulate oneself. Self-regulation provides a profession with the autonomy to govern licensed professionals within the boundaries of patient safety, while maintaining the profession by encouraging expertise in professional practice.

Six-Point Periodontal Charting: Six probing depths recorded on each tooth: mesial lingual, direct lingual, distal lingual, mesial buccal, direct buccal and distal buccal.

Sjogren Syndrome: An autoimmune disease that affects lachrymal and salivary glands. The decreased flow of fluids causes dry mouth and dry eyes. This is called Primary Sjogren Syndrome.

Smoking: A self-administered means of bringing nicotine into the body via the use of tobacco products (e.g., pipes, cigarettes, cigars, etc.) that requires combustion.

Snuff: Fire-cured, finely ground or powdered tobacco sold in both dry and moist forms; not chewed but a small amount ("pinch" or "quid") is placed and held between check and gingiva or lower lip, gingiva and mucosa; use associated with oral cancer. Also known as "spit tobacco."

Social Action: Challenging the system and changing the status quo through action to solve a social problem (e.g. access to care).

Societal Trust: The expectation of the public with regard to the healthcare professional in terms of ability and current knowledge in their field.

Software Systems: Systems that are provided either on a disc or downloaded; does not include any specific hardware.

Sonicare/RDH Mentor of the Year Award: An award to recognize an individual who has had the most impact on an individual's career as a dental hygienist.

Sonification: Sound vibrations strong enough to destroy bacterial cell walls.

Sound Technique: Used during instrumentation to test for sharpness. An experienced clinician will detect the sound of a sharp instrument (audible) versus one that is dull and provides no sound or the sound of sliding.

Spit Tobacco: Term synonymous with smokeless tobacco. Also known as snuff.

Stages of Change Theory (Transtheoretical Model): A non-linear theoretical model that supports the belief that individuals pass through specific stages of change before they are able to successfully adopt a new behavior.

Stafne Bone Cyst: Indentation on the lingual surface of the mandible within a portion of the submandibular gland.

Stakeholder: Any individual or group affected by an organization or course of action.

Standard Precautions: Set of precautions that combine the major features of universal precautions and body substance isolation and integrate and expand these elements into a standard of care designed to protect HCP and patients from pathogens that may be spread by blood or any other body fluid, excretion or secretion.

State Practice Act: A state law that defines rules and regulations for the dental hygienists within that state.

Statistically Significant: An interpretation of statistical data that indicates that an occurrence was probably the result of a causative factor and not simply a chance result. Statistical significance at the 1% level indicates a 1 in 100 probability that a result can be ascribed to chance.

Sterilization: A process that eliminates or kills all forms of microbial life, including bacterial spores that are the much more difficult to kill than are the common microbial contaminants found on patient-care items. Sterilization can be achieved by the use of heat, chemicals, high pressure or filtration.

Store-and-Forward Teleconsultation: In the store-and-forward teleconsultation, medical and dental history, clinical examination, radiographs, images and videos, etc., are collected by dentists, dental hygienists and other team members in a remote clinic. This information is stored in an EHR or electronic dental record and then forwarded to the dental specialist at the hub clinic via email attachments or FTP. The specialist reviews patient history and the clinical examination information, renders an opinion on diagnosis and treatment recommendations and informs the remote clinic via email report.

Strategic Plan: A planning device used as a road map for achieving outcomes of a social action movement.

Stress Interviews: A job interview where an individual is placed in a stressful situation and the interviewers see how this person copes under pressure.

Stroke: Interruption of blood supply to the brain.

Subjective Assessment Data: Observations of the patient presented by the patient.

Substantivity: A substance's ability to provide slow release of therapeutic activity by binding to hard and soft tissue surfaces while resisting dilution by saliva.

Superfloss®: Nylon strand with a threader at one end and variable width diameter spongy portion and a regular floss segment to clean around implants and under fixed bridges or appliances.

Supportive Periodontal Therapy (SPT): This is the maintenance procedure that the patient is placed on after active periodontal therapy is completed.

SWOT Analysis: A method used to analyze the strengths and weaknesses within an organization and the opportunities and threats external to the organization that affect the outcome of social action.

Syncope: Temporary loss of consciousness caused by sudden drop in blood pressure. Also known as fainting.

Synergy in Social Action Theory: The interaction within and among the key elements of (1) learning and educating, (2) situations and social interactions and (3) individual action and collective action that sustain social action through perpetual momentum.

Systematic Review: A literature review focused on a single research question designed to identify, appraise, select and synthesize all high quality research evidence relevant to that question. Systematic reviews of high-quality research studies such as randomized, controlled clinical trials are crucial to evidence-based practice.

Systemic Errors (Bias): External influences that may affect the accuracy of statistical measurements.

T

Tachycardia: Fast heart rate.

Tachypnea: Fast respiration rate.

Team Contribution: The act of contributing to the skills of a group of people.

Teledentistry: A rising new area of dentistry that applies telecommunication and information technologies to facilitate and improve oral health care with patients in access to care communities.

Telehealth: Telehealth refers to the delivery of information and healthcare related services, such as public health education and health promotion, prevention and clinical care and home care via telecommunication technologies.

Telephone Interviews: An interview that is conducted on the phone to screen individuals in order to narrow down the pool of job applicants, who will then be chosen for an in-person interview.

Tell/Show/Do: A technique used in dentistry to alleviate dental phobia, or the patient's fear, when the dentist explains to the patient what will be done (tell), shows the patient what will be done (show) and then conducts the dental procedure (do).

Tenacity: The quality of holding things together or being cohesive in nature.

Tension Neck Syndrome: Pain and tenderness in the cervical musculature, usually due to poor ergonomic conditions.

Terminal Shank: The part of the shank of the instrument that extends from the working end to the closest bend.

Test Stick: An acrylic stick used to test the sharpness of an instrument by engaging the blade of the instrument at a proper angulation to the test stick.

Therapeutic Diagnosis: A systematic method of identifying oral health issues by first prescribing therapies known to treat particular conditions. If the condition resolves with the prescribed therapy, the diagnosis is complete.

Third-Party Image Programs: Software developed by independent companies that is designed to supplement the functionality of existing software packages.

Thoracic Outlet Syndrome: A neurovascular disease causing compression of the nerves and artery that supply the arm and hand. Symptoms include numbness, weakness, pain, discoloration or coldness.

Tobacco Interventions: Provider actions and behaviors that prevent or stop patient tobacco use.

Tooth Abrasion: Loss of tooth structure or damage to it as a result of mechanical removal, frequently from toothbrushing.

Tori: Is an outgrowth of bone commonly found on the roof of the mouth and on either side of the mandible by the tongue area.

Traditional Interviews: A job interview where an individual will be asked a series of questions that have straight forward answers. The interviewer determines if an individual has the skills needed for the position.

Transtheoretical Model of Behavior Change: An approach to behavior change that suggests that people move through stages in order to modify and maintain new behaviors.

Trapezius Myalgia: Pain and tenderness in the upper trapezius muscle, often due to prolonged shoulder elevation or emotional stress.

Traumatic Bone Cyst: A pathologic cavity in bone that is not lined with epithelium. A traumatic bone cyst can also be known as a simple bone cyst.

Treatment Plan: A detailed written plan explaining the treatment to be performed during subsequent visits, and the length of time required for each visit or procedure.

Treatment/Patient Care Coordinator: An individual who works directly with the patients to understand their specific dental needs and goals, conduct dental radiographs (pending licensure) and work with the dentist to carry out their treatment plans and financial resources for dental treatment.

Trendelenburg's Position: In supine position inclined downward at a 45 – degree angle with heart higher than the head.

Triclosan: An organic compound, polychloro phenoxy phenol, and antibacterial chemical added to many household products, in this chapter specifically dentifrices, to combat bacteria associated with gingivitis.

U

U.S. Department of Health and Human Services: The governmental agency responsible for the health of the U.S. population.

Ultrasonic Scaler: A power driven scaling device that operates in a frequency range of 25,000 to 50,000 cycles per second to convert electrical current into mechanical vibrations.

Ultraviolet Toothbrush Devices: Sanitize a toothbrush using ultraviolet light.

Underserved Population: Underserved population refers to those with economic barriers (low-income or Medicaid-eligible populations), or cultural and/or linguistic access barriers to primary medical and dental care services.

Universal Curet: A periodontal instrument that is designed with two parallel cutting edges and a rounded toe that can be used anywhere in the dentition.

USB Camera Systems: Intraoral cameras that connect to the computer through a standard USB interface.

Utility Patent: A patent that is subdivided into three categories (mechanical, electrical and chemical) and protects the way an invention is used and works. This type of patent is for a new and useful method, device or chemical compound.

V

Vaccination: Process to induce immunity by the exposure of the immune system to a killed or weakened form of the disease organism (vaccine-induced immunity).

Validity: A term used to describe whether a test or technique actually measures what it is intended to measure and measures the accuracy of the measurement. Validity can refer to an individual measurement or to the design and approach taken in a clinical research study.

Values: Personal beliefs and attitudes.

VELScope®: Oral cancer screening device; a blue light is emitted into a patient's mouth, and on the basis of fluorescence determines if there are cellular changes indicating precancerous changes intraorally. VELScope® is manufactured by LED Dental, Inc.

Veracity: This relates to the virtue of truth and the responsibility of both the patient and the professional to be truthful in the patient doctor relationship.

Veterinary Dentistry: The field of dentistry that applies to the care of animals in the diagnosis, treatment and prevention of diseases of the oral cavity.

Visible Spectrum: Is the portion of the electromagnetic spectrum that the human eye can see . . . allowing people to see the colors that we do.

ViziLite®: Oral cancer screening device; patient rinses with a solution and a blue light is emitted into patient's mouth to emphasize cellular changes that can be used to detect oral cancer. ViziLite is manufactured by Zila, a Tolmar Company.

Vision Statement: A one or two sentence description of what an individual, company or organization wants to become or achieve in the future.

Volunteer Activities: An act in which an individual will provide complimentary services to assist others in a community or group.

W

Wellness Balanced-Life Element: One of the basic principles of a balanced, satisfying lifestyle. The Wellness element encompasses that portion of individuals' lives in which they spend time on creative, spiritual and other enjoyable activities.

Wellness: Physical well-being, especially when maintained or achieved through good diet, regular exercise and a personal healthcare program.

White Blood Cells (WBCs): A group of several cell types that circulate in the blood system in order to fight infection and provide a functioning immune system. A low white blood cell count, also known as leukopenia, is a decrease in disease-fighting cells (leukocytes) circulating in the blood. It has been shown that elevated white blood cells (WBCs) in the mouth reflect the presence and severity of periodontal disease; following periodontal treatment WBCs return to low levels.

Working End: The working end consists of three different parts (face, back and lateral surface). A critical part of the instrument and determines the use of the instrument.

Working Interviews: This type of interview occurs after the initial interview. The potential employer would ask job candidates whom they interview to work a half or full day in their work environment and the candidates are compensated for their time.

X

Xerostomia: Dry mouth is due to a significant reduction or lack of saliva, commonly caused by medications; various diseases, medical treatments such as chemotherapy, radiation therapy or surgery.

Xylitol: A sugar alcohol which helps to prevent caries by altering the metabolism of cariogenic bacteria, specifically S. mutans.

Index

Index

Subjective assessment data 339

Substantivity 339

Superfloss® 340

Supportive periodontal therapy 340

SWOT analysis 233-4, 340

Syncope 340

Synergy in social action theory 226, 237-8, 240, 340

T

Tachycardia 340

Tachypnea 340

Technology 23, 25, 27-8, 48, 140, 223, 294

Teledentistry 25, 340

    access to care 25, 46, 68, 70, 220, 226, 228-9,
      238, 240, 317, 338, 340

    real-time teleconsultation 336

    store-and-forward teleconsultation 339

    telehealth 340

Tell/Show/Do 340

Tenacity 341

Tension neck syndrome 341

Terminal shank 341

Test stick 341

Therapeutic diagnosis 341

Thoracic outlet syndrome 341

Tobacco cessation aar 25, 306, 328

    (ask, advise, refer) 306

    5 As 306

    spit tobacco 338

    tobacco interventions 341

Tooth abrasion 341

Toothpaste 74, 76, 213, 292, 316, 320, 336

Tori 341

Transtheoretical model of behavior change 341

Trapezius myalgia 341

Treatment/patient care coordinator 210-11, 342

Treatment plan 341

Trendelenburg's position 342

Triclosan 342

U

Ultrasonics 27, 294, 326-7, 332

    amplitude 308

    manually tune 326

    micro streaming or acoustic streaming 327

    micro ultrasonics 327

    microtrauma 328

    milliamperage 328

    sonification 338

    tuning 326

    ultrasonic scaler 342

Ultraviolet toothbrush devices 342

Underserved population 342

U.S. department of health and human services 238, 293, 342

USB camera systems 342

Utility patent 342

V

Vaccination 342

validity 342

Validity 342

Values 343

VELScope® 343

Veracity 343

Veterinary dentistry 126, 343

Visible spectrum 343

Vision statement 147, 343

ViziLite® 343

Volunteer activities 343

W

Wellness 309, 343

Wellness balanced-life element 343

White blood cells 343

X

Author Biography, SAVVY SUCCESS Textbooks and Faculty Guide and Continuing Education Opportunities with SAVVY SUCCESS

Biography

Christine A. Hovliaras, RDH, BS, MBA, CDE, President, Professional Savvy, LLC, an oral care consulting, professional marketing and continuing education company located in New Jersey. Christine is a dental hygiene professional with over 28 years of experience in clinical, educational and research experience in both academia and industry. Her expertise in industry includes dental clinical research, sales training, professional sales and professional marketing and relations at the Warner-Lambert Company from 1989-2001. She was Editor-in-Chief of ADHA's Access Magazine from 2005-2008 and Editor Emeritus during 2009-2010. She is a consultant, national and international speaker, professional writer and voiceover artist in the medical and dental professions.

Through Professional Savvy, LLC, Christine provides professional business marketing services and strategies to oral care companies, professional associations, and dental/specialty practices, speaking presentations at national and global professional meetings and career planning and business development opportunities for dental professionals. Christine has written numerous articles in dental peer-reviewed journals and professional dental hygiene magazines. Christine is a member of many professional dental hygiene and dental organizations. Christine also works part-time as a registered dental hygienist in New Jersey.

She received the VIP Division 2011/2012 Professional Woman of the Year for Outstanding Leadership and Commitment within the Dental Profession from the National Association of Professional Women, the 2009 New Jersey Dental Hygienists' Association Carol King Award, 2008 Certification as a Dental Editor, 2006 Sigma Phi Alpha Honorary member, a 2005 Recipient of the Pfizer/ADHA Award of Excellence in Dental Hygiene and is a recipient of the Who's Who in Business and Professional Executives in 2004.

Four Great Educational Tools For Dental Hygienists

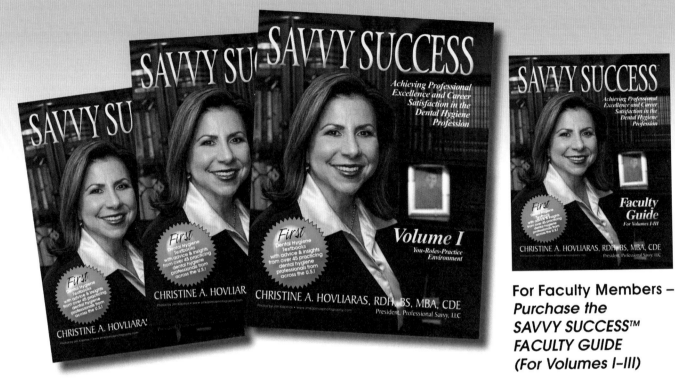

PROFESSIONAL SAVVY'S NEW
THREE VOLUME TEXTBOOKS & FACULTY GUIDE

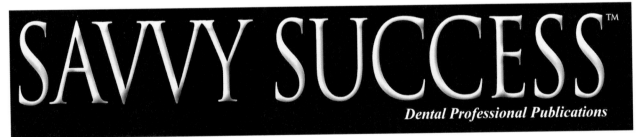

Achieving Professional Excellence and Career Satisfaction in the Dental Hygiene Profession

For Student Dental Hygienists and Practicing Dental Hygiene Professionals –

Don't Miss Purchasing

Volume II: Patient Care and
Volume III: Technology-Ethics-Career Success

Visit www.savvysuccessbooks.com or www.professionalsavvychd.com.

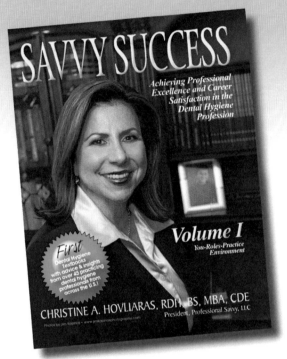
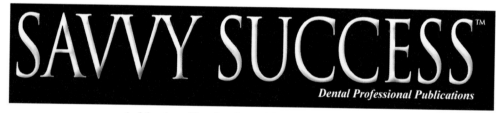

CPSIA information can be obtained
at www.ICGtesting.com
Printed in the USA
LVXC02n0203111115
461961LV00007B/14